Important Information

W9-BSN-308

Please fill out the information below and fax back or return it in the envelope provided with your order.
Your feedback is important in helping us provide you with quality courses which meet all your continuing education needs.

Print Clearly

Today's Date: _____

Name: _____

License Type: _____
(i.e. RN, LPN, LVN, APRN)

Address: _____

Order No.: _____
(located at the top of your FasTrax answer sheet)

City: _____ State: _____ Zip: _____

Day Phone: (_____) _____

Email: _____

Course Title: _____

Item No.: N _____
(located on the back cover of course book)

Comments: _____

_____

_____

_____

What topics would you like to see offered as future courses?

_____

_____

_____

_____

_____

How many contact hours are you most interested in? *(Please check one)*

❏ 1-5 hours   ❏ 10-12 hours   ❏ 15 hours   ❏ 20-24 hours   ❏ 25 hours   ❏ 30 hours   ❏ other_____
(specify)

What improvements can we make to our catalogs, products or services?

If you need more space, include an additional page (please do not staple).

_____

_____

_____

_____

_____

Thank you for taking the time to help us better understand your needs.

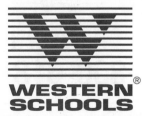

WESTERN® SCHOOLS

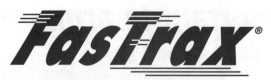

STOP! Read these instructions BEFORE starting your exam

Exam Grading Options

To send in your FasTrax answer sheet...

1 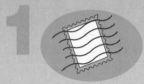 **Mail** to:
Western Schools, P.O. Box 1930
Brockton, MA 02303-1930

2 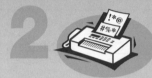 **Fax** to:
1-508-230-2679

Receive your certificate of completion free within 12 business days.

For Rush Service...

3 **2-Day Rush Fax** (1-508-238-0172)
$15 fee results by fax in 48 business hours

4 **1-Day Rush Fax** (1-508-238-0172)
$25 fee results by fax in 24 business hours

5 **Same Day Fax** (1-508-238-0172) **$35 fee**
Fax in by 2pm EST, results by fax by 6pm EST;
Monday-Friday (excludes holidays)

6 **2-Day Express Courier*** Mail or Fax
(1-508-238-0172) **$25 fee** add 48 business
hours for processing
*Cannot deliver to P.O. Boxes

7 **1-Day Express Courier*** Mail or Fax (1-508-238-0172)
$40 fee add 24 business hours for processing
*Cannot deliver to P.O. Boxes

- If selecting same day or 24 or 48-hour Rush Service via Fax or Express Courier, sign the FasTrax form at the top of your exam answer sheet and fill in your complete credit card information.
- To order any fax-back service, you must have a 24-hour dedicated fax line. DO NOT use a fax cover sheet.

- Keep the transmission confirmation from your fax machine until you receive your certificate of completion.
- Western Schools® accepts check, Visa, MasterCard, Discover/Novus, Diners Club, and American Express.
- All charges are per exam.

To help us process your exam quickly, please follow these steps:

A Answer all test questions by completely filling in your response on the FasTrax answer sheet. **Use blue or black ink.** FasTrax will not read pencil. You may use liquid paper to correct errors, or you may fill in with pencil – just remember to go over the pencil with ink when finished. The FasTrax answer sheet allows for up to 100 answers. For courses with fewer than 100 questions, fill in your answers in sequence and leave remaining spaces blank. Keep a copy of your answer sheet for your records.

B Select the FasTrax Grading Option on the answer sheet that best suits your needs (details above).

C Be sure to verify your name and address on the FasTrax sheet and indicate any changes.

Please note that Western Schools® courses are not transferable.
Certificates are dated with the date your final exam is received by Western Schools®

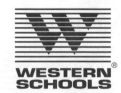

WESTERN® SCHOOLS

Please call Customer Service at 1-800-618-1670 with questions or comments

Rev: 07/05

FORM NO. CPC-MAX2 (4-03)

04/23/07 NCI5HSNUWDAZAZZ 04/23/07 0000315170 30 02

Thank You
Packed with Pride
Nancy

QTY	ITEM NO.	DESCRIPTION	UNIT PRICE	EXT. PRICE	WHSE. LOC.
1 N1115 HC 32		Cardiovascular Nursing: A Comprehensive Overview	39.95	39.95	51DD54

Net Product $		39.95
P & H		6.50
Total Shipment $		46.45
Amt Charged to VI		46.45

PACKING LIST

CUSTOMER SERVICE

For Customer Service see Toll-FREE number on front
Hours (EST): Monday-Friday 7:00 am - 10:00 pm
Saturday: 9:00 am - 6:00 pm

Our Return Policy

If you're not completely satisfied with your purchase, you may return it for an exchange or refund within 30 days of the original purchase(ship date). Returned merchandise must be in new condition, unmarked and should contain any original tags. Software, video, audio and hosiery products must be unopened. We do not refund shipping & handling charges. However, exchange orders are shipped to you free of charge(excluding the cost of rush service). If you return any of the items purchased as part of a discount or special offer, your refund will be adjusted accordingly.

Timing

You can expect your refund or exchange within three to four weeks from the time you mail your return back to us. For credit card orders, please allow up to two statements for your credit to appear. Any exchange you make will be treated as a new order and a new charge will be applied to your credit card.

Easy Exchange/Return Instructions

1. Detach the Merchandise/Return Form below. Keep the top portion for your records.
2. To the left of each item on the Exchange/Return Form, enter the reason code and the quantity you are returning.
3. If exchanging, enter the necessary information on the Exchage Order Form below.
4. Indicate Exchange or Refund on the Exchange/Return label on the other side of this form.
5. Enclose the Merchandise/Return Form with the merchandise in a well-sealed box. Attach the Exchange/Return Label to the outside and return through any UPS Shipper or Insured Mail. Keep your receipt.

TEAR ALONG PERFORATION

Merchandise Return Form: *Please include this with your package.*

TO MAKE AN EXCHANGE OR RECEIVE A REFUND, FOLLOW THESE INSTRUCTIONS

1. **Please tell us what you are returning** by checking either the "exchange" or "refund" box located below.

   Indicate Exchange or Refund on the Exchange/Return Label on the other side of this form.

2. **To place an exchange order,** list the new items you are ordering in the Exchange box located to the right. Fill out all columns and total the items. You will not be charged additional shipping and handling charges on items that are back ordered.

3. **Prepare your package** by including this Merchandise Return Form in your package. Affix the Exchange/Return label to your package. Ship via insured Parcel Post. Sorry, we cannot accept COD.

4. **Shipping on your exchange is FREE:** Standard delivery is 7-14 days. **For Rush Shipping:** add the desired amount to order: **3-4 Business Days $9.00 Overnight (Mon.-Fri.): $18.00 Overnight (Sat.): $22.00** Rush service available in US only.

RETURNED ITEMS

CHECK ONE Exchange	CHECK ONE Refund	Reason Code	Item No.	Product Name	Qty.	Total $ Returned

Total $ Returned

PLEASE ORDER YOUR EXCHANGE ITEM BELOW

Item No.	Product Name	Color	Size	Qty.	Unit Price	Total $ Exchange

Total $ Exchanged	
Minus Total $ Returned	
SUBTOTAL	
MA residents add 5% Sales Tax	
Add Rush Shipping Charges (if requested)	
TOTAL DUE/(total credit)	

Method of Payment: [ ]Check [ ]Discover/Novus [ ]VISA [ ]MC [ ]Amex

Card # _____ Exp. Date _____

Signature _____

REASON CODES

Quality/Satisfaction
81. Defective
82. Decided against course
83. Already took course

Service
84. Wrong item shipped
85. Shipped to wrong address
86. Received too late

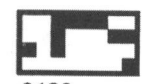
9120

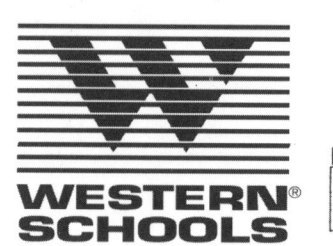

WESTERN SCHOOLS

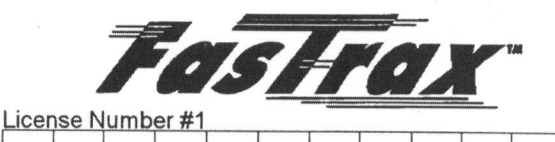

Account No: 0071611768
Order No: W0174375

Cardiovascular Nursing: A Comprehensive Overview

KIMBERLY MCCARTHY
248 EYLAND AVE
SUCCASUNNA, NJ 07876

License Number #1

State of License		Type of License (example: RN)		

Expiration Date: M M / D D / 2 0 Y Y Y

License Number #2 (if different from above)

State of License		Type of License (example: RN)		

Expiration Date: M M / D D / 2 0 Y Y Y

Must check one option as explained on the enclosed FasTrax instruction sheet:

☐ #1: **Mail in,** results by mail within 12 business days
☐ #2: **Fax in,** (1-508-230-2679), results by mail within 12 business days
☐ #3: **2-Day Rush Fax** (1-508-238-0172), results by fax in 48 business hours ($15 fee)
☐ #4: **1-Day Rush Fax** (1-508-238-0172), results by fax in 24 business hours ($25 fee)
☐ #5: **Same Day Fax** (1-508-238-0172), in by 2pm EST, results by fax by 6pm EST, Mon.-Fri. (excludes holidays) ($35 fee)
☐ #6: **2-Day Express Courier** Mail or Fax (1-508-238-0172), add 48 business hours for processing ($25 fee)
☐ #7: **1-Day Express Courier** Mail or Fax (1-508-238-0172), add 24 business hours for processing ($40 fee)

Dedicated Fax Number for Certificate

			-			-			

Credit Card Number:

Credit Card Expiration Date: /

Signature:

Exam

1 Ⓐ Ⓑ Ⓒ Ⓓ Ⓔ   26 Ⓐ Ⓑ Ⓒ Ⓓ Ⓔ   51 Ⓐ Ⓑ Ⓒ Ⓓ Ⓔ   76 Ⓐ Ⓑ Ⓒ Ⓓ Ⓔ
2 Ⓐ Ⓑ Ⓒ Ⓓ Ⓔ   27 Ⓐ Ⓑ Ⓒ Ⓓ Ⓔ   52 Ⓐ Ⓑ Ⓒ Ⓓ Ⓔ   77 Ⓐ Ⓑ Ⓒ Ⓓ Ⓔ
3 Ⓐ Ⓑ Ⓒ Ⓓ Ⓔ   28 Ⓐ Ⓑ Ⓒ Ⓓ Ⓔ   53 Ⓐ Ⓑ Ⓒ Ⓓ Ⓔ   78 Ⓐ Ⓑ Ⓒ Ⓓ Ⓔ
4 Ⓐ Ⓑ Ⓒ Ⓓ Ⓔ   29 Ⓐ Ⓑ Ⓒ Ⓓ Ⓔ   54 Ⓐ Ⓑ Ⓒ Ⓓ Ⓔ   79 Ⓐ Ⓑ Ⓒ Ⓓ Ⓔ
5 Ⓐ Ⓑ Ⓒ Ⓓ Ⓔ   30 Ⓐ Ⓑ Ⓒ Ⓓ Ⓔ   55 Ⓐ Ⓑ Ⓒ Ⓓ Ⓔ   80 Ⓐ Ⓑ Ⓒ Ⓓ Ⓔ
6 Ⓐ Ⓑ Ⓒ Ⓓ Ⓔ   31 Ⓐ Ⓑ Ⓒ Ⓓ Ⓔ   56 Ⓐ Ⓑ Ⓒ Ⓓ Ⓔ   81 Ⓐ Ⓑ Ⓒ Ⓓ Ⓔ
7 Ⓐ Ⓑ Ⓒ Ⓓ Ⓔ   32 Ⓐ Ⓑ Ⓒ Ⓓ Ⓔ   57 Ⓐ Ⓑ Ⓒ Ⓓ Ⓔ   82 Ⓐ Ⓑ Ⓒ Ⓓ Ⓔ
8 Ⓐ Ⓑ Ⓒ Ⓓ Ⓔ   33 Ⓐ Ⓑ Ⓒ Ⓓ Ⓔ   58 Ⓐ Ⓑ Ⓒ Ⓓ Ⓔ   83 Ⓐ Ⓑ Ⓒ Ⓓ Ⓔ
9 Ⓐ Ⓑ Ⓒ Ⓓ Ⓔ   34 Ⓐ Ⓑ Ⓒ Ⓓ Ⓔ   59 Ⓐ Ⓑ Ⓒ Ⓓ Ⓔ   84 Ⓐ Ⓑ Ⓒ Ⓓ Ⓔ
10 Ⓐ Ⓑ Ⓒ Ⓓ Ⓔ   35 Ⓐ Ⓑ Ⓒ Ⓓ Ⓔ   60 Ⓐ Ⓑ Ⓒ Ⓓ Ⓔ   85 Ⓐ Ⓑ Ⓒ Ⓓ Ⓔ
11 Ⓐ Ⓑ Ⓒ Ⓓ Ⓔ   36 Ⓐ Ⓑ Ⓒ Ⓓ Ⓔ   61 Ⓐ Ⓑ Ⓒ Ⓓ Ⓔ   86 Ⓐ Ⓑ Ⓒ Ⓓ Ⓔ
12 Ⓐ Ⓑ Ⓒ Ⓓ Ⓔ   37 Ⓐ Ⓑ Ⓒ Ⓓ Ⓔ   62 Ⓐ Ⓑ Ⓒ Ⓓ Ⓔ   87 Ⓐ Ⓑ Ⓒ Ⓓ Ⓔ
13 Ⓐ Ⓑ Ⓒ Ⓓ Ⓔ   38 Ⓐ Ⓑ Ⓒ Ⓓ Ⓔ   63 Ⓐ Ⓑ Ⓒ Ⓓ Ⓔ   88 Ⓐ Ⓑ Ⓒ Ⓓ Ⓔ
14 Ⓐ Ⓑ Ⓒ Ⓓ Ⓔ   39 Ⓐ Ⓑ Ⓒ Ⓓ Ⓔ   64 Ⓐ Ⓑ Ⓒ Ⓓ Ⓔ   89 Ⓐ Ⓑ Ⓒ Ⓓ Ⓔ
15 Ⓐ Ⓑ Ⓒ Ⓓ Ⓔ   40 Ⓐ Ⓑ Ⓒ Ⓓ Ⓔ   65 Ⓐ Ⓑ Ⓒ Ⓓ Ⓔ   90 Ⓐ Ⓑ Ⓒ Ⓓ Ⓔ
16 Ⓐ Ⓑ Ⓒ Ⓓ Ⓔ   41 Ⓐ Ⓑ Ⓒ Ⓓ Ⓔ   66 Ⓐ Ⓑ Ⓒ Ⓓ Ⓔ   91 Ⓐ Ⓑ Ⓒ Ⓓ Ⓔ
17 Ⓐ Ⓑ Ⓒ Ⓓ Ⓔ   42 Ⓐ Ⓑ Ⓒ Ⓓ Ⓔ   67 Ⓐ Ⓑ Ⓒ Ⓓ Ⓔ   92 Ⓐ Ⓑ Ⓒ Ⓓ Ⓔ
18 Ⓐ Ⓑ Ⓒ Ⓓ Ⓔ   43 Ⓐ Ⓑ Ⓒ Ⓓ Ⓔ   68 Ⓐ Ⓑ Ⓒ Ⓓ Ⓔ   93 Ⓐ Ⓑ Ⓒ Ⓓ Ⓔ
19 Ⓐ Ⓑ Ⓒ Ⓓ Ⓔ   44 Ⓐ Ⓑ Ⓒ Ⓓ Ⓔ   69 Ⓐ Ⓑ Ⓒ Ⓓ Ⓔ   94 Ⓐ Ⓑ Ⓒ Ⓓ Ⓔ
20 Ⓐ Ⓑ Ⓒ Ⓓ Ⓔ   45 Ⓐ Ⓑ Ⓒ Ⓓ Ⓔ   70 Ⓐ Ⓑ Ⓒ Ⓓ Ⓔ   95 Ⓐ Ⓑ Ⓒ Ⓓ Ⓔ
21 Ⓐ Ⓑ Ⓒ Ⓓ Ⓔ   46 Ⓐ Ⓑ Ⓒ Ⓓ Ⓔ   71 Ⓐ Ⓑ Ⓒ Ⓓ Ⓔ   96 Ⓐ Ⓑ Ⓒ Ⓓ Ⓔ
22 Ⓐ Ⓑ Ⓒ Ⓓ Ⓔ   47 Ⓐ Ⓑ Ⓒ Ⓓ Ⓔ   72 Ⓐ Ⓑ Ⓒ Ⓓ Ⓔ   97 Ⓐ Ⓑ Ⓒ Ⓓ Ⓔ
23 Ⓐ Ⓑ Ⓒ Ⓓ Ⓔ   48 Ⓐ Ⓑ Ⓒ Ⓓ Ⓔ   73 Ⓐ Ⓑ Ⓒ Ⓓ Ⓔ   98 Ⓐ Ⓑ Ⓒ Ⓓ Ⓔ
24 Ⓐ Ⓑ Ⓒ Ⓓ Ⓔ   49 Ⓐ Ⓑ Ⓒ Ⓓ Ⓔ   74 Ⓐ Ⓑ Ⓒ Ⓓ Ⓔ   99 Ⓐ Ⓑ Ⓒ Ⓓ Ⓔ
25 Ⓐ Ⓑ Ⓒ Ⓓ Ⓔ   50 Ⓐ Ⓑ Ⓒ Ⓓ Ⓔ   75 Ⓐ Ⓑ Ⓒ Ⓓ Ⓔ   100 Ⓐ Ⓑ Ⓒ Ⓓ Ⓔ

Shade circles like this: ●
Not like this: ⊗ ☒

USE BLUE OR BLACK INK ONLY! Do not use pencil!

0000315170-0030
N1115 HC 32

Evaluation

1 Ⓐ Ⓑ Ⓒ Ⓓ Ⓔ
2 Ⓐ Ⓑ Ⓒ Ⓓ Ⓔ
3 Ⓐ Ⓑ Ⓒ Ⓓ Ⓔ
4 Ⓐ Ⓑ Ⓒ Ⓓ Ⓔ
5 Ⓐ Ⓑ Ⓒ Ⓓ Ⓔ
6 Ⓐ Ⓑ Ⓒ Ⓓ Ⓔ
7 Ⓐ Ⓑ Ⓒ Ⓓ Ⓔ
8 Ⓐ Ⓑ Ⓒ Ⓓ Ⓔ
9 Ⓐ Ⓑ Ⓒ Ⓓ Ⓔ
10 Ⓐ Ⓑ Ⓒ Ⓓ Ⓔ
11 Ⓐ Ⓑ Ⓒ Ⓓ Ⓔ
12 Ⓐ Ⓑ Ⓒ Ⓓ Ⓔ
13 Ⓐ Ⓑ Ⓒ Ⓓ Ⓔ
14 Ⓐ Ⓑ Ⓒ Ⓓ Ⓔ
15 Ⓐ Ⓑ Ⓒ Ⓓ Ⓔ
16 Ⓐ Ⓑ Ⓒ Ⓓ Ⓔ
17 Ⓐ Ⓑ Ⓒ Ⓓ Ⓔ
18 Ⓐ Ⓑ Ⓒ Ⓓ Ⓔ
19 Ⓐ Ⓑ Ⓒ Ⓓ Ⓔ
20 Ⓐ Ⓑ Ⓒ Ⓓ Ⓔ
21 Ⓐ Ⓑ Ⓒ Ⓓ Ⓔ
22 Ⓐ Ⓑ Ⓒ Ⓓ Ⓔ
23 Ⓐ Ⓑ Ⓒ Ⓓ Ⓔ
24 Ⓐ Ⓑ Ⓒ Ⓓ Ⓔ
25 Ⓐ Ⓑ Ⓒ Ⓓ Ⓔ

W0174375   **1115**

Cardiovascular Nursing:
A Comprehensive Overview

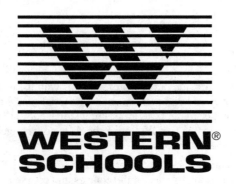

WESTERN® SCHOOLS

By
Karen M. Marzlin, RN, C, CCRN, BC, CVN
Cynthia L. Webner, RN, C, CCRN, BC, CVN

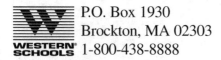 P.O. Box 1930
Brockton, MA 02303
1-800-438-8888

ABOUT THE AUTHORS

Karen M. Marzlin, RN, C, CCRN, BC, CVN, Legal Nurse Consultant has more than 18 years' experience in cardiac nursing. She has worked clinically in a wide variety of cardiac nursing areas. A portion of her career has been dedicated to nursing management and cardiovascular program administration. Her management experience includes the cardiac catheterization laboratory, stress testing center, and cardiac rehabilitation. Karen left her administrative position several years ago to return to clinical practice and focus on creating excellence at the bedside. Karen has a passion for excellence. She currently enjoys working in multiple roles, including bedside clinician, educator, and consultant.

Cynthia L. Webner, RN, C, CCRN, BC, CVN, Legal Nurse Consultant has more than 25 years of cardiac nursing experience. She has worked clinically in both medical and surgical cardiac nursing units. A portion of her career has been dedicated to cardiac nursing management and cardiovascular program administration, where her focus was developing programs to improve the care of cardiac patients. After more than a decade away from the bedside, Cindy left her administrative position to return to clinical practice. She has a passion for caring for cardiac patients and is committed to learning something new every day as she works as a bedside clinician, educator, and consultant.

Karen and Cindy, in addition to maintaining a part-time clinical practice, are co-owners of Key Choice, a training and consulting business. They are also partners with Carol Jacobson, RN, MSN, in Cardiovascular Nursing Education Associates (CNEA). CNEA is dedicated to providing cardiac education courses with a focus on cardiovascular and critical care certification. Linking knowledge to practice is the goal of every education program.

> **Karen Marzlin** and **Cynthia Webner** have disclosed that they have no significant financial or other conflicts of interest pertaining to this course book.

ABOUT THE SUBJECT MATTER REVIEWER

Susan L. Woods, PhD, RN, FAHA, FAAN, is a professor in the Biobehavioral Nursing and Health Systems Department and Associate Dean for Academic Services at the University of Washington, Seattle. She has been a registered nurse since 1967 and, since then, has held clinical and academic positions. She received the 1985 Distinguished Research Award from the American Association of Critical Care Nurses, the 1995 Oregon Health Sciences University Nursing Alumni Award, and the 1995 Katherine Lembright Award for Cardiovascular Nursing Research from the Council on Cardiovascular Nursing of the American Heart Association. She is the coeditor of *Cardiac Nursing,* 5th edition, published by Lippincott Williams & Wilkins.

> **Susan Woods** has disclosed that she has no significant financial or other conflicts of interest pertaining to this course book.

Nurse Planner: Amy Bernard, RN, BSN, MS

Copy Editor: Jaime Stockslager Buss

Indexer: Sylvia Coates

Western Schools' courses are designed to provide nursing professionals with the educational information they need to enhance their career development. The information provided within these course materials is the result of research and consultation with prominent nursing and medical authorities and is, to the best of our knowledge, current and accurate. However, the courses and course materials are provided with the understanding that Western Schools is not engaged in offering legal, nursing, medical, or other professional advice.

Western Schools' courses and course materials are not meant to act as a substitute for seeking out professional advice or conducting individual research. When the information provided in the courses and course materials is applied to individual circumstances, all recommendations must be considered in light of the uniqueness pertaining to each situation.

Western Schools' course materials are intended solely for *your* use and *not* for the benefit of providing advice or recommendations to third parties. Western Schools devoids itself of any responsibility for adverse consequences resulting from the failure to seek nursing, medical, or other professional advice. Western Schools further devoids itself of any responsibility for updating or revising any programs or publications presented, published, distributed, or sponsored by Western Schools unless otherwise agreed to as part of an individual purchase contract.

Products (including brand names) mentioned or pictured in Western School's courses are not endorsed by Western Schools, the American Nurses Credentialing Center (ANCC), or any state board.

ISBN: 978-1-57801-151-3

A dedication from the authors, Karen Marzlin and Cynthia Webner

Firstly, to our God and our creator –
by whom we are fearfully and wonderfully made.

To our Aultman Heart Center colleagues –
who continue to raise the bar for clinical and leadership excellence.

To Drs. Terry Tegtmeier and Milan Dopirak –
for always having time to share their clinical wisdom
with patience and with humor.

To our family and friends for supporting and encouraging us while we focused on this project.

Finally, to Nathan, the most wonderful gift from God.

IMPORTANT: Read these instructions *BEFORE* proceeding!

Enclosed with your course book, you will find the FasTrax® answer sheet. Use this form to answer all the final exam questions that appear in this course book. If you are completing more than one course, be sure to write your answers on the appropriate answer sheet. Full instructions and complete grading details are printed on the FasTrax instruction sheet, also enclosed with your order. Please review them before starting. *If you are mailing your answer sheet(s) to Western Schools, we recommend you make a copy as a backup.*

ABOUT THIS COURSE

A Pretest is provided with each course to test your current knowledge base regarding the subject matter contained within this course. Your Final Exam is a multiple choice examination. **You will find the exam questions at the end of each chapter.**

In the event the course has less than 100 questions, leave the remaining answer boxes on the FasTrax answer sheet blank. **Use a black pen to fill in your answer sheet.**

A PASSING SCORE

You must score 70% or better in order to pass this course and receive your Certificate of Completion. Should you fail to achieve the required score, we will send you an additional FasTrax answer sheet so that you may make a second attempt to pass the course. Western Schools will allow you three chances to pass the same course…*at no extra charge!* After three failed attempts to pass the same course, your file will be closed.

RECORDING YOUR HOURS

Please monitor the time it takes to complete this course using the handy log sheet on the other side of this page. See below for transferring study hours to the course evaluation.

COURSE EVALUATIONS

In this course book, you will find a short evaluation about the course you are soon to complete. This information is vital to providing Western Schools with feedback on this course. The course evaluation answer section is in the lower right hand corner of the FasTrax answer sheet marked "Evaluation," with answers marked 1–19. Your answers are important to us; please take a few minutes to complete the evaluation.

On the back of the FasTrax instruction sheet, there is additional space to make any comments about the course, the school, and suggested new curriculum. Please mail the FasTrax instruction sheet, with your comments, back to Western Schools in the envelope provided with your course order.

TRANSFERRING STUDY TIME

Upon completion of the course, transfer the total study time from your log sheet to question 19 in the course evaluation. The answers will be in ranges; please choose the proper hour range that best represents your study time. You **MUST** log your study time under question 19 on the course evaluation.

EXTENSIONS

You have two (2) years from the date of enrollment to complete this course. A six (6) month extension may be purchased. If after 30 months from the original enrollment date you do not complete the course, *your file will be closed and no certificate can be issued.*

CHANGE OF ADDRESS?

In the event you have moved during the completion of this course, please call our student services department at 1-800-618-1670, and we will update your file.

A GUARANTEE TO WHICH YOU'LL GIVE HIGH HONORS

If any continuing education course fails to meet your expectations or if you are not satisfied in any manner, for any reason, you may return it for an exchange or a refund (less shipping and handling) within 30 days. Software, video, and audio courses must be returned unopened.

Thank you for enrolling at Western Schools!

WESTERN SCHOOLS
P.O. Box 1930
Brockton, MA 02303
(800) 438-8888
www.westernschools.com

Cardiovascular Nursing:
A Comprehensive Overview

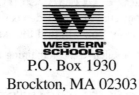

WESTERN®
SCHOOLS

P.O. Box 1930
Brockton, MA 02303

Please use this log to total the number of hours you spend reading the text and taking the final examination.

Date	Hours Spent
_____	_____
_____	_____
_____	_____
_____	_____
_____	_____
_____	_____
_____	_____
_____	_____
_____	_____
_____	_____
_____	_____
_____	_____
_____	_____

TOTAL [   ]

Please log your study hours with submission of your final exam. To log your study time, fill in the appropriate circle under question 19 of the FasTrax® answer sheet under the "Evaluation" section.

Cardiovascular Nursing:
A Comprehensive Overview

WESTERN SCHOOLS
CONTINUING EDUCATION EVALUATION

Instructions: Mark your answers to the following questions with a black pen on the "Evaluation" section of your FasTrax® answer sheet provided with this course. You should not return this sheet.

Please use the scale below to rate how well the course content met the educational objectives.

A Agree Strongly	**C Disagree Somewhat**
B Agree Somewhat	**D Disagree Strongly**

After completing this course, I am able to

1. Recall the basic structures of the heart and associate these structures with the physiologic functions of the heart.

2. Discuss the way pharmacology is used to manipulate the components of cardiac output and myocardial oxygen demand to improve myocardial performance.

3. Describe the key pharmacological agents used to preserve and increase myocardial oxygen supply.

4. Discuss the impact of risk factors on the development of coronary heart disease.

5. Verbalize a comprehensive understanding of the scope of coronary artery disease management throughout the continuum of presentation, from stable angina through acute myocardial infarction.

6. Discuss the indications for, benefits of, and potential complications of cardiac revascularization.

7. Describe current strategies for the management of heart failure.

8. Recognize the three main types of cardiomyopathy and their physiological differences.

9. Recognize aortic valve disease and identify its impact on the body.

10. Recognize mitral valve disease and identify its impact on the body.

11. Discuss the implications of atrial fibrillation and the current management strategies for it.

12. Recognize the indications for cardiac pacemakers and defibrillators and understand the impact of these devices on a patient.

13. The content of this course was relevant to the objectives.

14. This offering met my professional education needs.

15. The objectives met the overall purpose/goal of the course.

16. The course was generally well-written and the subject matter explained thoroughly. (If no, please explain on the back of the FasTrax instruction sheet.)

17. The content of this course was appropriate for home study.

18. The final examination was well-written and at an appropriate level for the content of the course.

19. **PLEASE LOG YOUR STUDY HOURS WITH SUBMISSION OF YOUR FINAL EXAM.**
    Please choose the response that best represents the total study hours it took to complete this 32-hour course.

    A. Less than 27 hours

    B. 27–30 hours

    C. 31–34 hours

    D. Greater than 34 hours

CONTENTS

FIGURES AND TABLES

PRETEST

1. Begin this course by taking the pretest. Circle the answers to the questions on this page, or write the answers on a separate sheet of paper. Do not log answers to the pretest questions on the FasTrax test sheet included with the course.

2. Compare your answers to the PRETEST KEY located in the back of the book. The pretest answer key indicates the course chapter where the content of that question is discussed. Make note of the questions you missed, so that you can focus on those areas as you complete the course.

3. Complete the course by reading each chapter and completing the exam questions at the end of the chapter. Answers to these exam questions should be logged on the FasTrax test sheet included with the course.

1. The heart has several layers, including the endocardium, myocardium, and epicardium. The myocardium is the

   a. inner surface of the heart chambers and valves.

   b. smooth outer layer of the heart that contains a network of coronary arteries and veins.

   c. thick middle layer of the heart that contains cardiac muscle fibers.

   d. thin fibrous sac that surrounds the heart.

2. The mitral valve is located between the

   a. aorta and the left ventricle.

   b. right atrium and the right ventricle.

   c. right ventricle and the pulmonary artery.

   d. left atrium and the left ventricle.

3. One of the primary types of medications used to decrease preload is

   a. diuretics.

   b. beta-blockers.

   c. calcium channel blockers.

   d. digoxin.

4. Preventing the conversion of angiotensin I to angiotensin II best describes the action of

   a. ACE inhibitors.

   b. angiotensin receptor blockers.

   c. calcium channel blockers.

   d. nitrates.

5. Nicotinic acid and fibric acid derivatives are most effective in lowering

   a. high-density lipoprotein cholesterol.

   b. low-density lipoprotein cholesterol.

   c. triglycerides.

   d. C-reactive protein.

6. Aspirin, glycoprotein IIb/IIIa inhibitors, and clopidogrel are all medications that can be utilized for

   a. thrombolytic therapy.

   b. antiplatelet therapy.

   c. fibrinolytic therapy.

   d. anticoagulation therapy.

7. People with known coronary heart disease have a risk of having a cardiac event over the next 10 years. That risk is

   a. 10%.

   b. 20%.

   c. 30%.

   d. 40%.

8. The single most important modifiable cardiovascular risk factor is

   a. hypertension.

   b. high cholesterol.

   c. diabetes mellitus.

   d. smoking.

9. Angina that is described as increasing in severity and frequency is referred to as

   a. unstable angina.

   b. stable angina.

   c. Prinzmetal's angina.

   d. new-onset angina.

10. The most reliable diagnostic test used to determine the presence of coronary artery disease is

    a. electrocardiography.

    b. cardiac angiography.

    c. stress testing.

    d. nuclear imaging.

11. The second most common cause of mortality related to cardiac bypass surgery is

    a. cardiac arrhythmias.

    b. sternal wound infection.

    c. postoperative stroke.

    d. intraoperative myocardial infarction.

12. National standards establish a time frame for achieving perfusion to the coronary artery with angioplasty when a patient with an acute myocardial infarction arrives at an emergency department. This time frame is

    a. 30 minutes.

    b. 60 minutes.

    c. 90 minutes.

    d. 120 minutes.

13. The most common cause of left ventricular dysfunction resulting in heart failure is

    a. hypertensive heart disease.

    b. valvular heart disease.

    c. rheumatic heart disease.

    d. ischemic coronary heart disease.

14. According to the New York Heart Association Classification, a patient with class III heart failure is described as

    a. comfortable at rest but less-than-ordinary activity results in fatigue, palpitations, dyspnea, or anginal pain.

    b. free from fatigue, palpitations, dyspnea, and anginal pain during ordinary activity.

    c. comfortable at rest but ordinary activity results in fatigue, palpitations, dyspnea, or anginal pain.

    d. having symptoms of cardiac insufficiency at rest.

15. Dilated cardiomyopathy is defined as

   a. rigidity of the cardiac walls resulting in a decreased ability of the chamber walls to expand during cardiac filling.

   b. enlarged cardiac chambers with an impaired ability to contract resulting in systolic dysfunction.

   c. an increase in muscle mass resulting in a decrease in ventricular filling and a decrease in cardiac output.

   d. enlarged cardiac chambers with an impaired ability to contract resulting in diastolic dysfunction.

16. The most common cause of aortic stenosis is

   a. rheumatic heart disease.

   b. infective endocarditis.

   c. senile degenerative calcification.

   d. congenital valve disease.

17. Mitral facies is a pinkish purple discoloration of the cheeks that is common in patients with

   a. severe mitral stenosis.

   b. severe mitral regurgitation.

   c. severe aortic stenosis.

   d. severe aortic regurgitation.

18. Atrial fibrillation that comes on spontaneously and terminates itself is called

   a. persistent atrial fibrillation.

   b. permanent atrial fibrillation.

   c. temporary atrial fibrillation.

   d. paroxysmal atrial fibrillation.

19. Class II antiarrhythmic medications used to control heart rate in patients with atrial fibrillation include

   a. calcium channel blockers.

   b. beta-blockers.

   c. potassium channel blockers.

   d. sodium channel blockers.

20. A patient with permanent pacemakers should be aware that

   a. the use of a microwave oven may damage the pacemaker.

   b. the use of a microwave oven by someone else in his or her presence is acceptable as long as the person with the pacemaker does not touch the microwave.

   c. the use of a microwave oven will not harm the pacemaker.

   d. he or she should leave the room when a microwave oven is running.

INTRODUCTION

The prevention of cardiovascular disease should begin at birth. From birth, the delicate inner layer of our vessels, the endothelium, begins the fight to combat a wide variety of insults that can damage cells and vessel walls. This damage begins a progression of cardiovascular disease that may disable and ultimately end life. Prevention is the first step to cardiovascular health. Unfortunately, too many people wait until disease progression is well under way before taking notice.

In February 2005, the National Center for Health Statistics released preliminary death statistics for 2003. Diseases of the heart remain the number one cause of death in the United States. Although the numbers for 2003 declined by 3.6%, heart disease remains at the top of the list for both men and women (National Vital Statistics Report, 2005). Although many advances have recently been made in cardiovascular medicine, they have not been enough to move cardiovascular death from the top of the list. Many people believe that intracoronary stenting and open-heart surgery can solve the problem of heart disease. Unfortunately, these procedures only resolve the end result of the problem. Without risk factor modification, the process continues. In many cases, before intracoronary stenting and open-heart surgery are options, irreversible damage to the heart occurs, resulting in a decline in cardiac activity. Damage to the myocardium can also result from processes that do not involve blockage of the coronary arteries, including hypertension and valvular disease.

Because of its prevalence, nurses commonly care for patients who have cardiovascular disease or are at risk for it. This book provides information to support nurses working in a variety of settings who care for patients with cardiovascular disease. The book is designed to provide a reference for nurses working in noncardiovascular specialties. It is also a good introductory text for nurses who desire to work in the cardiovascular arena. The curriculum begins with a foundation of cardiovascular anatomy and physiology. Once normal cardiovascular functioning is understood, the learner can then move forward to understanding pathophysiology. The content of the chapters on cardiovascular medications and risk factors is used throughout the rest of the text, as cardiovascular disease processes are discussed. Nursing application points are highlighted throughout the text to assist in identifying key issues in the care of patients with cardiovascular disease.

Heightened awareness is the first step toward impacting this devastating disease. Nurses with knowledge open the door to early recognition and treatment of cardiovascular disease. The astute nurse can make the difference between a life that is cut short by cardiovascular disease and one that is long and healthy.

CHAPTER 1

CARDIAC ANATOMY AND PRINCIPLES OF PHYSIOLOGY

CHAPTER OBJECTIVE

After completing this chapter, the reader will be able to recall the basic structures of the heart and associate these structures with the physiologic functions of the heart.

OBJECTIVES

After studying this chapter, the reader will be able to

1. identify the layers of the heart wall.

2. explain the structural difference between atrioventricular valves and semilunar valves.

3. describe systole and diastole and their purpose in the cardiac cycle.

4. decribe the anatomy of the coronary arteries.

5. recognize the components of the cardiac conduction system.

6. define the components of cardiac output.

7. describe how the heart and lungs form a cardiopulmonary circuit that delivers oxygen to body tissues.

8. explain the role of the autonomic nervous system in regulating the heart and blood pressure.

9. explain the role of the renin-angiotensin-aldosterone system in regulating blood pressure.

INTRODUCTION

Cardiac anatomy and physiology form a critical foundation for understanding cardiovascular nursing. All clinical application builds on this foundation. Even in the field of medicine, "in this technology driven era, a new appreciation of cardiac anatomy has emerged as the cornerstone for clinical cardiology" (Fuster, Alexander, et al., 2001, p. 45).

BASIC CARDIAC ANATOMY

The heart is a hollow, muscular, four-chambered organ. It is positioned in the mediastinum (middle of the thoracic cavity) between the lungs, just above the diaphragm. The heart is attached to the thorax by the great vessels. The great vessels include the aorta, pulmonary artery, inferior vena cava, and superior vena cava. The adult heart is approximately 5 inches by 3 1/2 inches by 2 1/2 inches (Dennison, 2000), or approximately the size of a person's fist. The tip of the left ventricle forms the apex (bottom) of the heart. The apex is located at approximately the fifth intercostal space, at the midclavicular line. The base, or top, of the heart is located at approximately the second intercostal space (see Figure 1-1).

Cardiac Chambers

The right and left atria (upper chambers) are separated by a mass of connective tissue called the *interatrial septum*. The right and left atria are low-

FIGURE 1-1: LOCATION OF HEART IN CHEST

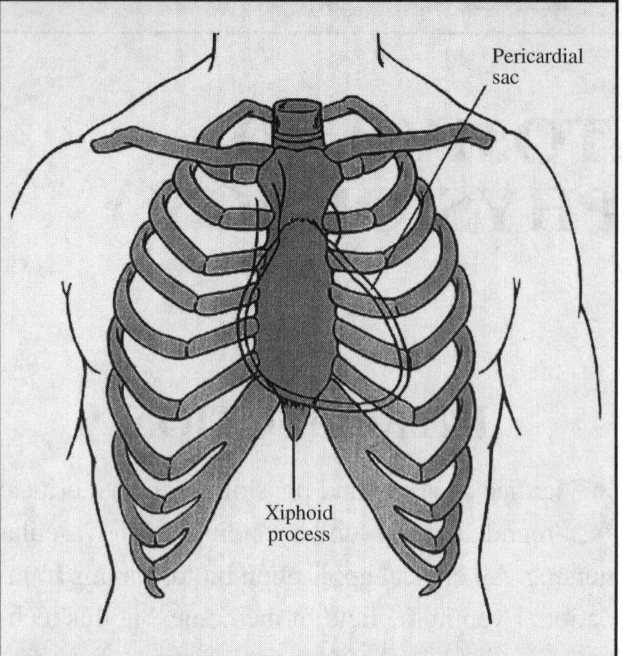

Pericardial sac

Xiphoid process

Note. From *Atlas of Anesthesia: Critical Care* by N. Yeston and R. Kirby. Edited by R. Miller (series editor) and R. Kirby. Copyright 1997 Current Medicine, Inc. Used with permission from Images.MD.

pressure, thin-walled chambers that receive blood and act as reservoirs. The right atrium receives deoxygenated blood from the venous system via the inferior and superior venae cavae, as well as from the coronary sinus (the primary coronary vein). The left atrium receives oxygenated blood from the pulmonary veins after the blood has traveled through the lungs (see Figure 1-2).

The right and left ventricles (lower chambers) are the pumping chambers of the heart and receive blood from the atria. The ventricles are separated by the interventricular septum. The right ventricle is a thin-walled, low-pressure pump that receives deoxygenated blood from the right atrium. This ventricle pumps blood into the pulmonary artery, which carries the blood to the lungs to exchange carbon dioxide for oxygen. The left ventricle is a thick-walled, high-pressure pump that receives oxygenated blood from the left atrium and pumps blood into the aorta for distribution throughout the circulatory system.

FIGURE 1-2: LEFT FRONTAL VIEW OF THE HEART

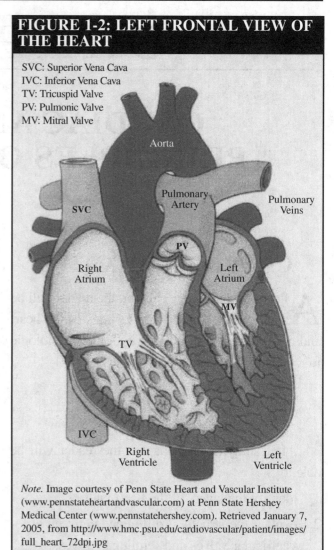

SVC: Superior Vena Cava
IVC: Inferior Vena Cava
TV: Tricuspid Valve
PV: Pulmonic Valve
MV: Mitral Valve

Aorta

Pulmonary Artery

Pulmonary Veins

SVC

PV

Right Atrium

Left Atrium

MV

TV

IVC

Right Ventricle

Left Ventricle

Note. Image courtesy of Penn State Heart and Vascular Institute (www.pennstateheartandvascular.com) at Penn State Hershey Medical Center (www.pennstatehershey.com). Retrieved January 7, 2005, from http://www.hmc.psu.edu/cardiovascular/patient/images/full_heart_72dpi.jpg

Clinical Application

Because the right ventricular wall is thinner than the left ventricular wall, the right ventricle fails more easily in response to elevated pulmonary pressures than the left ventricle does to elevated systemic pressures.

Layers of the Heart

The three layers of the heart are the endocardium, myocardium, and epicardium. The pericardium is an additional layer that surrounds the heart (see Figure 1-3).

Endocardium

The endocardium is a serous membrane consisting of connective tissue, elastic fibers, and a thin layer of epithelial cells that form a smooth surface for the movement of blood and prevention of clot formation. The endocardium is not only the inner surface of the

FIGURE 1-3: LAYERS OF THE HEART WALL

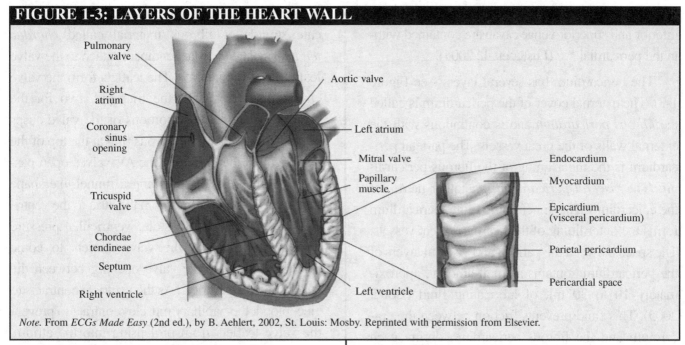

Note. From *ECGs Made Easy* (2nd ed.), by B. Aehlert, 2002, St. Louis: Mosby. Reprinted with permission from Elsevier.

heart chambers and valves but also continues on to cover the walls of the vessels of the entire vascular system, creating a closed circulatory system.

Clinical Application
Inflammation of the endocardium or heart valves is called endocarditis.

Myocardium

The myocardium is the thick middle layer of the heart. The largest layer of the heart, the myocardium contains cardiac muscle fibers that have the ability to contract as well as conduct electrical stimuli. The myocardium of the ventricles is thicker than the myocardium of the atria. The left ventricle has the thickest myocardium due to the high pressure in the aorta that the ventricle must pump against to eject its contents. As patients develop myocardial hypertrophy (increased cell size), this layer of the heart becomes larger.

Clinical Application
Damage to the myocardial layer of the heart results in a decreased ability for the heart to contract, resulting in an impaired ability to eject blood from the ventricles.

Epicardium

The epicardium is the smooth outer layer of the heart that contains the network of coronary arteries and veins, the autonomic nerves, the lymphatic system, and fat tissue. Coronary blood vessels that supply the myocardium and endocardium with oxygen-rich blood must cross the epicardium before passing through the myocardium, and finally, entering the endocardium. Increased age and obesity increase the amount of fat tissue in the epicardial layer, resulting in an increase in the amount of tissue that must be supplied with oxygen-rich blood before supplying the myocardium and endocardium (Fuster et al., 2004).

Clinical Application
An increasing amount of adipose tissue in the epicardium can increase a person's risk of myocardial rupture during or after an acute myocardial infarction (MI).

Pericardium

The thin sac surrounding the heart is called the *pericardium*. This fibrous sac protects the heart from infection and traumatic injury. The pericardium has little elastic tissue and cannot expand acutely. Almost the entire ascending aorta, the main pulmonary artery, all four pulmonary veins, and portions of the inferior and superior venae cavae are contained within the pericardial sac (Fuster et al., 2004).

The pericardium has several layers (see Figure 1-3). The external cover of the pericardium is called the *fibrous pericardium* and is continuous with the external walls of the great vessels. The parietal pericardium is the inner lining of the fibrous pericardium. The *visceral pericardium* is another name for the epicardium. This inner lining of the pericardium forms the outer lining of the heart and great vessels. The space between the parietal and visceral layers of the pericardium contains a small amount, approximately 10 to 30 ml, of lubricating fluid (Bond, 2005). This fluid prevents friction between the epicardium and the fibrous pericardium during each cardiac contraction. Pericardial disease can interfere with the ability of the ventricles to fill during diastole. Pericarditis is inflammation of the pericardium.

Clinical Application

If the aorta ruptures or dissects, the pericardium can rapidly fill with blood. Rapid filling of the pericardial sac can produce fatal results, including cardiac tamponade and death.

Cardiac Valves

The four cardiac valves located within the heart are designated as either *atrioventricular (AV) valves* or *semilunar valves* (see Figure 1-4). The valves located between the atria and ventricles are AV valves. The tricuspid valve is located between the right atrium and right ventricle, and the mitral valve is located between the left atrium and left ventricle. The two semilunar valves are located between the ventricles and the great vessels. The pulmonic valve is located between the right ventricle and the pulmonary artery, and the aortic valve is located between the left ventricle and the aorta.

Atrioventricular Valves

The AV valves are anatomically different from the semilunar valves. Papillary muscles project from the inner surface of the ventricle and attach to delicate strands of fibrous material called *chordae tendineae*. The chordae tendineae attach to the valve leaflets (see Figure 1-5). The leaflets form the valve cusps (three cusps for the tricuspid, two for the mitral). The uppermost portions of the valve cusps are joined together by a fibrous ring at the top of the valve, called the *annulus*. The AV valves open passively during diastole, forming a funnel-like shape that allows blood to flow from the atria to the ventricles. At the end of diastole, ventricular pressure increases and forces the valve leaflets to come together and close the valve opening between the atrium and the ventricle. As the ventricle contracts to eject blood, the papillary muscles contract to prevent the valve leaflets from prolapsing into the atrium. The closure of the leaflets prevents the backward flow of blood from the ventricle to the atrium. At the end of systole, when the ventricle relaxes, the AV valves open again and the cycle is repeated.

Clinical Application

During an acute MI of the left ventricle, the papillary muscle of the mitral valve can become weakened and potentially rupture. If the papillary muscle ruptures, the mitral valve can no longer maintain unidirectional blood flow. As a result, blood backs up into the left atrium during ventricular contraction, causing acute left-sided heart failure.

Semilunar Valves

Each semilunar valve consists of an annulus and three cusps (see Figure 1-6). The pulmonic and aortic valves have the same structure; however, the aortic valve leaflets are heavier and thicker due to the increased pressure system in the left side of the heart. The pulmonic valve is located between the right ventricle and the pulmonary artery, and the aortic valve is located between the left ventricle and the aorta. These valves function by pressure changes in the heart and the great vessels. During diastole, the semilunar valves are closed as the ventricles fill with blood from the atria. As the AV valves close and sys-

FIGURE 1-4: VALVES AND CHAMBERS OF THE HEART

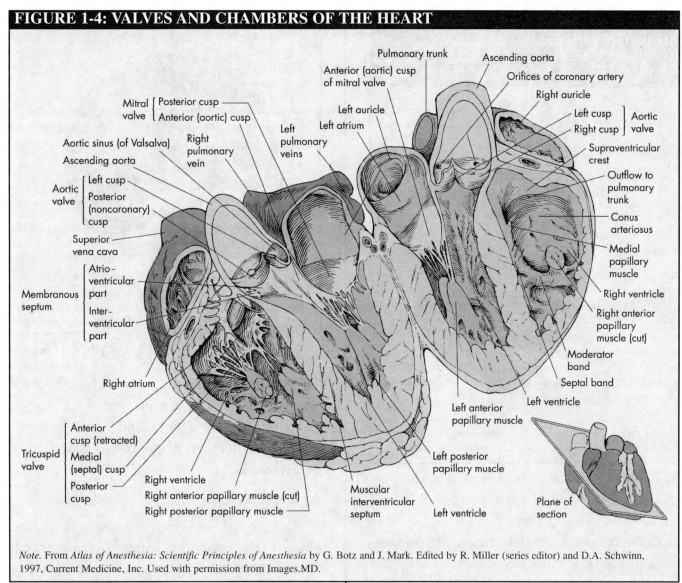

Note. From *Atlas of Anesthesia: Scientific Principles of Anesthesia* by G. Botz and J. Mark. Edited by R. Miller (series editor) and D.A. Schwinn, 1997, Current Medicine, Inc. Used with permission from Images.MD.

tole begins, the ventricles begin to contract. Once the pressure in the ventricles is greater than the pressure on the other side of the semilunar valves, the valves force open and blood is ejected out of the ventricles into the great vessels. When ventricular ejection is complete, the pressure in the ventricles is less than the pressure in the great vessels, and the semilunar valves close tightly. Tight closure prevents the backward flow of blood from the great vessels to the ventricles. The cycle then begins again.

Clinical Application

When auscultating the heart, the first heart sound (S_1), referred to as "lub," is associated with closure of the AV valves. The second heart sound (S_2), referred to as "dub," is associated with closure of the semilunar valves. These two sounds together form the "lub-dub" heard during cardiac auscultation.

Clinical Application

S_1 ("lub") represents the beginning of ventricular systole, or contraction, and S_2 ("dub") represents the beginning of ventricular diastole, or relaxation.

When cardiac valves function correctly, they permit forward flow of blood when they are open

FIGURE 1-5: MITRAL VALVE AND THE RELATIONSHIPS OF THE CUSPS, CHORDAE TENDINEAE, AND PAPILLARY MUSCLES

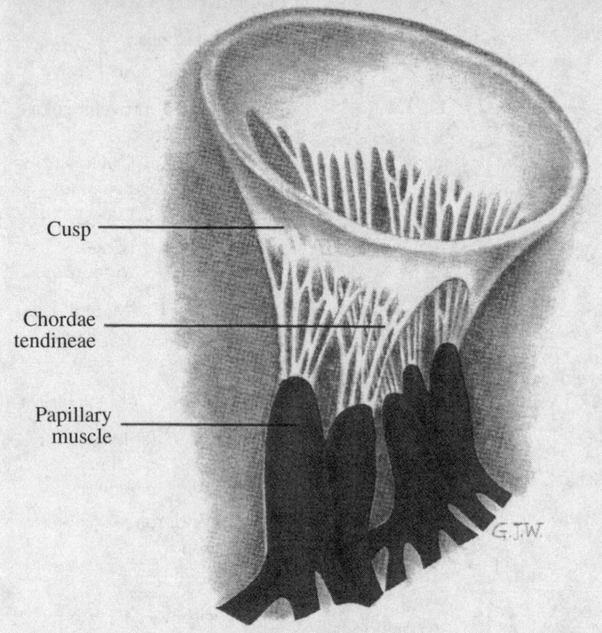

Cusp

Chordae
tendineae

Papillary
muscle

Note. From *Critical Care Nursing: Diagnosis and Management* (2nd ed.), by L.A. Thelan, J.K. Davie, L.D. Urden, and M.E. Lough, 1994, St. Louis: Mosby. Reprinted with permission from Elsevier.

and prevent backward flow of blood when they are closed. During ventricular systole, the tricuspid and mitral valves close to prevent backward flow of blood from the ventricles into the atria. During ventricular systole, all blood forced from the ventricles during ejection is propelled forward through open pulmonic and aortic valves into the pulmonary and systemic vascular beds. During ventricular diastole, the tricuspid and mitral valves open, allowing filling of the ventricles from the atria. When the pulmonic and aortic valves close properly during ventricular diastole, they prevent the backward flow of blood from the pulmonary and systemic vascular beds into the ventricles.

Clinical Application

An aortic valve that does not close properly results in a backward flow of blood from the aorta into the left ventricle, reducing the stroke volume of the previous contraction.

FIGURE 1-6: NORMAL AORTIC VALVE

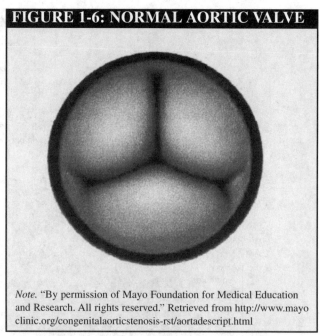

CIRCULATORY SYSTEM

The heart and blood vessels work together for one primary purpose: the delivery of oxygen and other nutrients to the cellular level. The capillaries are the location where oxygen and nutrients are exchanged.

Arterial System

Oxygenated blood leaves the left ventricle and travels to the tissue level via the systemic arterial system. Arteries are made up of elastic tissue that allows them to respond to the high pressures associated with the force of left ventricular contraction. Large arteries also contain smooth muscle.

All arteries have three layers of tissue that surround the open lumen (see Figure 1-7). The inner layer, called the *intima,* has a thin lining of endothelium that contains epithelial cells. The intima decreases resistance to flow and minimizes the chance of platelet aggregation. The *media,* the middle layer, is composed of smooth muscle and elastic connective tissue. The media is responsible for changes in the diameter of the vessel as needed to assist with blood pressure control. The fibrous outer layer, called the *adventitia,* is designed to protect the vessel and provide connection to other internal struc-

FIGURE 1-7: CROSS-SECTION OF AN ARTERY AND A VEIN

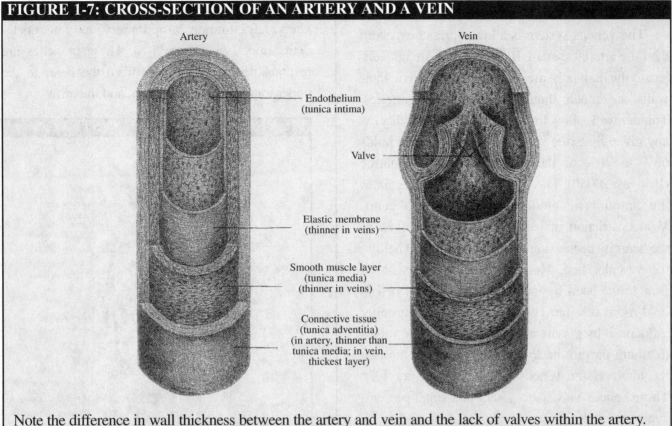

Artery   Vein

Endothelium
(tunica intima)

Valve

Elastic membrane
(thinner in veins)

Smooth muscle layer
(tunica media)
(thinner in veins)

Connective tissue
(tunica adventitia)
(in artery, thinner than
tunica media; in vein,
thickest layer)

Note the difference in wall thickness between the artery and vein and the lack of valves within the artery.

Note. From *Critical Care Nursing: Diagnosis and Management* (2nd ed.), by L.A. Thelan, J.K. Davie, L.D. Urden, and M.E. Lough, 1994, St. Louis: Mosby. Reprinted with permission from Elsevier.

tures. Arteries have the ability to expand or contract in response to the body's cardiac output needs.

Arterioles

The large arteries carry blood from the aorta to the rest of the body. The arteries divide and become smaller as they move away from the aorta. The smallest arteries branch into arterioles. Arterioles connect to the capillary bed. At the arteriole level of the capillary is smooth muscle that is referred to as the *precapillary sphincter*. The arterioles and the precapillary sphincter regulate blood flow to the capillaries. This regulation of blood flow is primarily determined by the oxygen needs of the tissue through a process called *autoregulation*. When oxygen needs increase, the arterioles dilate. This dilatation decreases resistance to flow and results in increased flow to the capillaries (Darovic, 2002).

Capillary System

When oxygenated blood reaches the capillary level, oxygen and other nutrients are exchanged. Because capillary walls are only one cell thick, gases and nutrients pass through the walls easily. Miles of capillaries are located near almost all body cells. The capillaries contain no smooth muscle (Bridges, 2005b). Therefore, capillary tone depends on the tone of the vessel just before and after the capillary. Four pressures influence the movement of fluids across capillary membranes: capillary hydrostatic pressure, interstitial hydrostatic pressure, capillary oncotic pressure, and interstitial colloidal oncotic pressure (Opie, 2004). Once oxygen and nutrients are exchanged for waste products, deoxygenated blood is returned to the right atrium from the capillaries via the venous system.

Venous System

The venous system is a lower-pressure system than the arterial system. Because veins are not subject to the high pressures of the arterial system, their walls are much thinner than those of arteries. Thinner walls allow for much more distensibility. At any given time, the venous system generally holds 65% to 70% of the body's total blood volume (Bridges, 2005b). The venous system also regulates the amount of blood returning to the heart. Vasoconstriction of veins increases blood flow to the heart by decreasing the amount of blood held in the vascular bed. Vasodilatation decreases blood flow to the heart by increasing the vascular bed to hold more volume. The venous system is strongly influenced by gravity and relies on one-way valves that help prevent backward flow of blood through the low-pressure venous system (see Figure 1-7). These venous valves are absent in a small percentage of people and can be damaged by age or by catheter insertion (Fuster et al., 2004). Venous return is also augmented by contraction of skeletal muscles, which compress veins and help to propel blood forward.

Clinical Application
Weakened vein valves cause varicose (dilated) veins. Age, prolonged standing, and pregnancy contribute to varicose veins.

Clinical Application
In right-sided heart failure, venous valves are important in maintaining the unidirectional flow of blood back to the right side of the heart.

Normal Circulatory Patterns

The thoracic aorta arises from the aortic valve, which is divided into three segments: ascending aorta, aortic arch, and descending thoracic aorta. The origin of the coronary arteries is located in the ascending aorta immediately above the aortic valve. The location of the origin of the coronary arteries allows them to receive blood that is rich in oxygen.

The aortic arch has three branches: brachiocephalic artery, left common carotid artery, and left subclavian artery (see Figure 1-8). These branches are responsible for blood flow from the heart to the upper torso, neck, head, brain, and the arms.

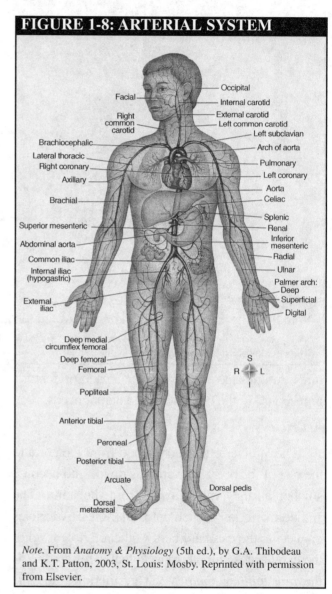

FIGURE 1-8: ARTERIAL SYSTEM

Note. From *Anatomy & Physiology* (5th ed.), by G.A. Thibodeau and K.T. Patton, 2003, St. Louis: Mosby. Reprinted with permission from Elsevier.

The thoracic aorta, which is located below the aortic arch, branches off to supply blood to the torso, including the thoracic cavity and the lungs. The abdominal aorta supplies blood to the abdominal organs and the kidneys. At approximately the fourth lumbar vertebra, the aorta divides into the internal iliac arteries. The structures of the lower trunk, including the reproductive organs and the legs, receive their blood supply from the internal iliac arteries.

The venous system mimics the arterial system in returning blood to the heart. Prior to entering the heart, the entire venous system enters into the superior vena cava or the inferior vena cava. The superior vena cava receives venous blood returning from the head, neck, upper extremities, and thorax. The inferior vena cava receives blood from below the level of the diaphragm, including the abdomen, pelvis, and lower extremities. The superior and inferior venae cavae empty the returning deoxygenated blood into the right atrium. The coronary veins also drain into the coronary sinus, which then empties directly into the right atrium.

Circulation through the Heart

Once deoxygenated blood is received by the right atrium, it moves to the right ventricle through the tricuspid valve during ventricular diastole. After the right ventricle fills, the tricuspid valve closes and the ventricle contracts and ejects the blood through the open pulmonic valve into the pulmonary artery. The pulmonary artery divides into the right and left pulmonary arteries and carries blood to the pulmonary capillaries, where gas exchange occurs. Blood leaving the right ventricle is low in oxygen and high in carbon dioxide. When gas exchange occurs, oxygen enters the blood and carbon dioxide leaves the blood and is exhaled.

The pulmonary veins return oxygenated blood to the left side of the heart via the left atrium. The blood in the left atrium moves through the open mitral valve into the left ventricle during ventricular diastole. At the end of diastole, the mitral valve closes and the left ventricle contracts, forcing the aortic valve open and ejecting the oxygenated blood into the aorta for participation in systemic circulation. (See Figure 1-9.)

THE CARDIAC CYCLE

*S*ystole, contraction of the heart muscle, results in ejection of blood from the chamber. *Diastole,*

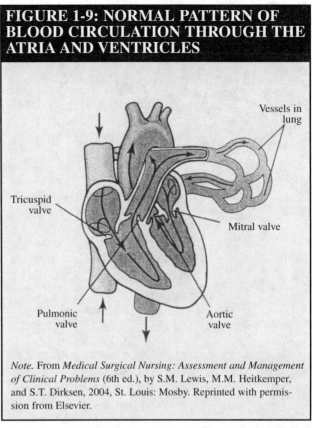

FIGURE 1-9: NORMAL PATTERN OF BLOOD CIRCULATION THROUGH THE ATRIA AND VENTRICLES

Vessels in lung

Tricuspid valve

Mitral valve

Pulmonic valve

Aortic valve

Note. From *Medical Surgical Nursing: Assessment and Management of Clinical Problems* (6th ed.), by S.M. Lewis, M.M. Heitkemper, and S.T. Dirksen, 2004, St. Louis: Mosby. Reprinted with permission from Elsevier.

relaxation of the heart muscle, allows the chamber to fill. Each of the atria and ventricles undergoes systole and diastole. In a resting adult, each cardiac cycle lasts approximately 0.8 second (Opie, 2004). The efficiency of the cardiac cycle depends on the health of the cardiac muscle, valves, and conduction system. The heart's conduction system provides the timing of events for atrial and ventricular systole (see Figure 1-10).

Ventricular Diastole

Ventricular diastole begins when ventricular contraction is complete. When the pressure in the pulmonary vascular bed and the aorta exceeds the pressure in the right and left ventricles, the semilunar valves close. Simultaneously, the pressure in the filled atria exceeds the pressure in the nearly empty ventricles and the AV valves (tricuspid and mitral valves) open. Once the tricuspid and mitral valves open, a rapid, passive filling of the ventricles occurs as blood moves from the atria through the open valves into the ventricles. Approximately 75% of ventricular filling occurs during this passive filling

FIGURE 1-10: THE CARDIAC CYCLE

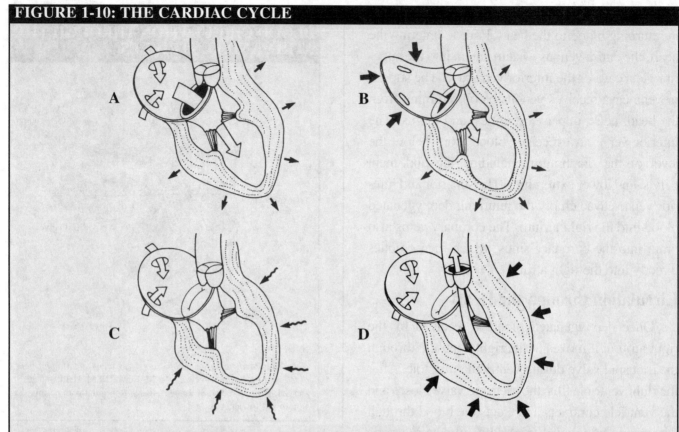

Drawings A and B: Ventricular diastole. A. Passive filling of ventricle. B. Active filling of ventricle (atrial kick). Drawings C and D: Ventricular systole. C. Isovolumic contraction. D. Ventricular ejection.

Note. From *Hemodynamic monitoring: Invasive and noninvasive clinical application* (3rd ed.), by G.O. Darovic, 2002, Philadelphia: Saunders. Reprinted with permission from Elsevier.

phase. The remainder of ventricular filling occurs with atrial contraction. This contraction of the atria is also known as *atrial systole*. Atrial systole is commonly referred to as *atrial kick* and contributes as much as 25% of the ventricular volume (Bond, 2005).

Clinical Application

When a person is in atrial fibrillation, he or she loses the atrial kick contribution to left ventricular volume. This loss of atrial kick can result in enough decrease in stroke volume to cause a decrease in cardiac output and, ultimately, symptoms of decreased perfusion.

Ventricular Systole

After atrial contraction, the pressures in the atria and ventricles equalize, the AV valves partially close, and ventricular systole begins. Ventricular systole has two phases. The first phase is *isovolu-*

mic, or *isovolumetric, contraction* (Darovic, 2002; Thibodeau & Patton, 2003), so named because the volume of blood in the ventricles does not change during this phase. During isovolumic contraction, the ventricular walls tense and press toward the center of the ventricular cavity. This tensing of the walls increases the pressure in the ventricles. When the pressure in the ventricles exceeds that in the atria, the AV valves close quickly, preventing backward flow of blood into the atria. In order for ejection of the ventricular contents to occur, the myocardial walls of the ventricles must develop enough pressure to force the semilunar (aortic and pulmonic) valves open. Once the pressure in the ventricles exceeds the pressure in the aorta and pulmonary artery, the aortic and pulmonic valves open.

The second phase of systole is *ejection*, during which blood is ejected into the systemic and pulmonary circulation. The semilunar valves close at the end of systole, when the pressure in the arteries exceeds the pressure in the ventricles. Normally, ventricular diastole (ventricular filling) is two times longer than ventricular systole (ventricular emptying).

Clinical Application

As heart rate increases, ventricular diastolic time shortens while ventricular systolic time essentially stays the same. Therefore, an increased heart rate decreases the time available to fill the ventricles and the coronary arteries.

Contractility

The atria and ventricles have contractile muscle cells called *myocytes*. Without functioning myocytes, the myocardium cannot contract. The remainder of the cardiac cells are either pacemaker cells or cells capable of excitability and conductivity. The adult heart has approximately 19 billion cardiac cells (Bond, 2005). Millions of cardiac cells are lost with each year of life. If a person lives to age 100, he or she will have lost approximately two thirds of his or her original heart cells (Opie, 2004). Cardiac muscle cells differ from skeletal muscle cells in that they are shorter, broader, and more interconnected. Intercalated disks form junctions between cardiac muscle cells, allowing them to function as integrated units. The junctions serve as electrical connections, joining muscle fibers in a single unit capable of rapidly conducting an impulse. These connections allow both atria and ventricles to contract almost simultaneously.

Cardiac muscle cells are also more metabolically active, require more energy, and experience more prolonged contractions than do skeletal muscle cells. This prolonged contraction prevents impulses from coming rapidly enough to produce a sustained contraction, thereby, preventing cardiac muscle from running low on adenosine triphosphate (ATP) and becoming fatigued (Opie, 2004). The process of myocardial contraction utilizes the ATP molecules for energy.

The contractile property of the cardiac muscle cell comes from the myofibril. Myofibrils consist of repeating units called *sarcomeres* and contain protein units responsible for contraction (Bond, 2005). Cardiac muscle fibers contain transverse tubules, also called *T tubules,* that are extensions of the cell membranes. A significant amount of calcium enters the cell through the T tubules from the interstitial fluid surrounding the cells. Without this additional calcium coming through the T tubules, the force of myocardial contraction would be greatly reduced (Opie, 2004).

Clinical Application

The amount of extracellular calcium ions affects the availability of calcium to enter the cardiac cells via the T tubules. Low extracellular calcium ions can therefore affect the force of myocardial contraction.

CORONARY ARTERIES

The coronary arteries begin in the epicardial layer of the heart. These arteries then travel through the myocardium and ultimately to the endocardium to provide oxygen-rich blood to the entire cardiac musculature (see Figure 1-3). During systole, as the heart contracts, blood flow through the coronary arteries is markedly reduced due to compression on the vessels. Therefore, coronary artery perfusion occurs primarily during diastole, when the ventricles are relaxed. Also during diastole, oxygenated blood just ejected from the left ventricle to the aorta enters the coronary arteries through two small openings, just above the closed aortic valve. These small openings are located in the right aortic sinus and left aortic sinus. From the openings flow the left and right coronary artery systems (see Figure 1-11).

Clinical Application

Coronary circulation begins with the epicardium and reaches the endocardium last; therefore, myocardial ischemia and infarction begin in the endocardium.

FIGURE 1-11: AORTIC VALVE

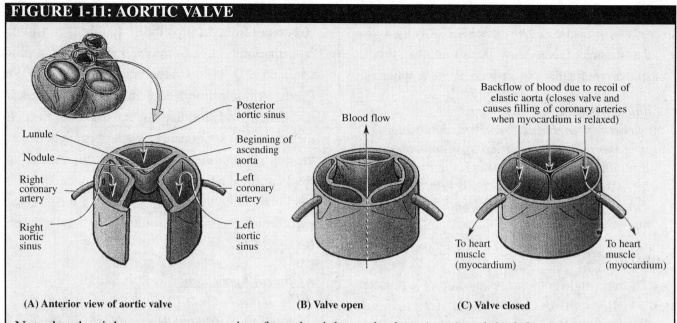

(A) Anterior view of aortic valve

Posterior aortic sinus

Lunule

Nodule

Beginning of ascending aorta

Right coronary artery

Left coronary artery

Right aortic sinus

Left aortic sinus

(B) Valve open

Blood flow

(C) Valve closed

Backflow of blood due to recoil of elastic aorta (closes valve and causes filling of coronary arteries when myocardium is relaxed)

To heart muscle (myocardium)

To heart muscle (myocardium)

Note that the right coronary artery arises from the right aortic sinus (cusp) and the left coronary artery arises from the left aortic sinus (cusp).

Note. From *Clinically Oriented Anatomy* (4th ed.), by K.L. Moore and A.F. Dalley, 1999, Philadelphia: Lippincott Williams & Wilkins. Reprinted with permission from Lippincott Williams & Wilkins.

Clinical Application

A thickened myocardial wall (hypertrophy) results in decreased flow of oxygen-rich blood to the deep myocardium and endocardial layer.

Left Coronary Artery System

The left main coronary artery, which supplies oxygenated blood to the largest portion of the myocardium, travels a short distance before dividing into the *left anterior descending artery* (LAD) and *left circumflex artery* (LCX) (see Figure 1-12).

Left Anterior Descending Artery

The LAD supplies oxygenated blood to the anterior wall of the left ventricle, with some perfusion of the right ventricle as well. The septal perforating branches of the LAD supply oxygenated blood to the septum and the bundle branches, whereas the diagonal branches supply oxygenated blood to the anterior left ventricular free wall (see Figure 1-12 and Table 1-1).

Left Circumflex Artery

The LCX supplies oxygenated blood to the lateral wall of the left ventricle and the left atrium. The

FIGURE 1-12: ANTERIOR VIEW OF THE HEART SHOWING THE LOCATIONS OF THE CORONARY ARTERIES

Superior vena cava

Aorta

Aortic semilunar valve

Right atrium

Right coronary artery

Right marginal artery

Right ventricle

Pulmonary trunk

Left coronary artery

Left atrium

Circumflex artery

Anterior descending artery

Left ventricle

Posterior descending artery

Note. From *ECGs Made Easy* (2nd ed.), by B. Aehlert, 2002, St. Louis: Mosby. Reprinted with permission from Elsevier.

LCX may also supply oxygenated blood to the inferior wall of the left ventricle in some people. The sinoatrial (SA) node receives oxygenated blood from the LCX in 45% of the population (Bond, 2005; Fuster et al., 2004), and the AV node receives its oxy-

TABLE 1-1: CORONARY ARTERY SUPPLY	
Coronary Artery	**Circulation Supplied To**
Left anterior descending artery	Anterior left ventricle Anterior two-thirds of septum Bundle of His and bundle branches
Left circumflex artery	Left atrium SA node (45% of population) AV node (10% of population) Lateral left ventricle Posterior left ventricle Posterior septum (20% of population)
Right coronary artery	Right atrium SA node (55% of population) AV node (90% of population) Inferior left ventricle Posterior septum (80% of population) Right ventricle Posterior left ventricle Left posterior bundle branch

genated blood from the LCX in 10% of the population (Bond, 2005) (see Figure 1-12 and Table 1-1).

Right Coronary Artery System

The right coronary artery (RCA) comes from the right side of the aorta. The RCA supplies oxygenated blood to the right atrium and right ventricle as well as the inferior and posterior walls of the left ventricle in most people. A branch of the RCA supplies oxygenated blood to the SA node in 55% of the population (Bond, 2005; Fuster et al., 2004), and the AV nodal branch of the RCA supplies oxygenated blood to the AV node in about 90% of the population (Bond, 2005). The posterior branch of the left bundle branch system receives oxygenated blood from the RCA and the LAD (see Figure 1-12 and Table 1-1).

Dominance

The term *right* or *left dominance* refers to the vessel (LCX or RCA) from which the posterior descending artery (PDA) arises. In 70% of the population, the PDA arises from the RCA (Fuster et al., 2004). In the remainder of the population, the PDA

arises from the LCX. The PDA supplies oxygenated blood to the posterior portions of the right and left ventricles as well as the posterior one third of the septum.

Collateral Circulation

Collateral circulation provides communication between the major coronary arteries and their branches. When stenosis of one artery produces a pressure gradient, the collateral vessels can dilate with time and provide a natural bypass for blood flow beyond the stenosis.

The coronary arterioles lie within the myocardium and supply blood to the capillaries. The capillary system is also referred to as the *microcirculation*. Abnormalities in microcirculation can cause cardiac symptoms in the presence of normal epicardial coronary arteries.

Clinical Application

The location of occlusion of a coronary artery provides important information about the structures of the myocardium affected by the occlusion. For example, a total occlusion of the LAD produces a left ventricular anterior wall MI with potential for right and left bundle branch blocks.

Clinical Application

Occlusion of the RCA commonly produces AV heart blocks because the RCA supplies the AV node in approximately 90% of the population (Dennison, 2000).

Cardiac Veins

The cardiac veins drain into the coronary sinus, which empties into the right atrium. In nearly all people, the coronary veins run parallel to the coronary arteries.

ACTION POTENTIAL AND THE CARDIAC CONDUCTION SYSTEM

Action Potential

The action potential is a series of events that results in a change of the electrical charge inside a cell from negative (resting) to positive (stimulated), and back to negative. This change in electrical charge is the result of a difference in the concentration of ions across the cell membrane. The ions primarily responsible for cardiac function are sodium, potassium, and calcium. The cardiac action potential consists of *polarization* (resting state), *depolarization* (stimulation of the cardiac muscle cell), and *repolarization* (return of the cell to a resting state). As depolarization occurs, normal healthy cardiac muscle cells respond with contraction of the muscle. However, depolarization does not guarantee contraction. If a cardiac muscle cell has been damaged, normal contraction might not occur, even when the cell is stimulated. Additionally, an abnor-

mal level of sodium, potassium, or calcium can adversely affect the action potential.

Conduction System

Contraction of the chambers of the heart in a coordinated fashion is necessary for normal function of the heart. The cardiac conduction system allows for this systematic approach (see Figure 1-13).

SA Node

Stimulation of cardiac muscle cells is normally initiated in a small group of pacemaker cells located in the center of the SA node. The SA node is the natural pacemaker of the heart and sets a heart rate of 60 to 100 beats per minute. External nervous system stimulation is not necessary for SA node activity but can impact it. The SA node is located near the coronary sinus and close to the junction between the superior vena cava and the right atrium (Opie, 2004). The SA node is supplied by the RCA in 55% of the population. The LCX supplies the SA node in the remaining 45% of the population. From the SA node, depolarization travels through the right atrial tissue via internodal pathways and through the left atrial tissue via Bachmann's bundle. From the internodal pathways, the impulse travels to the AV node.

AV Node

The AV node slows conduction from the atria to the ventricles. Conduction is slowed to assure that the ventricles are relaxed at the time of atrial contraction, allowing them to fill completely before contracting. The AV node is located in the right atrium, just above the insertion of the tricuspid valve (Jacobson & Gerity, 2005; Opie, 2004).

AV Junction

From the AV node, the electrical impulse travels along the bundle of His. The AV node and the bundle of His are surrounded by tissue known as the *AV junction*. The AV junction contains pacemaker cells and will initiate a heart rate of 40 to 60 beats per minute if no impulse is received from the SA node.

FIGURE 1-13: NORMAL CARDIAC CONDUCTION SYSTEM

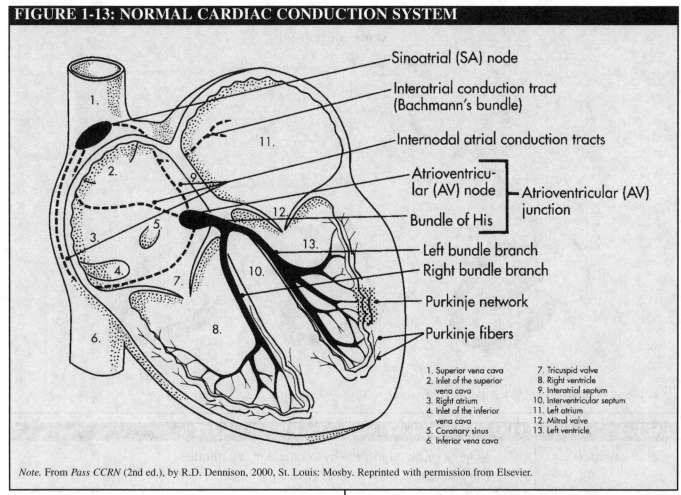

Sinoatrial (SA) node

Interatrial conduction tract (Bachmann's bundle)

Internodal atrial conduction tracts

Atrioventricu-lar (AV) node — Atrioventricular (AV) junction

Bundle of His

Left bundle branch

Right bundle branch

Purkinje network

Purkinje fibers

1. Superior vena cava
2. Inlet of the superior vena cava
3. Right atrium
4. Inlet of the inferior vena cava
5. Coronary sinus
6. Inferior vena cava
7. Tricuspid valve
8. Right ventricle
9. Interatrial septum
10. Interventricular septum
11. Left atrium
12. Mitral valve
13. Left ventricle

Note. From *Pass CCRN* (2nd ed.), by R.D. Dennison, 2000, St. Louis: Mosby. Reprinted with permission from Elsevier.

Bundle Branches

The bundle of His divides into the right and left bundle branches. The *right bundle branch* carries the impulse to the right ventricle. The *left bundle branch* divides into the left posterior bundle branch and the left anterior bundle branch. The left posteri-or bundle branch carries the impulse to the posteri-or and inferior left ventricle; the left anterior bundle branch carries the impulse to the anterior and supe-rior left ventricle.

Purkinje Fibers

From the bundle branches, the impulse travels to the Purkinje fibers, where depolarization is car-ried through the subendocardial layers of the heart. The Purkinje network is also the location of the heart's third group of pacemaker cells. If no impulse is received through the normal conduction patterns, the Purkinje system will initiate a heart rate of 20 to 40 beats per minute.

HEMODYNAMIC PRINCIPLES AND VENTRICULAR FUNCTION

Cardiac Output

Perfusion of the body with oxygenated blood is dependent on cardiac output. *Cardiac output* is the amount of blood ejected by the left ventricle every minute. Heart rate and stroke volume are the primary determinants of cardiac output (see Figure 1-14). It has three components: *preload*, *afterload*, and *con-tractility*. Changes in heart rate, preload, afterload, or contractility change cardiac output (see Table 1-2). Additionally, increasing any one of these factors increases myocardial oxygen demand. *Stroke volume* is the volume of blood ejected by the left ventricle with each beat. Each ventricle holds about 150 ml when full and ejects about 50% to 60% of its volume with each beat (Dennison, 2000). The percentage of

FIGURE 1-14: DETERMINANTS OF CARDIAC OUTPUT

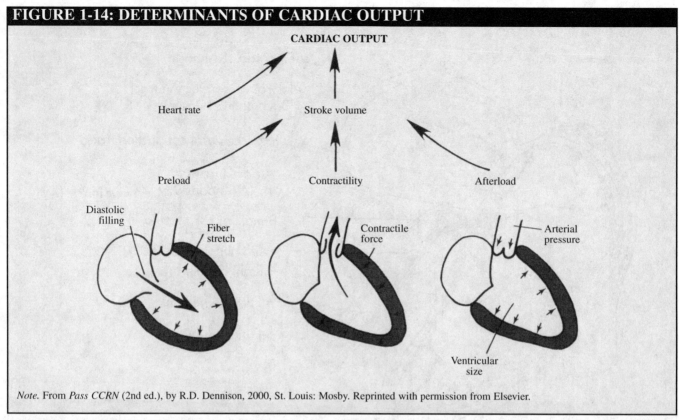

Note. From *Pass CCRN* (2nd ed.), by R.D. Dennison, 2000, St. Louis: Mosby. Reprinted with permission from Elsevier.

TABLE 1-2: KEY DEFINITIONS RELATING TO CARDIAC OUTPUT

Cardiac output	Volume of blood ejected by ventricle every minute Cardiac output = Heart rate x Stroke volume
Stroke volume	Volume of blood ejected by ventricle each beat Stoke volume = Preload + Afterload + Contractility
Ejection fraction	Percent of volume in ventricle ejected with each beat
Preload	Stretch on the ventricular myocardial fibers at the end of ventricular diastole; determined by the volume in the ventricle at the end of diastole
Afterload	Pressure the ventricle must overcome to eject its contents
Contractility	Ability of the ventricle to pump independent of preload or afterload

volume ejected with each beat is termed the *ejection fraction*.

Clinical Application

Patients with decreased contractility from a previous MI have lower ejection fractions and reduced stroke volumes.

Determinants of Cardiac Output

Heart Rate

Heart rate is defined as the number of times the heart beats every minute. Normal heart rate in an adult ranges from 60 to 100 beats per minute. During exercise, heart rate naturally increases to meet the increased metabolic needs of the body. Heart rate also decreases as the body's needs decrease, such as during sleep. However, extremely slow heart rates (less than 40 beats per minute) and extremely high heart rates (greater than 150 beats per minute) experienced over a prolonged period can negatively affect cardiac output. High heart rates do not allow adequate time for ventricular filling, and low heart rates do not provide an adequate volume of ejected blood per minute.

Preload

Preload, one of the determinants of stroke volume, is defined as the stretch on the ventricular myocardial fibers at the end of ventricular diastole. The volume of blood filling the ventricles causes the myocardium to stretch. According to Starling's law, the larger the volume of blood in the ventricle at the end of diastole (within physiologic limits), the greater the energy of the subsequent contraction (Opie, 2004). Therefore, as the filling of the ventricle increases, the strength of the subsequent contraction also increases, resulting in a greater stroke volume.

Venous return to the heart determines the amount of blood that enters the ventricles and stretches myocardial fibers. The amount of venous blood returned to the right atrium ultimately enters the right and left ventricles. It is this volume of blood that produces the stretch in the ventricles during diastole. If venous return decreases, as with hypovolemia, preload decreases. When preload decreases, stroke volume decreases.

Clinical Application
Evaluation of a patient's fluid status gives a clinician a good indication of preload. A patient experiencing extracellular fluid deficit will have a decreased preload, whereas a patient with extracellular fluid overload will have an increased preload.

Afterload

Afterload, another component of stroke volume, is the workload of the ventricle, or the pressure the ventricle must overcome to eject its contents. Afterload is affected by both anatomical structures and physiological changes that may impede the ejection of ventricular contents. These structures and changes include aortic or pulmonic valve function, arterial or pulmonary arterial pressures (vascular resistance), compliance of vascular walls, and diastolic pressure in the great arteries. If the ventricular contents are to be ejected, the pressure in the ventricles must become great enough to force the aortic and pulmonic valves open. A stenotic valve is much more difficult to open due to the abnormalities in the valve. Therefore, aortic or pulmonic stenosis increases afterload.

The overall resistance the left ventricle must pump against, known as *systemic vascular resistance,* is determined primarily by the systemic arterioles (Opie, 2004). When the arterioles dilate, systemic vascular resistance decreases; when they constrict, systemic vascular resistance increases. Arterioles respond to systemic changes and vasoconstrict or vasodilate depending on the hemodynamic needs of the body. Noncompliant vascular walls, as exist in hypertension, do not relax easily and increase afterload. The vascular resistance the right ventricle must pump against is the *pulmonary vascular resistance.* It is determined by the pulmonary artery pressures.

Blood pressure is not equal to systemic vascular resistance. It is a product of cardiac output and systemic vascular resistance. However, blood pressure is a noninvasive method of evaluating systemic vascular resistance. Generally, as diastolic pressure rises, so does systemic vascular resistance.

Clinical Application
Patients with untreated hypertension have a continuous increase in afterload, resulting in increased left ventricular workload. Sustained increased workload eventually causes the left ventricle to fail.

Contractility

The third and final component of the stroke volume equation is *contractility.* Contractility is the ability of the ventricle to contract independent of preload or afterload. Contractility is referred to as the *inotropic state of the myocardium* and is a major component of systole. During ventricular contraction, the sarcomere (repeating unit of the myofibril), or cardiac muscle, shortens (Bond, 2005). The extent of myofibril shortening determines the velocity of the ejection of the myocardial contents. Damage to the myocardial muscle cells, as occurs in MI, decreases the ability of the myofibrils to shorten and impairs the ability of the ventricle to contract. Overstretch of the myofibrils also results in myofibrils that can no longer shorten effectively.

Additional Factors Contributing to Cardiac Output

The shape of the left ventricle is designed to provide a contraction that is generally an inward movement. This inward movement occurs simultaneously among all walls of the ventricle. This normal inward contraction of the ventricle is referred to as *normal muscular synergy* (Darovic, 2002). This normally coordinated contraction may become uncoordinated due to a variety of conditions. For example, the ventricle may become damaged due to ischemic heart disease or aneurysms. Abnormalities in conduction, such as bundle branch blocks and ventricular ectopy, can also alter normal contraction patterns. Finally, changes in ventricular size caused by dilatation or fibrosis can also alter normal muscular synergy. Dysynergy can result in an increase in the energy needed for contraction and a decrease in cardiac output.

Additionally, both ventricles are designed to contract simultaneously. Ventricular dysynchrony occurs when the right and left ventricles do not contract at the same time. This dysynchrony is commonly demonstrated by a bundle branch block pattern on an electrocardiogram. If the right and left ventricles do not contract in unison, cardiac output and performance are compromised.

Clinical Application

Dilated cardiomyopathy results from myocardial fibrils that have been overstretched and can no longer shorten normally. Therefore, patients with dilated cardiomyopathy have decreased contractility.

THE CARDIOPULMONARY CIRCUIT AND DELIVERY OF OXYGEN

The heart and lungs work together to form the cardiopulmonary circuit (see Figure 1-15). The purpose of the cardiopulmonary circuit is to deliver oxygen to all the tissues of the body. The amount of oxygen delivered to the tissues is determined by three factors:

- cardiac output
- hemoglobin level
- oxygen saturation.

Under normal conditions, approximately 1,000 ml of oxygen are delivered to the tissues each minute via the arterial system and the tissues of the body extract approximately 25% of the oxygen delivered to them (Dennison, 2000), leaving approximately a 75% reserve. If the cardiopulmonary circuit fails to deliver enough oxygen to meet the needs of the tissues, the amount left in the reserve diminishes. The oxygen reserve is measured by assessing the percent of oxygen saturation of venous blood.

Myocardial Oxygenation

The balance of myocardial oxygen supply and demand is key in providing cardiac muscle with the proper amount of oxygen to maintain optimum function (Figure 1-16). The ability of the myocardium to contract effectively is directly related to the amount of oxygen that is supplied to the heart. The myocardium is unique because the left ventricle extracts approximately 75% of the oxygen that is delivered, as opposed to the 25% that is normally extracted by other tissues (Darovic, 2002). Two thirds of oxygen

FIGURE 1-15: SCHEMATIC OF THE CARDIOPULMONARY CIRCUIT

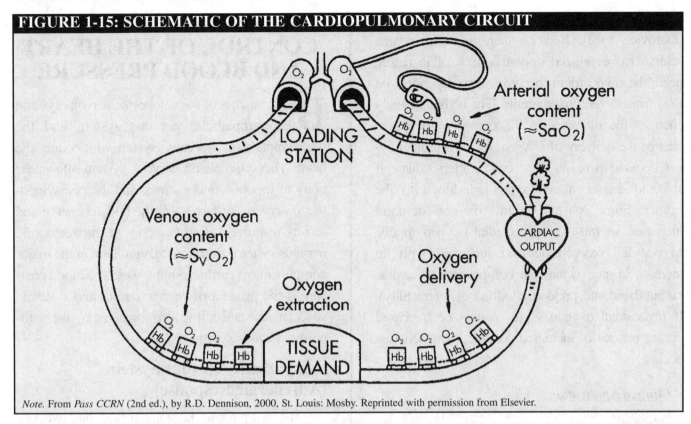

Note. From *Pass CCRN* (2nd ed.), by R.D. Dennison, 2000, St. Louis: Mosby. Reprinted with permission from Elsevier.

FIGURE 1-16: FACTORS INFLUENCING MYOCARDIAL SUPPLY AND DEMAND

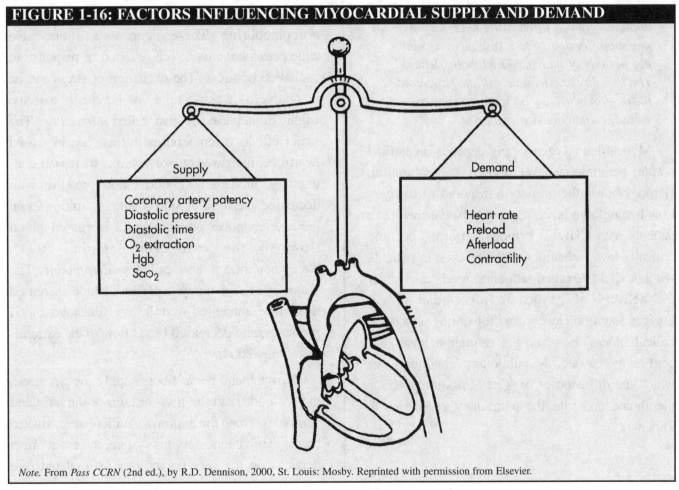

Note. From *Pass CCRN* (2nd ed.), by R.D. Dennison, 2000, St. Louis: Mosby. Reprinted with permission from Elsevier.

extraction occurs during isovolumic contraction (Darovic, 2002). Because there is little oxygen reserve to be utilized during periods of increased need, the myocardium becomes very dependent on flow from the coronary arteries. The body inherently changes the diameter of the coronary arteries to change the delivery of oxygen. As myocardial oxygen demand increases, the coronary arteries dilate, if able, to deliver more oxygen-rich blood to the myocardium. As myocardial oxygen demand increases, so must the myocardial oxygen supply. Myocardial oxygen demand increases with an increase in any of the four components of cardiac output (heart rate, preload, afterload, or contractility). If myocardial oxygen supply cannot be increased during periods of increased demand, then ischemia occurs.

Clinical Application

In patients with coronary heart disease (CHD), narrowed blood vessels are often unable to dilate enough to provide the necessary oxygen supply and, therefore, angina occurs during periods of increased metabolic demand. The inability to adequately dilate is why stable angina generally occurs with activity and subsides when activity is stopped.

Myocardial oxygen supply depends on cardiac output, hemoglobin level, and oxygen saturation. Hemoglobin is the primary transporter of oxygen. Low hemoglobin levels can exacerbate ischemia in patients with CHD. If hemoglobin levels become critically low, ischemia can occur, even in patients without CHD. Oxygen saturation levels also affect the delivery of oxygen to myocardial tissue. Oxygen saturation levels can drop during periods of critical illness. Low oxygen saturation levels are commonly caused by pulmonary conditions, in which the diffusion of oxygen across the alveolar membrane and into the pulmonary capillaries is impaired.

NEUROLOGICAL CONTROL OF THE HEART AND BLOOD PRESSURE

Both branches of the autonomic nervous system, the sympathetic nervous system and the parasympathetic nervous system, innervate the heart. The sympathetic nervous system allows the body to function under stress, and the parasympathetic nervous system helps the body conserve and restore resources. Both branches of the autonomic nervous system contribute to regulation of the major components of cardiac output. Because blood pressure is the product of cardiac output and systemic vascular resistance, it is also impacted by the autonomic nervous system.

Sympathetic Nervous System (Adrenergic Response)

The sympathetic nervous system has two key neurotransmitters, or messengers: epinephrine and norepinephrine. These neurotransmitters, also called *catecholamines,* are released in response to excitation or stress. The excitation or stress can be as simple as waking up to as severe as extreme fright. Epinephrine is also called *adrenaline.* The major effects of epinephrine release are increased heart rate, increased stroke volume, increased contractility, increased systolic blood pressure with decreased diastolic blood pressure (resulting in an increase in pulse pressure), and increased blood flow to the extremities (Opie, 2004). Norepinephrine is also called *nonadrenaline.* The major effects of norepinephrine include increased heart rate, increased systolic and diastolic blood pressures, and decreased blood flow to the extremities (Opie, 2004).

Sympathetic nerve fibers supply the SA node, the AV node, and the myocardium of the atria and ventricles. Once the neurotransmitters are activated by the sympathetic nervous system, the exact effect depends on the specific receptors stimulated (see

Table 1-3). Beta$_1$-adrenergic receptors are located in the heart and, when stimulated, cause an increase in heart rate, conductivity, and contractility. Beta$_2$-adrenergic receptors are located in the lungs and periphery and, when stimulated, cause bronchial and peripheral vasodilatation. Alpha$_1$-adrenergic receptors are located in the vessels of vascular smooth muscle and affect the tone of the small arterioles responsible for determining systemic vascular resistance. Stimulation of alpha receptors results in arterial vasoconstriction and ultimately an increase in blood pressure. Alpha$_1$ and beta$_2$ stimulation oppose each other in the periphery and oppositely affect systemic vascular resistance. The net result of sympathetic nervous system stimulation on alpha- and beta-receptors depends on the degree to which each receptor is stimulated. In general, alpha-receptors are more sensitive to norepinephrine and beta-receptors are more sensitive to epinephrine (Clinical Pharmacology Database, 2004). The renal, mesenteric, and coronary blood vessels also contain dopaminergic receptors. Stimulation of dopaminergic receptors results in vasodilatation.

Clinical Application
The high sensitivity of beta-receptors to epinephrine is the reason epinephrine is used during cardiac resuscitation in patients with pulseless rhythms.

Parasympathetic Nervous System (Vagal Response)

The parasympathetic nervous system innervates the SA node, AV node, AV junction, and myocardium of the atria (Dennison, 2000). There is minimal parasympathetic innervation of the ventricles. When the parasympathetic nervous system is stimulated, the response is called a *cholinergic,* or *vagal,* response. Acetylcholine is the neurotransmitter that is released when parasympathetic nerve fibers are stimulated. It binds to parasympathetic receptors. Cholinergic receptors are classified into two types: nicotinic and muscarinic (Bond, 2005). Parasympathetic receptors located in the heart and smooth muscles are called *muscarinic receptors.*

Clinical Application
Atropine interferes with the effects of the parasympathetic nervous system. Therefore, atropine will only have an effect on low heart rates that are the result of parasympathetic stimulation, such as a vagal response.

Stimulation of the parasympathetic nervous system decreases heart rate and slows conduction. It has very little effect on the force of ventricular contraction because of the minimal innervation of the parasympathetic nervous system in the ventricles. When the parasympathetic nervous system is stimulated, acetylcholine is released, resulting in a cholinergic, or vagal, response. Acetylcholine

TABLE 1-3: ADRENERGIC RECEPTOR LOCATION AND RESPONSE		
Receptor	**Location of Receptor**	**Response to Stimulation**
Alpha$_1$	Vascular smooth muscles	Vasoconstriction
Beta$_1$	SA node, AV node, and myocardium	Increased heart rate Increased conduction Increased contractility
Beta$_2$	Vascular and bronchial smooth muscles	Bronchodilatation Vasodilatation
Dopaminergic	Vascular smooth muscle (renal, coronary, and mesenteric)	Vasodilatation

directly inhibits the SA node, thus decreasing heart rate. Stimulation of the parasympathetic nervous system also causes vasodilatation due to nitric oxide release from the endothelium (Opie, 2004). Venous vasodilatation decreases preload, and arterial vasodilatation decreases afterload. Vagal tone is more pronounced during sleeping hours. When blood pressure is elevated, the feedback from the baroreceptors (discussed below) causes parasympathetic stimulation, which results in a slower heart rate, decreased force of contraction, and vasodilatation. These effects result in lower cardiac output and blood pressure.

Clinical Application

The activation of the parasympathetic nervous system during an acute hypertensive crisis explains the reflex bradycardia commonly seen in this clinical situation. Conversely, low blood pressure causes reflex tachycardia.

Baroreceptors

Baroreceptors are specialized nerve tissues located in the aortic arch and carotid sinus (the origin of the internal carotid artery) (Thibodeau & Patton, 2003). They function as sensors in the nervous system and are sensitive to wall tension within the arterial vessels. An increase or decrease in wall tension and pressure sends signals to the medulla, the vasomotor center in the brain stem via the *afferent pathways* (Opie, 2004). The medulla interprets the information it receives from the baroreceptors and transmits information back to the heart and blood vessels via motor nerves called *efferent pathways* (Opie, 2004). Impulses from this center control the diameter of blood vessels. When blood pressure is increased, baroreceptors recognize the increased wall tension and send a message to inhibit the sympathetic nervous system and stimulate the parasympathetic nervous system. Heart rate slows and veins and arteries dilate throughout the system. These changes result in decreased blood pressure. When blood pressure decreases, wall tension

decreases. The opposite effects, increased heart rate and vasoconstriction, occur with stimulation of the sympathetic nervous system.

Clinical Application

When the vagal maneuver of carotid massage is performed, baroreceptors in the carotid arteries are stimulated to slow conduction from the SA node through the AV node and, therefore, heart rate is decreased.

Chemoreceptors

The carotid arteries also contain chemoreceptors. These receptors respond to changes in blood chemistry, including arterial oxygen content, arterial carbon dioxide levels, and arterial pH (Opie, 2004). As blood pressure lowers to a critical point, the delivery of oxygen also decreases to a critical point. As oxygen delivery decreases, carbon dioxide levels increase. When stimulated by an elevated arterial carbon dioxide level, chemoreceptors send a message to the vasomotor center to stimulate cardiac activity via the sympathetic nervous system. Heart rate increases and vasoconstriction occurs, causing an increase in blood pressure with a resultant increase in oxygenation.

Role of the Renin-Angiotensin-Aldosterone System

Renin is released from the kidneys in response to low circulating volume, low cardiac output, or poor kidney perfusion. Activation of the sympathetic nervous system and increased catecholamines stimulate renin release. In response to renin, angiotensin I is converted to angiotensin II in the presence of angiotensin-converting enzyme (ACE). ACE is found in the capillary bed of the lungs and other tissues. The important end results of the renin-angiotensin-aldosterone system (RAAS) are caused by the effects of circulating angiotensin II. Angiotensin II has three primary effects:

1. arterial vasoconstriction

2. stimulation of thirst

3. stimulation of the adrenal cortex to secrete aldosterone (aldosterone increases sodium and water reabsorption).

As the blood vessels constrict and water is reabsorbed and retained, blood pressure increases and perfusion to the body, including the kidneys, improves. This increased perfusion then decreases the production of renin by the kidneys.

Clinical Application

The end results of stimulation of the RAAS include arterial vasoconstriction and aldosterone secretion. Arterial vasoconstriction increases afterload, and aldosterone secretion increases preload. These effects are clinically important in patients with heart failure who have chronic stimulation of the RAAS.

CONCLUSION

An understanding of basic anatomy and physiology of the heart is essential for all health care professionals. The heart is a complex, intricate pump with one purpose: the forward propulsion of blood to perfuse the body and remove waste products. Many anatomical and physiological factors can impact how well the heart fulfills its purpose. Even in people without heart disease, the cardiovascular system may not always work optimally. It is the responsibility of all health care professionals to recognize the impact of treatments, medications, and other interventions on this carefully designed system.

EXAM QUESTIONS

CHAPTER 1
Questions 1-9

1. The inner layer of the heart that is contiguous with the cardiac valves and great vessels is the

   a. pericardium.

   b. epicardium.

   c. myocardium.

   d. endocardium.

2. AV valves are anatomically different than semilunar valves in that they have

   a. two cusps instead of three cusps.

   b. three cusps instead of two cusps.

   c. papillary muscles and chordae tendineae.

   d. a valve annulus.

3. During ventricular diastole, the

   a. AV valves are open as the ventricles fill from the atria.

   b. AV valves are closed as the ventricles fill from the atria.

   c. semilunar valves are open as the ventricular contents are ejected.

   d. semilunar valves are closed as the ventricular contents are ejected.

4. In most people, the coronary artery that supplies the inferior wall of the left ventricle and the AV node is the

   a. left main coronary artery.

   b. LCX.

   c. LAD.

   d. RCA.

5. In normal cardiac conduction, depolarization begins at the SA node. One fact about the SA node is that

   a. it is located in the left ventricle and is damaged to some extent during every MI.

   b. sudden cardiac death occurs if the SA node is blocked.

   c. the natural rate of SA node firing is 60 to 100 times per minute.

   d. the SA node receives its blood supply from the LAD in approximately 90% of the population.

6. The major determinants of cardiac output include

   a. heart rate, preload, afterload, and contractility.

   b. heart rate, blood pressure, arterial oxygen saturation, and contractility.

   c. blood pressure, contractility, arterial oxygen saturation, and preload.

   d. afterload, preload, contractility, and blood pressure.

7. The actual delivery of oxygen to tissues is determined not only by cardiac output but also by the amount of

   a. glucose in the blood.

   b. hemoglobin and the oxygen saturation of the hemoglobin.

   c. white blood cells interfering with delivery of oxygen.

   d. cholesterol in the blood.

8. The autonomic nervous system increases blood pressure through many mechanisms, including

     a. activation of the parasympathetic nervous system in the ventricles.

     b. stimulation of $alpha_1$ receptors in the vessels, causing venous vasodilatation.

     c. stimulation of $beta_1$ receptors, causing arterial vasoconstriction.

     d. stimulation of $alpha_1$ receptors, causing arterial vasoconstriction.

9. The RAAS helps the regulation of blood pressure by producing

     a. angiotensin II and causing dilatation when blood pressure is high.

     b. angiotensin II and causing vasoconstriction when blood pressure is low.

     c. vasopressin and causing dilatation when blood pressure is high.

     d. vasopressin and causing vasoconstriction when blood pressure is low.

CHAPTER 2

CARDIOVASCULAR PHARMACOLOGY AND HEMODYNAMIC FUNCTION

CHAPTER OBJECTIVE

After completing this chapter, the reader will be able to discuss the way pharmacology is used to manipulate the components of cardiac output and myocardial oxygen demand to improve myocardial performance.

LEARNING OBJECTIVES

After studying this chapter, the reader will be able to

1. list pharmacological options available to increase or decrease the major components of cardiac output and myocardial oxygen demand, including:
   - preload,
   - afterload,
   - contractility,
   - heart rate.

2. define the mechanism of action, key indications, and key considerations for the following groups of medications:
   - sympathomimetics,
   - parasympatholytics,
   - angiotensin-converting enzyme inhibitors,
   - aldosterone antagonists,
   - beta-blockers,
   - calcium channel blockers,
   - other venous and arterial vasodilators,
   - digoxin.

INTRODUCTION

Cardiovascular pharmacology is a complex subject, and one that grows and changes daily with the addition of each new body of research. This chapter looks at how cardiovascular pharmacology affects hemodynamic function in two distinctly different ways to provide a comprehensive understanding of the subject. Pharmacology specific to the treatment of certain cardiac conditions will be discussed in later chapters.

This chapter is divided into two subsections. Section one provides an overview of pharmacological options to manipulate the major determinants of cardiac output and myocardial oxygen demand. The section surveys the options available to manipulate preload, afterload, contractility, and heart rate. The purpose of this section is to provide a "big picture" look at the effects of pharmacological agents on these determinants of myocardial performance.

Section two takes a closer look at the major groups of cardiovascular medications and, in some cases, individual medications. This section presents more information about the mechanism of action, results, and key nursing considerations of these medications.

The final goal of cardiovascular pharmacology is to improve cardiac performance. This goal is achieved in a variety of ways by manipulating the major components of cardiac output and myocardial oxygen demand. In clinical practice, these four components (heart rate, preload, afterload, and contractility) are sometimes manipulated with intravenous agents in emergency situations, such as cardiogenic shock; however, they are most commonly manipulated in chronic disease management with oral medications, such as in heart failure.

OVERVIEW OF CARDIOVASCULAR PHARMACOLOGY

Preload

Preload is the stretch on the ventricle at the end of diastole. The volume of blood in the ventricle causes this stretch.

Increasing Preload

When preload is too low, cardiac output decreases. Hypovolemic shock is an example of a clinical situation in which preload drops acutely. Preload is also low when an extracellular fluid deficit or excessive venous vasodilatation occurs. When venous vasodilatation occurs, blood is pulled away from the heart and preload decreases. The pharmacological options for increasing preload are outlined in Table 2-1.

Decreasing Preload

When preload is too high, a stretch beyond normal physiologic limits can cause a decrease in the force of contraction. In addition, increased preload causes an increase in myocardial oxygen demand. Patients with heart failure are at risk for having extracellular fluid overload and may need therapy both acutely and on a continual basis to decrease preload. Table 2-2 outlines the pharmacological options for decreasing preload.

Afterload

Afterload is the resistance that the ventricle must overcome to eject its contents. Systemic vascular resistance measures left ventricular afterload. Systemic vascular resistance also plays a major role in maintaining blood pressure.

Increasing Afterload

An increase in afterload is not a desired effect in patients with heart disease; therefore, medications to increase afterload are only given in emergency situations. For example, medications to increase afterload are indicated when hypotension is unresponsive to fluids or other treatment and blood pressure is dangerously low. Pharmacological options for increasing afterload are listed in Table 2-3. *Vasopressor* is the term given to medications used to increase afterload.

Decreasing Afterload

High afterload increases myocardial oxygen demand. Decreasing afterload is a goal of therapy for all patients with left ventricular dysfunction, heart failure, and hypertension. Table 2-4 lists a variety of pharmacological options used in the reduction of afterload.

Contractility

Contractility is the ability of the ventricle to contract independently of preload or afterload.

TABLE 2-1: PHARMACOLOGICAL CONSIDERATIONS FOR INCREASING PRELOAD	
Options	**Specific Agents/Key Information**
• Administer extracellular fluid expanders	• Isotonic crystalloids, such as 0.9% saline and lactated Ringer's solution • Colloids, such as albumin, dextran, and hetastarch • Blood or blood products
• Decrease dose or stop drugs that cause venous vasodilatation	• Nitroglycerin, nesiritide, and morphine sulfate (venous vasodilatation pools blood away from the heart and decreases preload)

TABLE 2-2: PHARMACOLOGICAL CONSIDERATIONS FOR DECREASING PRELOAD

Options	Specific Agents/Key Information
1. Stop or decrease fluid	
2. Diuretics	• A loop diuretic, such as furosemide, reduces extracellular circulating volume
3. Angiotensin-converting enzyme (ACE) inhibitors	• Interfere with the physiologic response of the renin-angiotensin-aldosterone system (RAAS) (aldosterone secretion decreases, as do sodium and water retention) • ACE inhibitors end in "pril," such as captopril
4. Aldosterone antagonists	• Spironolactone and eplerenone • Directly block aldosterone and decrease sodium and water retention
5. Venous vasodilators	• Intravenous (IV) nitroglycerin, nesiritide, and morphine sulfate Venous vasodilatation pools blood away from the heart and decreases preload.

TABLE 2-3: PHARMACOLOGICAL CONSIDERATIONS FOR INCREASING AFTERLOAD

Options	Specific Agents/Key Information
1. Sympathomimetics to stimulate the alpha receptors of the sympathetic nervous system	• Dopamine • Norepinephrine • Phenylephrine • Epinephrine
2. Arginine vasopressin (antidiuretic hormone [ADH])	• Vasoconstrictive and antidiuretic effect • Promotes reabsorption of water • Restores catecholamine sensitivity

Because preload, afterload, and contractility all impact cardiac output, it is sometimes difficult to readily determine the exact cause of low cardiac output. Contractility is known to be impaired in cardiac patients who have left ventricular dysfunction and low ejection fractions.

Increasing Contractility

Inotropes are medications that increase contractility. Patients suffering from significant left ventricular dysfunction may need the support of an intravenous inotrope to increase contractility if they are unable to maintain a cardiac output sufficient to meet the demands of the body. Patients in acute cardiogenic shock or patients in end-stage heart failure have known left ventricular dysfunction. Because inotropic agents substantially increase myocardial oxygen demand, it is important to correct problems with preload or afterload before administering an inotropic agent to improve cardiac output.

Table 2-5 outlines agents used to increase myocardial contractility.

Decreasing Contractility

Oral medications are commonly prescribed to decrease contractility and, therefore, decrease myocardial oxygen demand. A common indication for this is angina. Options for decreasing contractility are listed in Table 2-6.

Heart Rate

Cardiac output is heart rate multiplied by stroke volume. Increasing heart rate mathematically increases cardiac output. However, if heart rate becomes too rapid, the ventricles do not have time to adequately fill, and cardiac output decreases.

TABLE 2-4: PHARMACOLOGICAL CONSIDERATIONS FOR DECREASING AFTERLOAD

All therapies involve arterial vasodilatation.

Options	Specific Agents/Key Information
1. Smooth muscle relaxants	• Nitroprusside • Hydralazine
2. Calcium channel blockers	• Dihydropyridine calcium channel blockers (ending in "ine"), such as amlodipine, have strong arterial vasodilator properties
3. Alpha receptor blockers	• Labetalol (combination alpha- and beta-blocker) • Prazosin and terazosin
4. ACE inhibitors	• Interrupt the RAAS and limit production of angiotensin II, a potent arterial vasoconstrictor • Medications ending in "pril"
5. Angiotensin II receptor blockers (ARBs)	• Directly block the effects angiotensin II • Medications ending in "sartan," such as valsartan
6. Phosphodiesterase (PDE) inhibitors	• Milrinone (used as an IV inotrope but also has arterial vasodilator properties)

TABLE 2-5: PHARMACOLOGICAL CONSIDERATIONS FOR INCREASING CONTRACTILITY

Options	Specific Agents/Key Information
1. Sympathomimetics that stimulate the beta$_1$ (β1) receptors of the sympathetic nervous system	• Dobutamine (most commonly used because it is a predominant β1 stimulator) • Other sympathomimetics may have inotropic properties even if not used primarily for an inotropic purpose
2. PDE inhibitors	• Milrinone (used as an IV inotrope but also has arterial and venous vasodilator properties)
3. Cardiac glycosides	• Digoxin (weak inotrope and is never used IV to support left ventricular dysfunction; exerts weak inotropic properties when given orally)

TABLE 2-6: PHARMACOLOGICAL CONSIDERATIONS FOR DECREASING CONTRACTILITY

Options	Specific Agents/Key Information
1. Beta-blockers that block the β1 receptors of the sympathetic nervous system	• Metoprolol • Carvedilol • "olol" medications * *Note:* Medications that block β1 receptors may also have properties that cause β2 and alpha-receptor blockade
2. Calcium channel blockers	• Diltiazem • Verapamil

Increasing Heart Rate

In clinical practice, heart rate is only intentionally increased to improve cardiac output when it is below the normal rate and the patient is symptomatic. If heart rate is normal, it is not increased to a faster rate to increase cardiac output because an increase in heart rate also produces an increase in myocardial oxygen demand. Pharmacological options for increasing heart rate are listed in Table 2-7.

Decreasing Heart Rate

During an arrhythmia in which heart rate is dangerously high, medications are used to decrease ventricular response and thus heart rate. Medications that decrease heart rate are also given to patients with normal heart rates when there is a desire to further decrease myocardial oxygen demand. Table 2-8 describes the pharmacological options for decreasing heart rate.

Clinical Application

The majority of the options for manipulating the components of cardiac output and myocardial oxygen demand are oral agents. Nurses should consider the hemodynamic impact of oral medications as well as the hemodynamic impact of intravenous medications.

A CLOSER LOOK AT CARDIOVASCULAR MEDICATIONS

Sympathomimetics

Sympathomimetics are medications that stimulate the sympathetic nervous system and can be used to increase heart rate, contractility, and afterload. Different sympathomimetics have different dominant actions, depending on the receptors they stimulate:

- ß1 receptors are located in the heart. ß1 stimulation increases heart rate and contractility.

- ß2 receptors are located in the lungs and periphery. ß2 stimulation causes bronchial and peripheral vasodilatation in skeletal muscle.

- Alpha receptors are located in the arterioles. Alpha stimulation causes arteriole vasoconstriction and increases afterload.

- Dopaminergic receptors are located in the renal and mesenteric beds. When stimulated, these receptors dilate the renal and mesenteric arteries.

Boxes 2-1 to 2-3 list specific sympathomimetics by purpose and receptor stimulation. Tables 2-9 to 2-12 take a closer look at four of the most common sympathomimetics used in cardiovascular nursing.

TABLE 2-7: PHARMACOLOGICAL CONSIDERATIONS FOR INCREASING HEART RATE	
Options	**Specific Agents/Key Information**
1. Parasympatholytics (lysis of the parasympathetic nervous system)	• Atropine (most commonly used pharmacological agent to increase heart rate)
2. Sympathomimetics that stimulate the ß1 receptors of the sympathetic nervous system	• Epinephrine • Dopamine
Note: The nonpharmacological intervention of pacing the heart with either an external, temporary, or permanent pacemaker is commonly the preferred method of increasing heart rate to a set and controlled rate.	

TABLE 2-8: PHARMACOLOGICAL CONSIDERATIONS FOR DECREASING HEART RATE

Options	Specific Agents/Key Information
1. Beta-blockers that block the ß1 receptors of the sympathetic nervous system	• Metoprolol and cardvedilol • "olol" medications • Class II antiarrhythmics*
2. Calcium channel blockers	• Diltiazem and Verapamil • Class IV antiarrhythmics*
3. Cardiac glycosides	• Digoxin
4. Unclassified antiarrhythmics	• Adenosine (slows or stops conduction through the atrioventricular [AV] node)
5. Other antiarrhythmics	• Class I and class III antiarrhythmics* • Used to establish or maintain a normal rhythm and therefore control heart rate

* Vaughan Williams classification system

BOX 2-1: ALPHA RECEPTOR STIMULATORS USED TO INCREASE AFTERLOAD

• Dopamine
• Norepinephrine
• Phenylephrine
• Epinephrine

BOX 2-2: ß1 RECEPTOR STIMULATORS USED TO INCREASE CONTRACTILITY

• Dobutamine (most commonly used sympathomimetic for inotropic purposes)
• Epinephrine
• Norepinephrine (used primarily as a vasopressor but also has inotropic properties)
• Dopamine (used primarily as a vasopressor but also has inotropic properties)

BOX 2-3: ß1 RECEPTOR STIMULATORS USED TO INCREASE HEART RATE

• Epinephrine
• Dopamine

Medications That Affect The Renin-Angiotensin-Aldosterone System

Three groups of medications directly affect the RAAS: ACE inhibitors, ARBs, and aldosterone antagonists.

ACE Inhibitors

ACE inhibitors prevent the conversion of angiotensin I to angiotensin II by inhibiting ACE. Angiotensin II is a potent arterial vasoconstrictor, therefore, ACE inhibitors promote arterial vasodilatation by preventing the formation of angiotensin II. This arterial vasodilatation reduces afterload.

The formation of angiotensin II also stimulates the release of aldosterone from the renal cortex. Aldosterone informs the body to retain sodium and, therefore, water while excreting potassium. Angiotensin II also stimulates the release of arginine vasopressin (ADH), which causes additional vasoconstriction and water reabsorption. When angiotensin II formation is inhibited, the release of aldosterone and vasopressin decrease and preload and afterload further decrease.

Because of the positive effects of decreasing afterload and preload, ACE inhibitors decrease the workload of the left ventricle. These medications are central to the management of patients with heart fail-

TABLE 2-9: EPINEPHRINE

What receptors are stimulated?	• ß1 and ß2 (at low doses) • Alpha receptors (at high doses)
What are the resultant actions?	• Increased contractility (positive inotrope) • Increased automaticity • Bronchodilatation • Selective vasoconstriction
When and why is it used?	• Advanced cardiac life support; first-line drug for cardiac standstill • Anaphylactic shock • Hypotension or profound bradycardia
What are special nursing considerations?	• Instant onset • Peak 20 minutes • 1 mg IV every 3 to 5 minutes during cardiac standstill

(Clinical Pharmacology Database, 2004; Cummins, 2003)

TABLE 2-10: DOBUTAMINE

What receptors are stimulated?	• Primarily ß1 • Some Alpha receptor stimulation • Modest ß2 (more ß2 than alpha)
What are the resultant actions?	• Increased contractility (positive inotrope) • Increased AV node conduction • Modest vasoconstriction
When and why is it used?	• Used as an inotrope with modest afterload reduction
What are special nursing considerations?	• Onset 1 to 2 minutes • Peak 10 minutes • Blood pressure is variable: ß2 causes vasodilation • Increased cardiac output increases blood pressure

(Clinical Pharmacology Database, 2004; Cummins, 2003)

ure. They are also used after myocardial infarction (MI) and in patients with coronary artery disease to prevent heart failure development. ACE inhibitors can decrease mortality in post-MI patients with an ejection fraction of less than 40% by decreasing left ventricular remodeling (Calclasure, Kozlowski, Highfill, & Loghin, 2001). The process of left ventricular remodeling will be discussed further in chapter 7. Additionally, ACE inhibitors are used to treat hypertension in diabetic and renal patients.

ACE inhibitors also promote a more antithrombotic environment through their impact on endothelial function and have an overall cardioprotective and vasculoprotective effect. They reduce left ventricular mass in hypertrophy and can decrease the progression rate of renal failure, especially in insulin-dependent diabetics (Gibbons et al., 2002). ACE inhibitors have known vasculoprotective effects in high-risk patients, and current research is evaluating the impact of ACE inhibitors on lower-

TABLE 2-11: DOPAMINE

What receptors are stimulated?	• Dopaminergic and some ß1 at low doses • ß1 at moderate doses • Pure alpha stimulation at high doses (> 10 mcg/kg/min)
What are the resultant actions?	• Increased contractility at small and moderate doses • Increased conduction • Vasoconstriction at high doses • Does not treat or prevent renal failure at low doses*
When and why is it used?	• Refractory hypotension • Shock
What are special nursing considerations?	• IV onset 1 to 2 minutes • Peak 10 minutes • Maximal effects at 20 mcg/kg/min • Large IV line or central line • Phentolamine (alpha blocker) for infiltrate

(Clinical Pharmacology Database, 2004; Cummins, 2003)

TABLE 2-12: NOREPINEPHRINE

What receptors are stimulated?	• Primarily alpha stimulation • Some ß1
What are the resultant actions?	• Potent vasoconstriction (vasopressor) • Some increased contractility (positive inotrope)
When and why is it used?	• Refractory hypotension • Shock • Used as vasopressor but has inotropic properties
What are special nursing considerations?	• Rapid IV onset • Duration 1 to 2 minutes (blood pressure checks every 2 minutes while titrating) • Large IV line or central line • Phentolamine (alpha blocker) for infiltration of IV site

(Clinical Pharmacology Database, 2004)

risk patients. The positive effects of ACE inhibitors commonly take weeks to months to be seen.

In addition to interfering with the formation of angiotensin II, ACE inhibitors enhance the action of kinins. This action has a positive effect in the management of heart failure. Eighty-five to 90% of patients can tolerate long-term ACE inhibitor therapy (Hunt et al.,

2005). However, a small percentage of patients develop an intractable cough related to kinin production, requiring them to stop taking ACE inhibitors. ACE inhibitors cannot be used in patients who have had life-threatening oral angioedema or in patients with severe renal failure. Great caution must be used when administering ACE inhibitors in the following situations:

- systolic blood pressure < 80 mm Hg
- creatinine > 3 mg/dl
- presence of bilateral renal artery stenosis
- elevated serum potassium.

(Hunt et al., 2005)

Although ACE inhibitors have a renoprotective effect in patients with diabetes or renal insufficiency, they can cause renal problems in patients with low cardiac outputs who have been relying on the activation of the RAAS for improved renal perfusion. ACE inhibitors also predispose patients to hyperkalemia because they decrease the release of aldosterone. For this reason, renal function and electrolyte levels must be monitored closely. ACE inhibitors end with "pril." Box-2-4 lists available ACE inhibitors.

BOX 2-4: ACE INHIBITORS	
Benazepril	Lisinopril
Captopril	Quinapril
Enalapril	Ramipril
Fosinopril	

Angiotensin II Receptor Blockers

ARBs directly block angiotensin II after it is formed. Current guidelines indicate the use of ARBs when ACE inhibitors are unable to be tolerated due to intractable cough or angioedema. ARBs have side effects and precautions similar to ACE inhibitors.

However, ARBs do not produce a cough because they do not enhance kinin production. Although this action is beneficial in eliminating the side effect of cough, it may also decrease effectiveness in the management of heart failure because kinins are responsible for vasodilator effects beneficial in the treatment of heart failure. Research comparing the benefits of ACE inhibitors and ARBs is ongoing. There is also ongoing research regarding the possible added benefits of concomitant ARB and ACE inhibitor use (Heart Failure Society of America, 2004). However, current heart failure guidelines still recommend ACE inhibitors as the preferred medications. In certain patients with mild to moderate heart failure, however, ARBs may be used in place of ACE inhibitors as first-line agents. These guidelines may change as new evidence compares the benefits of ACE inhibitors and ARBs. ARBs end with "sartan." Candesartan was the first ARB approved by the FDA for the use in the treatment of heart failure (Hunt et al., 2005). Box 2-5 lists available ARBs.

BOX 2-5: ANGIOTENSIN II RECEPTOR BLOCKERS	
Candesartan	Losartan
Eprosartan	Telmisartan
Irbesartan	Valsartan

Aldosterone Antagonists

Aldosterone is a mineralocorticoid hormone released from the adrenal cortex as part of the end result of the action of the RAAS. Aldosterone informs the body to hold onto sodium, and therefore water, and to excrete potassium. For this reason, aldosterone antagonists are sometimes referred to as *potassium-sparing diuretics*. ACE inhibitors indirectly affect the release of aldosterone, whereas aldosterone antagonists directly block aldosterone. The end result is a decrease in sodium and water retention and, therefore, a decrease in preload.

In addition to these effects, aldosterone is thought to play an even larger role in cardiovascular function. Some additional effects of aldosterone include:

- potentiation of catecholamines
- inhibition of the parasympathetic nervous system
- decreased arterial compliance
- enhancement of thrombosis
- promotion of vascular inflammation and injury.

(Hunt et al., 2005)

Two aldosterone antagonists are available: spironolactone and eplerenone. Spironolactone is a nonselective agent that blocks aldosterone and also exhibits an antiandrogenic effect in both men and women. This antiandrogenic effect can cause gynecomastia in men (Clinical Pharmacology Database, 2004). Low-dose spironolactone has been shown to decrease mortality in patients with severe heart failure who are already taking an ACE inhibitor (Laurent, 2005).

Eplerenone is a selective aldosterone antagonist and, therefore, does not have the associated side effect of gynecomastia in men. Eplerenone is indicated in patients with left ventricular dysfunction after MI and those with diabetes to prevent progression of heart failure, recurrent MI, and sudden cardiac death (Antman et al., 2004; Clinical Pharmacology Database, 2004). Both spironolactone and eplerenone can cause hyperkalemia, especially when given with an ACE inhibitor.

Beta-Blockers

Beta-blockers can block the ß1 or ß2 receptors of the sympathetic nervous system. When beta-blockers block ß1 receptors, a decrease in heart rate and contractility results. When they block ß2 receptors, bronchial and peripheral vasoconstriction occur. Therefore, caution should be used when administering beta-blockers to patients with restrictive airway disease or peripheral vascular disease.

Clinical Application
Many patients with cardiac disease have coexisting peripheral vascular disease. If a nonselective blocker is prescribed, the patient may experience an increase in intermittent claudication associated with the peripheral vascular disease. This effect is related to the blockage of ß2.

Beta-blockers are widely prescribed in cardiovascular medicine and are indicated for a number of cardiovascular disorders. Box 2-6 lists cardiovascular indications for the use of beta-blockers. Beta-blockers are included in the practice guidelines for the management of heart failure, stable angina, and acute coronary syndromes. Their use in these disorders will be discussed in more detail in later chapters.

BOX 2-6: CARDIOVASCULAR INDICATIONS FOR BETA-BLOCKERS

Acute MI

Angina

Aortic dissection

Digoxin-induced ventricular arrhythmias

Heart failure

Hypertension

Hypertrophic cardiomyopathy (HCM)

Mitral valve prolapse

Post-myocardial infarction

Prolonged QT syndrome

Supraventricular arrhythmias

Ventricular arrhythmias

(Adair & Fuenzalida, 2001)

Beta-blockers decrease myocardial oxygen demand by decreasing contractility and heart rate. They also help increase coronary perfusion by increasing diastolic filling time. There is a potential negative effect of increased left ventricular wall tension due to decreased heart rate. This increased wall tension may actually increase myocardial oxygen demand. Nitrates are commonly prescribed with beta-blockers to prevent this adverse effect (Gibbons et al., 2002).

When used to treat hypertension, beta-blockers prevent reflex tachycardia associated with other vasodilators. Although beta-blockers do not cause direct arterial vasodilatation, they decrease contractility and heart rate, which decreases cardiac output. A decrease in cardiac output lowers blood pressure. Some beta-blockers are cardioselective, meaning they predominantly block ß1; others are noncardioselective blocking both ß1 and ß2.

Cardioselective beta-blockers

- Acebutolol

- Metoprolol

- Atenolol

- Esmolol

Noncardioselective beta-blockers

- Propranolol
- Timolol
- Nandolol
- Sotolol
- Carvedilol (also has alpha blockade)

Contraindications to beta-blocker initiation include severe bradycardia, high-degree AV block, sick sinus syndrome, and acute decompensated heart failure (Gibbons et al., 2002). Caution must be exercised when using beta-blockers in patients with coexisting depression, asthma, or peripheral vascular disease. Caution is particularly important when using noncardioselective beta-blockers in patients with with asthma or peripheral vascular disease. Diabetic patients should exercise caution when taking beta-blockers because beta-blockers can mask the symptoms of hypoglycemia. Side effects of beta-blockers include lethargy, fatigue, insomnia, nightmares, impotence, worsening asthma, and worsening claudication (Gibbons et al., 2002).

Beta-blockers are sometimes combined with alpha-blockers. Alpha-blockers produce vasodilatation and are indicated in the treatment of hypertension.

Calcium Channel Blockers

Calcium channel blockers decrease the flux of calcium across cell membranes. Calcium channel blockers can be used to decrease heart rate, contrac-

tility, and afterload. The mechanisms of action of these three potential effects are:

- Decreased contractility: Blocks inward flow of calcium in phase two of the cardiac action potential and decreases the force of contractions
- Decreased heart rate: Depresses automaticity and velocity and decreases heart rate
- Decreased afterload: Relaxes vascular smooth muscle.

All calcium channel blockers have some common effects. For example, they all have some degree of negative inotropic effect. They also reduce both coronary and systemic vascular resistance. For these reasons, calcium channel blockers are effective in decreasing myocardial oxygen demand. However, not all calcium channel blockers are created equal and, therefore, they do not all have the same effects or degree of effect. There are three distinct groups of calcium blockers. Table 2-13 defines the differences between these groups.

Short- and intermediate-acting dihydropyridine calcium channel blockers are not used in the treatment of angina or hypertension because of their questionable safety profile. Nifedipine, an older generation dihydropyridine calcium channel blocker, is contraindicated in unstable angina because of its predominant peripheral arterial vasodilatory effects (Mendoza & Loghin, 2001). Sublingual use of nifedipine has not been acceptable since 1995, when it was shown to have adverse effects related to

TABLE 2-13: CALCIUM CHANNEL BLOCKERS

	Verapamil	Dihydropyridine calcium channel blockers	Diltiazem
Heart rate	↓	↑ (reflex tachycardia)	↓
AV nodal conduction	↓	Neutral	↓
Contractility	↓	↓	↓
Arterial vasodilatation	↑	↑	↑

(Clinical Pharmacology Database, 2004)

its unpredictable and sometimes dangerous hemo-dynamic response (Gibbons et al., 2002).

Newer generation, longer acting dihydropyridine calcium channel blockers, such as amlodipine, have more coronary vasodilatory properties and are better tolerated in patients with decreased left ventricular dysfunction. Amlodipine, a coronary vaso-elective dihydropyridine calcium channel blocker, is the best-tolerated calcium channel blocker in patients with ischemic cardiomyopathy (Gibbons et al., 2002).

Decompensated heart failure is a contraindication to the administration of calcium channel blockers. In patients with heart block or bradyarrhythmias, the calcium channel blockers that affect heart rate should not be used. Adverse effects of calcium channel blockers include peripheral edema, worsening heart failure, hypotension and constipation (Clinical Pharmacology Database, 2004). In addition, verapamil and diltiazem can cause bradycardia and heart block.

Primary indications for calcium channel blockers include:

- atrial fibrillation or flutter, paroxysmal supraventricular tachycardia: diltiazem or verapamil

- angina (including vasospastic angina), diltiazem or verapamil with nitrates; dihydropyridine ("ine") calcium channel blockers with beta-blockers (to prevent reflex tachycardia)

- hypertension: dihydropyridine ("ine") calcium channel blockers.

Additional indications include:

- HCM: diltiazem and verapamil (avoid dihydropyridine calcium channel blockers)

- treatment and prevention of coronary spasm: dihydropyridine calcium channel blockers.

Other Medications that Promote Arterial and Venous Vasodilatation

Nitroglycerin and Nitrates

When administered IV in low doses, nitroglycerin is a primary venous vasodilator. The dose of a sublingual nitroglycerin tablet is high enough to produce both venous and arterial vasodilatation. Low-dose IV nitroglycerin is effective in alleviating chest pain, even though it acts primarily as a venous vasodilator. It works by reducing preload and, therefore, myocardial oxygen demand. This reduction in myocardial oxygen demand can be sufficient to relieve chest pain associated with angina. Higher doses of nitroglycerin produce direct dilatation of the large coronary arteries and arterioles. Nitroglycerin also exhibits antithrombotic and antiplatelet effects.

Patients taking oral or topical nitrates can develop a tolerance. To prevent this tolerance, allow a nitrate-free period of 8 to 10 hours per day, preferably during the night (Calagan, Schachter, Kruger, Cameron, & Loghin, 2001). Some patients develop headaches as a result of the vasodilatation associated with nitroglycerin.

Clinical Application
Headaches should be treated immediately, because pain increases sympathetic nervous system stimulation and myocardial oxygen demand, potentially worsening ischemia.

Because nitrates decrease preload, they are contraindicated in patients with HCM, who are dependent on adequate preload to maintain their cardiac output. Nitrates and other vasodilators should also be used with extreme caution in patients with aortic stenosis because these patients have a limited ability to increase cardiac output in response to hypotension. Nitrates can cause some reflex tachycardia; administration with a beta-blocker can prevent this side effect.

Nitrates also should not be prescribed to men taking sildenafil. Rarely, the administration of sublingual nitroglycerin can produce bradycardia and hypotension due to activation of the Bezold-Jarisch reflex (Gibbons et al., 2002). When triggered, this reflex causes a vasovagal response (Bridges, 2005a).

Nitroprusside

Nitroprusside has mixed venous and arterial vasodilative properties; however, it is predominantly an arterial vasodilator. Nitroprusside is indicated in hypertensive crisis and acute heart failure to reduce afterload. Hypotension is the number one side effect and nursing consideration. Continuous blood pressure monitoring via an arterial line is preferred. Although thiocyanate toxicity can occur, it is not an initial nursing consideration because patients are not at risk unless they have been receiving nitroprusside for several days at high doses (Dennison, 2000).

Nesiritide

Nesiritide is a synthetic brain natriuretic peptide (BNP). BNP is naturally released from the ventricles in heart failure to promote vasodilatation and counteract the effects of the RAAS. Nesiritide is a newer vasodilator that has both venous and arterial vasodilative effects. It is used in the management of acute decompensated heart failure to decrease both preload and afterload. Nesiritide is administered as a short-term infusion (24 to 48 hours) for heart failure patients demonstrating signs of extracellular fluid overload. Because nesiritide also lowers blood pressure, the patient must have a blood pressure greater than 90 mm Hg systolic or evidence of high systemic vascular resistance (Clinical Pharmacology Database, 2004).

Digoxin

Digoxin is a cardiac glycoside that has very complex mechanisms of action. It has weak inotropic properties and also some parasympathetic properties. These parasympathetic properties decrease sympathetic outflow and decrease renin production, which are particularly beneficial when used in the treatment of heart failure.

Digoxin has a narrow therapeutic range, and toxicity can occur at therapeutic levels. Signs and symptoms of toxicity include

- nausea and vomiting

- headache

- confusion

- vision disturbances, such as the appearance of halos or a change in color perception.

To avoid toxicity, low doses of digoxin (0.125 mg per day) are now used in most patients (Hunt et al., 2005). Amiodarone, a class III antiarrhythmic, increases serum digoxin concentrations. Digoxin doses should be reduced if amiodarone is ordered (Chebaclo & Loghin, 2001). Prior to initiation of digoxin, the patient should have a normal potassium level. Hypokalemia increases the risk of digoxin toxicity. Because digoxin has multiple other medication interactions, careful assessment of the patient's medication profile is an important nursing intervention.

Dialysis is not effective in treating digoxin toxicity because of the high tissue-binding property of digoxin. Untreated digoxin-toxicity-induced arrhythmias can be fatal (Dennison, 2000). Arrhythmias seen with toxicity usually involve increased automaticity with impaired conduction, for example, paroxysmal atrial tachycardia with heart block.

Clinical Application
Digoxin should be withheld in a patient with clinical signs of digoxin toxicity, even in the presence of a therapeutic digoxin level, until the patient's clinical condition can be thoroughly discussed with the physician.

CONCLUSION

Cardiovascular pharmacology is rapidly changing. New pharmacological agents are under investigation in nearly all classes of medications and for all cardiovascular conditions. However, a solid understanding of the hemodynamic impact of pharmacology can be the foundation upon which to build new knowledge.

Cardiovascular drugs are commonly used to maximize hemodynamic performance in patients with poor left ventricular function. In addition, many of the same pharmacological agents are used in secondary prevention efforts to interrupt physiological responses leading to disease progression. Nurses play a tremendous role in assisting patients with achieving compliance with their prescribed pharmacological treatment plans. Increased compliance can be achieved when patients truly understand the physiologic benefits of therapy.

EXAM QUESTIONS

CHAPTER 2
Questions 10-19

10. The condition that warrants using medications to decrease preload is

    a. volume depletion from excessive diuretic use.

    b. volume excess from heart failure.

    c. low blood pressure.

    d. any heart condition.

11. Pharmacological options that can be used to increase preload include

    a. IV fluids and cessation of venous vasodilators.

    b. diuretics and venous vasodilators.

    c. any medication that lowers blood pressure.

    d. any medication that increases afterload.

12. Systemic afterload reduction is a primary goal in

    a. septic shock and heart failure.

    b. pneumonia and chronic obstructive pulmonary disease.

    c. septic shock and pneumonia.

    d. heart failure and hypertension.

13. Medications used to reduce afterload include

    a. arterial vasodilators.

    b. venous vasodilators.

    c. arterial vasoconstrictors.

    d. venous vasoconstrictors.

14. A nursing consideration when administering medications to increase contractility or heart rate is

    a. these medications can also cause severe bleeding.

    b. these medications also increase myocardial oxygen demand.

    c. these medications have a very high rate of allergic reactions.

    d. these medications cannot be given to anyone over age 60.

15. Medications that mimic the sympathetic nervous system can cause

    a. increased platelet count, increased red blood cell count, and increased fibrinogen level.

    b. decreased heart rate, decreased afterload, and decreased contractility.

    c. decreased platelet count, decreased red blood cell count, and decreased fibrinogen level.

    d. increased heart rate, increased afterload, and increased contractility.

16. The action of ACE inhibitors is best described as

    a. preventing the initial release of renin.

    b. directly blocking the effects of angiotensin II.

    c. preventing the conversion of angiotensin I to angiotensin II.

    d. directly blocking the effects of aldosterone.

17. A key nursing assessment for a patient taking both an ACE inhibitor and an aldosterone antagonist is monitoring the lab values for

    a. potassium.

    b. glucose.

    c. white blood cell count.

    d. phosphorus.

18. Beta-blockers should be used cautiously in patients with reactive airway disease and peripheral vascular disease because blocking of

    a. ß1 receptors can cause bronchial and peripheral vasodilatation.

    b. ß2 receptors can cause bronchial and peripheral vasodilatation.

    c. ß1 receptors can cause bronchial and peripheral vasoconstriction.

    d. ß2 receptors can cause bronchial and peripheral vasoconstriction.

19. When using a calcium channel blocker to help control heart rate, you would anticipate giving

    a. verapamil and carvedilol.

    b. amlodipine and diltiazem.

    c. diltiazem and verapamil.

    d. amlodipine and captopril.

CHAPTER 3

PHARMACOLOGY TO INCREASE MYOCARDIAL OXYGEN SUPPLY

CHAPTER OBJECTIVE

After completing this chapter, the reader will be able to describe the key pharmacological agents used to preserve and increase myocardial oxygen supply.

LEARNING OBJECTIVES

After studying this chapter, the reader will be able to

1. describe the benefits of low-density lipoprotein cholesterol (LDL-C) reduction and define the lipid-lowering agents most effective in reducing LDL-C.

2. list lipid-lowering agents used to reduce triglycerides and increase high-density lipoprotein cholesterol.

3. discuss the key side effects of and patient education criteria for lipid-lowering therapy.

4. describe the purpose of, indications for, and potential complications of thrombolytic and fibrinolytic therapy.

5. compare and contrast unfractionated heparin and low-molecular-weight heparin.

6. define the three main groups of antiplatelet agents used in the treatment of cardiovascular disease.

INTRODUCTION

Medications used to protect myocardial oxygen supply can be grouped into two categories: those aimed at the long-term prevention of atherosclerotic coronary artery disease and those aimed at the prevention or disruption of clot formation. These medications play a major role in the prevention and treatment of cardiovascular disease.

LIPID-LOWERING MEDICATIONS

Low-Density Lipoprotein Cholesterol

A 1% reduction in total cholesterol reduces the incidence of cardiac events by 2% (Gibbons et al., 2002). In addition, a 1% increase in high-density lipoprotein cholesterol (HDL-C) reduces the risk by 2% to 4% (U.S. Department of Health and Human Services [DHHS], 2001). Therefore, reduction of low-density lipoprotein cholesterol (LDL-C) is a primary goal in the management of coronary heart disease. In the presence of established coronary artery disease, lipid-lowering therapy should be prescribed with even mild elevations of LDL-C. The effects of various groups of medications on LDL-C levels are outlined in Table 3-1.

Of the available lipid-lowering drugs, the HMG-CoA reductase inhibitors (statins) are the most potent for reducing LDL-C. Other agents that substantially lower LDL-C are bile acid resins and nicotinic acid.

TABLE 3-1: EFFECTS OF LIPID-LOWERING THERAPY ON LDL-C LEVELS

Class of Medications	% Reduction
HMG-CoA reductase inhibitors (statins)	18-60%
Bile acid sequestrants	15-30%
Nicotinic acid	15-30%
Fibrates	5-20%
Intestinal absorption inhibitors	18%
(DHHS, 2001; Fair & Berra, 2005)	

TABLE 3-2: EFFECTS OF LIPID-LOWERING THERAPY ON TRIGLYCERIDE AND HDL-C LEVELS

Class of Medications	HDL-C	Triglycerides
Nicotinic acid	↑ 15-35%	↓ 20-50%
Fibrates	↑ 10-20%	↓ 20-50%
HMG-CoA reductase inhibitors (statins)	↑ 5-15%	↓ 7-37%
Bile acid sequestrants	↑ 3-5%	does not decrease, may even increase
Intestinal absorption inhibitors	↑ 1%	↓ 8%
(DHHS, 2001; Fair & Berra, 2005)		

All three of these drug classes have a dose-dependent effect on LDL-C.

In contrast, the effect of fibrates on LDL-C depends not on dose but on the patient's triglyceride level. If triglyceride level is normal, fibrates decrease LDL-C; however, if triglyceride levels are elevated, fibrates can potentially increase LDL-C level (Levine, 2002). Among the fibrates, fenofibrate has a greater effect on LDL-C reduction than clofibrate or gemfibrozil. However, fibrates tend to normalize LDL-C particle composition, changing the small, dense, atherogenic LDL particles to a larger, less dense, less atherogenic type. This increase in LDL particle size may contribute to an increase in LDL-C level, while still reducing the risk of coronary atherosclerosis (Clinical Pharmacology Database, 2004).

Triglycerides and High-Density Lipoprotein Cholesterol

Table 3-2 details the effects of lipid lowering medications on triglyceride and HDL-C levels.

The most effective agents for improving triglyceride and HDL-C levels are nicotinic acid (niacin) and the fibrates. Nicotinic acid has a dose-dependent effect; however, side effects may prevent patients from taking a sufficient dose. Fibrates have a fixed-dose effect and do not have the irritating side effects associated with nicotinic acid. Statins, especially simvastatin and atorvastatin, also lower triglycerides and increase HDL-C. Bile acid resins increase HDL-C but may also increase triglycerides.

Clinical Application
Helping patients understand the expected, quantifiable improvements in lipid levels associated with drug therapy may encourage compliance with the therapeutic regime.

Bile Acid Sequestrants

Bile acid sequestrants, also called *resins,* include:

• cholestyramine (Questran)

• colestipol (Colestid)

• colesevelam (WelChol).

These drugs combine with bile acids in the intestine and form an insoluble complex that is excreted in feces (Levine, 2002). The low level of bile acids provides feedback to the hepatic circulation to stimulate the production of more bile acids. Because cholesterol is used in the production of bile acids, the liver is also stimulated to produce more cholesterol.

Cholesterol, specifically the oxidation of cholesterol from LDL-C, is a major precursor for the formation of bile acids. The body breaks down cholesterol to make bile acids and then compensates by increasing LDL-C receptors to remove LDL-C from circulation (Fair & Berra, 2005). Although the liver is stimulated to produce more cholesterol, this new cholesterol is used to produce more bile acids. A net decrease in total cholesterol and LDL-C results. Bile acid sequestrants have minimal effects on HDL-C and can actually increase triglyceride levels.

Clinical Application

Bile acid sequestrants should be taken with the largest meal of the day because intestinal bile acids are greatest at this time.

The cholesterol-lowering effects usually begin in 24 to 48 hours, and peak effects are achieved within a 2- to 4-week time period (Clinical Pharmacology Database, 2004). Cholestyramine is one of the oldest medications used to treat hyperlipidemia; the U.S. Food and Drug Administration (FDA) first approved it in 1966 (Clinical Pharmacology Database, 2004). Colesevelam is approved for use with statins and produces a synergistic effect.

Side effects of bile acid sequestrants include gastrointestinal (GI) distress and constipation. Constipation is the most common and troublesome side effect. Bile acid sequestrants can bind with other substances (including other medications) in addition to binding to bile acids. Because of this binding potential, bile acid sequestrants interfere with the absorption of fat-soluble vitamins (A, D, and K). It may also accelerate their clearance and lower their effective plasma levels.

Clinical Application

Because of their binding property, bile acid sequestrants should not be taken at the same time as other medications. Advise patients to take other medications 1 hour before or 4 hours after taking bile acid sequestrants.

The use of these medications is contraindicated in patients with biliary obstruction or abnormal intestinal function. Because bile acid sequestrants can increase triglyceride levels, they are also contraindicated in patients with elevated triglycerides. The powder forms of bile acid sequestrants should be mixed with fluids. Bile acid resins are insoluble and form a gritty solution. This may not be pleasing to some patients and can affect compliance with the therapeutic regime. Tablets should not be cut, chewed, or crushed because they are designed to break down in the GI track. Colestipol is not absorbed and therefore has less toxic potential, making it safer for use in children and pregnant women (Clinical Pharmacology Database, 2004).

Niacin (Nicotinic Acid)

Also called *niacin,* nicotinic acid is a B complex vitamin. Because niacin is used in the enrichment of refined flour, niacin deficiency is rare in our country today. Dietary requirements for niacin can be met by the intake of either nicotinic acid or nicotinamide. As vitamins, both of these substances have identical functions. However, as pharmacological agents, they are very different. In addition to being a vitamin, niacin has additional dose-related pharmacological effects not seen with nicotinamide (Clinical Pharmacology Database, 2004).

In peripheral circulation, niacin dilates the cutaneous blood vessels and increases blood flow to the face, neck, and chest. Niacin may cause a release of histamine or prostacyclin that is responsible for this vasodilatation and the classic "flush" associated with niacin use. This vasodilatation can also produce pruritus, headaches, or other pain. Histamine can also increase gastric acid secretion, increasing the likelihood of GI side effects.

Niacin was the first lipid-lowering agent shown to decrease mortality in myocardial infarction (MI) patients (Clinical Pharmacology Database, 2004).

Nicotinic acid-related agents include:

• Niacor

- Slo-Niacin

- Niaspan

Decreased very-low-density lipoprotein cholesterol (VLDL-C) production is one of the primary actions of niacin (Fair & Berra, 2005). One explanation for this result is that niacin decreases the lipolysis of triglycerides in adipose tissue, thereby reducing the transport of free fatty acids to the liver and decreasing hepatic triglyceride synthesis (Clinical Pharmacology Database, 2004). Decreased triglyceride synthesis results in a reduction of VLDL-C production. Lowered LDL-C cholesterol can be a result of decreased VLDL-C production; alternatively, niacin may promote increased clearance of LDL-C precursors.

Niacin also raises HDL-C levels through a mechanism that is not fully understood but is related to increased levels of apo A-I and lipoprotein A-I and a decrease in levels of Apo-B. Women may have better results than men when taking niacin at the same dose (Clinical Pharmacology Database, 2004.)

The effects of niacin on the reduction of cholesterol are unrelated to its role as a vitamin. Therapeutic dosing is 1 to 2 g of niacin per day; therefore, the amount of niacin in vitamin supplements does not affect lipid levels (Levine, 2002). Side effects of niacin include flushing, GI distress, hyperglycemia, gout, and liver toxicity. Flushing and dyspepsia are likely to limit compliance with therapy. Flushing usually subsides within 2 weeks on a stable dose. When given 30 minutes before niacin, aspirin may also blunt the flushing response (Fair & Berra, 2005). Niacin should be administered with food to minimize GI side effects.

Fibrates

Also called *fibric acid agents,* fibrates include:

- clofibrate (Atromid-S)

- fenofibrate (Tricor)

- gemfibrozil (Lopid)

The mechanism of action for these medications is complex and not fully understood. However they stimulate lipoprotein lipase activity, which increases catabolism and clearance of triglycerides. They also decrease hepatic triglyceride production. In addition, they may also decrease cholesterol synthesis, increase the mobilization of cholesterol from tissues, enhance the removal of cholesterol from the liver, and increase cholesterol excretion in feces. They decrease VLDL-C synthesis and significantly reduce triglycerides. Fibrates also raise HDL-C levels (Clinical Pharmacology Database, 2004).

Fibrates are the drug of choice for type III hyperlipidemia and hypertriglyceridemia (DHHS, 2001). They decrease triglycerides by 25% to 50% and increase HDL-C in the presence of hypertriglyceridemia. However, they have variable effects on LDL-C. Despite this, fibrates, particularly fenofibrate, may increase the production of larger, less-dense LDL particles, which help promote LDL metabolism and reduce the number of smaller, more-dense particles associated with atherosclerosis. Fenofibrate also reduces lipoprotein (a) and serum fibrinogen, which is an independent risk factor for thrombosis (Clinical Pharmacology Database, 2004). Serum triglyceride levels begin to fall within 2 to 5 days, with maximal effects achieved within 3 weeks (Clinical Pharmacology Database, 2004.)

Side effects of fibrates include dyspepsia, rash, alopecia, fatigue, headache, impotence, anemia, myositis flulike syndrome, cholelithiasis, and abnormal liver function test results (Levine, 2002). Because fibrates are renally excreted, they are contraindicated in patients with severe renal disease. They are also contraindicated in patients with hepatic disease or preexisting gallbladder disease.

Combining a fibrate with a statin raises safety concerns because of the potential for myopathy and overt rhabdomyolysis. One fibrate, fenofibrate, however, does not interfere with the catabolism of statins (DHHS, 2001). Concomitant use of gemfibrozil with a statin increases the risk of rhabdomyolysis (Levine, 2002). However, almost all reports of such adverse effects have occured in situations in which the drug combination should have been avoided. Fibrates and statins should not be combined in the following situations:

- when high doses of statins, particularly simvastatin 80 mg per day or atorvastatin 80 mg per day, are used

- in patients with renal insufficiency because (fibrates are renally excreted and plasma levels are increased in patients with renal insufficiency, thereby increasing the risk for drug-drug interactions)

- in patients taking any agent that interferes with clearance of statins (for example, the immunosuppressive agent tacrolimus has this effect)

- in patients older than age 70 because of general increased problems with renal and hepatic function (DHHS, 2001).

HMG-CoA Reductase Inhibitors

Also known as *statins,* HMG-CoA reductase inhibitors have been widely studied in various clinical trials. Statins have been shown to decrease mortality and reduce the risk of major coronary events by 30% (Levine, 2002). They work by stimulating plaque regression. Examples of HMG-CoA reductase inhibitors include:

- lovastatin (Mevacor)

- simvastatin (Zocor)

- pravastatin (Pravachol)

- fluvastatin (Lescol)

- atorvastatin (Lipitor).

Lovastatin was the first HMG-CoA reductase inhibitor introduced (Clinical Pharmacology Database, 2004). Both lovastatin and simvastatin are administered in an inactive form and require hydrolysis to be activated. The mechanism of action of statins involves the inhibition of HMG-CoA reductase. HMG-CoA reductase catalyzes an early step in cholesterol synthesis. These inhibitors reduce the quantity of mevalonic acid, a precursor to cholesterol. Cholesterol levels in liver cells are reduced, and the body responds with increased hepatic uptake of LDL-C from the circulation. The result is a decrease in total cholesterol, LDL-C, and triglycerides.

The effect of HMG-CoA reductase inhibitors is dose dependent. The most active time for cholesterol biosynthesis is during the very early morning hours. For this reason, it is generally recommended to give statins late in the evening, prior to bedtime. However, not all medications in this group are clinically affected by the administration time. For example, the effects of atorvastatin on LDL-C reduction are not impacted by the time of day it is adminstered (Clinical Pharmacology Database, 2004). Higher doses of the most potent statins are generally needed to decrease triglyceride levels.

All medications in this group have been shown to reduce the risk of cardiovascular disease in clinical trials. In the 5-year Heart Protection Study, simvastatin was associated with a decrease in stroke, MI, and all-cause mortality. Benefits occurred regardless of initial cholesterol levels. This study also showed that diabetic patients had a lower rate of first-time vascular events (Clinical Pharmacology Database, 2004; Grundy et al., 2004).

Atorvastatin at the maximal dose has the greatest LDL-C lowering effect of all the HMG-CoA reductase inhibitors. Atorvastatin has a longer half-life and greater hepatic selectivity than the other HMG-CoA reductase inhibitors, which might explain its greater LDL-C lowering ability. At maximal doses, LDL-C can be lowered by 60% (Clinical Pharmacology Database, 2004). Clinical benefits of atorvastatin have been seen in patients with acute coronary syndrome (ACS), high-risk hypertensive patients, and patients with type II diabetes.

Fluvastatin has some properties that differ from other medications in its class. For example, it has a short half-life, is highly bound to proteins, and does not cross the blood-brain barrier. Some researchers claim that fluvastatin is less likely than other HMG-CoA reductase inhibitors to cause systemic side effects (Clinical Pharmacology Database, 2004).

Side effects of HMG-CoA reductase inhibitors range in their severity. Minor effects include:

*   headache

*   GI effects

*   potential worsening of cataracts.

Serious effects include:

*   myopathy or rhabdomyolysis (both associated with myalgia and fatigue)

*   hepatic failure.

Grapefruit juice contains an agent that slows the activity of the liver enzyme that metabolizes some of the agents in this class, particularly simvastatin and atorvastatin. Therefore, grapefruit juice consumption can increase the expected drug levels for a given dose and increase the risk of rhabdomyolysis. Patients should be instructed not to consume large quantities of grapefruit juice when taking these drugs.

Clinical Application

Coadministration of certain medications with HMG-CoA reductase inhibitors can also cause rhabdomyolysis. Instruct patients to report all medications they are taking to each prescribing physician.

Rhabdomyolysis can result in acute renal failure and even death. Patients must be instructed to immediately report the following signs and symptoms to their physician:

*   muscle aching or weakness

*   decreased or brown urine

*   fever blistering or loosening of the skin

*   skin rash or itching

*   yellowing of the skin or eyes.

Statins are contraindicated in patients with acute or chronic liver disease. Liver enzymes should be assessed after 6 weeks of therapy and every 6 months thereafter.

Statins can be combined with nicotinic acid, fibrates, and bile acid sequestrants, if necessary. Caution must be used, however, due to the increased risk of rhabdomyolysis with certain drug combinations. Overall, the HMG-CoA reductase inhibitors are the best-tolerated and most-effective agents used to lower lipid levels.

Intestinal Absorption Inhibitors

Intestinal absorption inhibitors are the newest class of lipid-lowering medications. These medications can be used alone or in combination with HMG-CoA reductase inhibitors. In 2002, ezetimibe was the first intestinal absorption inhibitor to be approved by the FDA. Ezetimibe blocks the absorption of cholesterol in the small intestine and therefore decreases the delivery of intestinal choelsterol to the liver. This results in a decrease of cholesterol stores in the liver and a subsequent increase in blood clearance of cholesterol (Clinical Pharmacology Database, 2004).

DRUGS THAT AFFECT COAGULATION

Coagulation Overview

The coagulation system has two primary purposes:

*   to protect the integrity of the vessels and prevent harmful bleeding

*   to maintain the fluid state of the blood.

These two goals must be achieved simultaneously to maintain health.

Clotting can be initiated by activation of either the intrinsic or extrinsic pathways of the clotting cascade. The intrinsic pathway is initiated by vessel injury and direct exposure to collagen. The extrinsic pathway is triggered by the endothelial release of tissue factor. Both the intrinsic and extrinsic pathways initiate the common pathway, through which a fibrin stable clot is produced.

In the common pathway:

- Prothrombin is converted to thrombin.

- Thrombin permits the conversion of fibrinogen to fibrin.

- A fibrin stable clot forms.

This fibrin stable clot, sometimes called a *red clot,* is the cause of most ST-segment elevation myocardial infarctions (STEMIs).

Platelets also respond to vessel injury through the processes of adhesion, activation, and aggregation. Platelet aggregation can be large enough to form a platelet plug, a white clot that seals a damaged vessel. This white clot is a primary culprit in unstable angina. In addition to the independent formation of a platelet plug, platelets also release components necessary for the clotting process in the intrinsic pathway. Platelets also contain a fibrin-stabilizing factor that is important in the final stage of the common pathway, prior to stable clot formation. Platelets cross-link with fibrinogen via the glycoprotein (GP) IIb/IIIa receptors to form a fibrin mesh, which gives a clot more substance.

Thrombolytics and Fibrinolytics

Two main categories of medications are used to dissolve clots that have already formed: medications that are nonfibrin specific (thrombolytics) and those that are fibrin specific (fibrinolytics). Both types are IV administered. Table 3-3 lists agents used to dissolve clots during acute STEMIs. For maximum effectiveness, these medications should be administered within 30 minutes of symptom onset (Antman et al., 2004). Indications and contraindications for these medications are discussed in greater detail in chapter 5.

Streptokinase was the earliest "clot busting" medication used to dissolve clots during an acute MI. It is a nonenzyme protein made from hemolytic streptococci that works by combining with circulating plasminogen and forming complexes that catalyze plasmin formation. The resultant increase in circulating plasmin creates a systemic lytic state, dissolving recent clots.

Because it is a foreign protein, streptokinase can cause allergic reactions. The most common indications of an allergic reaction include pruritus, urticaria, fever, nausea, flushing, headache, and malaise (Bene & Vaughan, 2005). In response to receiving streptokinase, patients also produce anti-streptokinase antibodies. Patients with antibodies to streptokinase may not receive the full benefit of the medication; therefore, it is contraindicated in these patients. Patients with antistreptokinase antibodies include those who have received streptokinase within the last 6 months and those who have had recent streptococcal infection (Bene & Vaughan, 2005).

TABLE 3-3: THROMBOLYTIC AND FIBRINOLYTIC AGENTS		
Type	**Actions/Physiologic Effects**	**Agents**
Fibrin specific	• Plasminogen activation • Rapid clot lysis • Clot specific	• Tissue plasminogen activators (t-PAs) • Alteplase (recombinant t-PA) • Reteplase (bolus dose recombinant t-PA) • Tenecteplase (single bolus dose recombinant t-PA)
Nonfibrin specific	• Systemic lysis • Slow clot lysis • More prolonged, systemic effect	• Streptokinase • Anistreplase (also known as *anisoylated plasminogen streptokinase activator complex,* or APSAC)

Anistreplase is a chemically altered form of streptokinase. It converts circulating plasminogen into plasmin and has systemic lytic effects similar to those of streptokinase. Able to be given in a bolus dose, anistreplase has demonstrated higher initial patency rates than streptokinase in clinical trials (Bene & Vaughan, 2005). Although the reasons are not fully understood, hypotension is a side effect of both anistreplase and streptokinase.

Tissue plasminogen activator (t-PA), a fibrin-specific lytic agent, is a serine protease produced by vascular endothelial cells. It is produced for clinical use using recombinant deoxyribonucleic acid (DNA) techniques. It has a particular affinity for fibrin; specifically, it activates the plasminogen that is bound to fibrin. Alteplase (recombinant t-PA), uses an accelerated dose to achieve more rapid reperfusion. The newer drugs derived from t-PA, reteplase (r-PA) and tenecteplase (TNK-t-PA), are designed for bolus dosing to eliminate medication errors associated with the administration of these types of medications. In the GUSTO I clinical trial involving both streptokinase and t-PA, there was an approximate 12% to 13 % rate of error in the administration of these drugs. In the group of patients in which an administration error was made, the mortality at 30 days was higher (Bene & Vaughan, 2005).

Reteplase and tenecteplase also have very short half-lives. The benefit of a short half-life is decreased risk of bleeding; the disadvantage is an increased likelihood of reocclusion after administration. Tenecteplase is a very fibrin-specific medication that causes minimal systemic bleeding, including intracranial bleeding. Allergic response and hypotension can also occur with t-PA and t-PA-related medications.

All medications in this group have a very narrow window of therapeutic effect. If dosing is too low, clot lysis does not occur and there is no interruption of the MI. If the dose is too high, systemic bleeding can occur. Bleeding commonly occurs at vascular access sites. However, intracranial bleeding can also occur and have devastating effects. The risk of bleeding is weighed against the potential benefit when making decisions about the administration of these medications. Contraindications for these medications are discussed in chapter 5. t-PA agents have better initial results with rapid reperfusion; however, they also have higher rates of intracranial hemorrhage. t-PA agents also have a substantially higher cost than streptokinase. In various studies using thrombolytics or fibrinolytics for reperfusion during an acute MI, the mortality reduction has been approximately 27% (Bene & Vaughan, 2005).

Clinical Application

Because thrombolytics and fibrinolytics must be administered within a very short time frame and have specific indications and contraindications, it is important for emergency departments to have clearly written protocols and checklists to guide nurses through the rapid and accurate administration of these medications.

Anticoagulants

Unfractionated Heparin

Commercially produced heparin is derived from porcine or bovine tissue. Heparin was discovered in 1916 and approved by the FDA for use in 1936 (Clinical Pharmacology Database, 2004). Unfractionated heparin (UFH) is the anticoagulant of choice for many conditions, including acute MI, pulmonary emboli, and deep vein thrombosis. In the pathophysiological processes of atherosclerosis and ACSs, endothelial injury results in thrombi, platelet aggregation, and vasoconstriction. Fibrinogen is ultimately converted to fibrin to produce a fibrin stable clot. The role of heparin in these conditions is to prevent thrombus formation.

Heparin is an antithrombotic agent but does not lyse existing clots. It works in the intrinsic and common pathways of the clotting cascade to prevent further development of thrombi. In higher doses, heparin also interferes with platelet aggregation. Heparin prevents the conversion of prothrombin to thrombin (factor IIa) by accelerating the action of antithrombin III. Antithrombin III naturally inhibits thrombin. The net result is the neutralization of the clotting capabilities of thrombin. However, heparin does not inactivate fibrin-bound thrombin. Heparin also inactivates clotting factors IXa and Xa.

Heparin binds to plasma proteins, blood cells, and endothelial cells. This nonspecific binding to plasma proteins and endothelial cells limits the bioavailability of UFH at low doses and also contributes to its variable response between patients. UFH is commonly administered intravenously (IV) using a weight-based protocol to help control anticoagulation response. Weight-based heparin dosing reaches the therapeutic goal more consistently than standard therapy (Braunwald et al., 2002). Heparin can also be administered subcutaneously. It is not absorbed from the GI track, so it cannot be given orally.

The anticoagulation effects of IV heparin are almost instant. Activated partial thromboplastin time (aPTT) is used to monitor the therapeutic effectiveness and safety range of heparin. A baseline aPTT, prothrombin time (PT), International Normalized Ratio (INR), platelet count, hemoglobin level, and hematocrit should be drawn before UFH is started. The goal is to have aPTT at 1½ times the control. A therapeutic aPTT should be reached within 24 hours of the initiation of therapy. aPTT results should be measured 6 hours after the dose is initiated and again 6 hours after any dose change. After two therapeutic aPTTs have been achieved, measurements can be obtained every 24 hours (Braunwald et al., 2002).

In addition to weight, other patient variables affect aPTT. The aPTT response for a given dose of UFH increases with age and decreases in smokers and diabetic patients (Braunwald et al., 2002).

Bleeding is an obvious potential complication of heparin administration. The optimal period of time that heparin can be continued is not yet defined. Most clinical trials involving heparin have continued it for 2 to 5 days. An aPTT should be drawn with any change in patient condition, and heparin should be immediately discontinued when bleeding is the suspected cause. Hemoglobin level, hematocrit level, and platelet count are drawn on a daily basis. Heparin can cause mild to severe thrombocytopenia (platelet count less than $150,000/mm^3$) (Fischbach, 2004). Heparin should be discontinued if platelets fall below $100,000/mm^3$.

Mild thrombocytopenia occurs in 10% to 20% of patients, whereas more severe thrombocytopenia occurs in only 1% to 2% of patients (Braunwald et al., 2002). Thrombocytopenia generally occurs 4 to 14 days after initiation of heparin therapy. A very rare but very severe form of thrombocytopenia due to an autoimmune immune response can occur, resulting in thrombosis. Patients with this type of response should never receive heparin, not even the small doses of heparin used in solutions to flush invasive lines.

Low-molecular-weight Heparin

Low-molecular-weight heparin (LMWH) is smaller in size than UFH. It works by accelerating the activity of antithrombin III. LMWH has a more potent effect on factor Xa than on factor IIa, although both are inhibited. LMWH also produces less inhibition of platelets than does UFH.

LMWH binds less to plasma proteins and endothelial cells than does UFH. It also has a longer half-life, which helps to produce a sustained and more predictable anticoagulation effect. For this reason, clotting times do not need to be monitored as they do with use of UFH. At recommended doses, PT and aPTT are not greatly impacted. LMWH is also associated with a lower incidence of heparin-induced thrombocytopenia but a higher rate of minor bleeding than is UFH (Bene & Vaughan, 2005).

LMWH is administered subcutaneously in a twice-a-day dosing. Patients can be taught self-administration. Enoxaparin, a form of LMWH, was first approved by the FDA for deep vein thrombosis (DVT) prevention in patients undergoing orthopedic surgery. In 1998, enoxaparin received approval for use in the treatment of unstable angina and non-STEMI. Some studies have demonstrated beter outcomes in treating ACSs with enoxaparin than with UFH (Clinical Pharmacology Database, 2004). The use of LMWH and UFH continues to be studied in the ACS population undergoing early invasive treatment.

Direct Thrombin Inhibitors

Direct thrombin inhibitors are indicated for the treatment of thrombosis in patients with heparin-induced thrombocytopenia. Direct thrombin inhibitors also have an advantage over heparin because they have the ability to inactivate fibrin-bound thrombin, thereby improving the antithrombotic effect. These medications also bind less to plasma proteins and produce a more reliable anticoagulant effect. Direct thrombin inhibitors include lepirudin and desirudin, recombinant forms of hirudin. Anaphylactic reactions have been observed with the use of lepirudin (Greinacher, Lubenow, & Eichler, 2003). Argatroban is a synthetic direct thrombin inhibitor indicated for the treatment and prevention of heparin-induced thrombocytopenia and associated thromboembolic events (GlaxoSmithKline, 2005). Bivalirudin is a synthetic direct thrombin inhibitor indicated for patients with unstable angina undergoing percutaneous coronary intervention. This medication is indicated as an alternative to heparin in all patients, not just patients with, or at risk for, heparin-induced thrombocytopenia (The Medicines Company, 2004). As with all anticoagulants, direct thrombin inhibitors are contraindicated with major active bleeding.

Indirect Factor Xa Inhibitors

Indirect factor Xa inhibitors are a new class of anticoagulants. Fondaparinux was the first FDA-approved medication in this class. Fondaparinux is approved for DVT and pulmonary embolism (PE) prophylaxis in patients undergoing hip or abdominal surgery. It is also approved for the treatment of DVT

or PE in conjunction with warfarin (Clinical Pharmacology Database, 2004). Clinical trials are also evaluating the use of fondaparinux in the treatment of ACSs.

Indirect factor Xa inhibitors produce antithrombotic action by neutralizing factor Xa and interrupting the clotting cascade that leads to thrombin formation. This class of medications does not however inhibit thrombin (factor IIa). Administration is via subcutaneous injection and there is no need for laboratory monitoring because bleeding time is not greatly altered. There is no antidote yet available for factor Xa inhibitors (Clinical Pharmacology Database, 2004).

Warfarin

Warfarin (Coumadin) is an oral anticoagulant agent. Like heparin, warfarin does not affect existing clots. One of the important actions of warfarin is the inhibition of the synthesis of factor II (prothrombin). Warfarin acts indirectly through the liver by altering the synthesis of other vitamin–K–dependent factors in the extrinsic pathway. These vitamin–K–dependent factors are left biologically inactive. Vitamin K is essential for the liver to manufacture several clotting factors, including factors II, VII, IX, and X.

Warfarin is primarily bound to albumin in the blood; very little of it circulates freely. It is, however, the freely circulating amount that produces a therapeutic value. The number of potential drug interactions is high due to the large amount of protein-bound warfarin.

There is a lag time of anywhere from 2 to 5 days, most typically 3 to 4 days, to reach a therapeutic level. The reason for this lag time is gradual disappearance of the clotting factors involved. At full therapeutic doses, vitamin K–dependent clotting factors decrease by 30% to 50% (Clinical Pharmacology Database, 2004). PT and INR should be monitored to evaluate effectiveness and safety. INR was developed to correct problems with standardization of anticoagulation intensity. INR relates the patient's PT to the intensity of actual coagulation. Hemorrhagic complications of warfarin use have decreased with the use of INR as the standard to monitor PT and guide dosing. Baseline PT and INR should be drawn prior to initiation of therapy.

Dosing usually starts at 5 mg per day. Loading doses are not recommended because time is required to gradually deplete existing clotting factors. Bolus dosing initially may result in excessive anticoagulation after clotting factors are depleted. PT and INR are monitored daily until a therapeutic level is reached. The dosage may need adjustment after 4 to 6 days due to individual sensitivity. After a therapeutic response (INR of 2.0 to 3.0 in most situations) is achieved, PT and INR are usually drawn twice weekly during the first 2 weeks of therapy. They are then drawn on a weekly basis for the remaining first 2 months of therapy and are monitored every 4 to 6 weeks on an ongoing basis for the duration of therapy. Patients with mechanical prosthetic valves need INRs of 2.5 to 3.5. It takes approximately 4 days to return to normal coagulation once the drug is discontinued.

Chronic conditions, such as atrial fibrillation, require lifelong therapy. Warfarin reduces the risk of embolic stroke in patients with atrial fibrillation by 65% to 70% (Clinical Pharmacology Database, 2004). Acute conditions, such as PE and DVT, usually require at least 6 months of therapy. A patient who had an acute MI with a resultant left ventricular thrombus also needs to be on warfarin for at least 6 months.

Patients who have malignant hypertension, coagulopathies, or history of bleeding are not candidates for warfarin therapy. Those who abuse alcohol or engage in activities with a high risk of trauma also are not candidates. Many drugs interact with warfarin to alter clotting time. Patients need to be instructed to inform every physician they see, including their dentists, that they are taking warfarin. They also need to be instructed to avoid the use of over-the-counter medications, unless approved by a physician. Over-the-counter medications containing aspirin, ibuprofen, or naprosyn should always be avoided by those taking warfarin.

Patients taking warfarin should include this information in their personal identification. Consistency in diet is important, especially with foods that are known to be high in vitamin K. Foods with a moderate to high content of vitamin K are listed in Box 3-1. Patient education regarding warfarin use is very important, and patient compliance is critical. Patients who are not reliable with medication administration may not be acceptable candidates for warfarin therapy. Patients should be taught to recognize less-obvious signs and symptoms of bleeding, such as black, tarry stools. They should also be instructed to report any signs of bleeding, including bleeding gums, epistaxis, and increased bruising. Patients should also be instructed about necessary safety precautions to avoid bleeding. These include:

- using an electric shaver
- using a soft-bristle toothbrush
- wearing protective gear while working outside (full shoes and gardening gloves)
- avoiding contact sports.

BOX 3-1: FOODS WITH MODERATE TO HIGH CONTENT OF VITAMIN K		
Brussels sprouts	Lettuce	Avocado
Kale	Cabbage	Green tea
Broccoli	Green onions	Liver
Collard greens	Cauliflower	Soybeans
Mustard greens	Certain peas	Soybean oil
Certain beans	Parsley	Turnip greens
	Spinach	
(Clinical Pharmacology Database, 2004)		

Warfarin should be stored in a cool, dry place away from light. It loses its potency when exposed to high heat. Warfarin does cross the placenta and is a known teratogen that can cause birth defects. Women of childbearing age should be counseled about effective birth control and potential risks to the unborn child if pregnancy should occur.

ANTIPLATELET THERAPY

Glycoprotein IIb/IIIa Inhibitors

The three GP IIb/IIIa inhibitors currently used include:

1. abciximab (ReoPro)

2. eptifibatide (Integrilin)

3. tirofiban (Aggrastat).

All three of these medications interfere with the final pathway of platelet aggregation. They inhibit GP IIb/IIIa receptors, where platelets and fibrinogen bind to form a fibrin mesh. GP IIb/IIIa receptors are abundant on platelet surfaces; there are approximately 50,000 to 80,000 receptors per platelet (Clinical Pharmacology Database, 2004). When platelets are activated, a change occurs in their receptors that increases their affinity to bind to fibrinogen. Fibrinogen links to these receptors and simultaneously binds receptors on two separate platelets. Platelet cross-linking occurs, leading to platelet aggregation. These medications actually occupy the receptors and prevent fibrinogen binding, thereby inhibiting platelet aggregation.

GP IIb/IIIa inhibitors are administered IV and may be administered concomitantly with aspirin, clopidogrel, and heparin. UFH is typically used, and doses are reduced when given with GP IIb/IIIa inhibitors. GP IIb/IIIa inhibitors prevent platelet aggregation regardless of the source of platelet stimulation (Braunwald et al., 2002). For example, they are effective in blocking thrombin-induced platelet aggregation.

Abciximab (ReoPro) was the first FDA-approved GP IIb/IIIa inhibitor. It has a short half-life, which is balanced by a very strong affinity for receptors. Abciximab can block more than 80% of GP IIb/IIIa receptors. It also blocks other receptors and can produce an anticoagulation effect. Some of

its receptor occupation can last for up to 10 days. Platelet aggregation gradually returns to normal 24 to 48 hours after the medication is discontinued (Braunwald et al., 2002). Eptifibatide and tirofiban generally exhibit effects consistent with their plasma levels. Their half-lives are approximately 2 to 3 hours, and platelet aggregation returns to normal within 4 to 8 hours of stopping the medication. When given alone, eptifibatide and tirofiban have no effect on PT or aPTT (Braunwald et al., 2002).

GP IIb/IIIa inhibitors increase the risk of bleeding, which typically occurs at the vascular access site. Platelet count and hemoglobin level should be monitored during the use of GP IIb/IIIa inhibitors. However, thrombocytopenia is not a common complication.

GP IIb/IIIa inhibitors are indicated in the treatment of unstable angina and non-STEMI because they reduce the incidence of ischemic complications (Braunwald et al., 2002). Their use with primary coronary interventions has also improved the results and safety of these procedures. They are alsoeffective in reducing the rate of reocclusion of reperfused vessels.

Adenosine Diphosphate Inhibitors

Clopidogrel (Plavix) is a thienopyridine derivative that is approved by the FDA for prevention of atherosclerotic events. It prevents adenosine diphosphate (ADP)–mediated activation of platelets. ADP activates the GP IIb/IIIa receptors. Clopidogrel irreversibly inhibits the binding of ADP to platelet receptors and thereby prevents ADP from activating the GP IIb/IIIa receptors (Gibbons et al., 2002). Clopidogrel causes platelet inhibition for the life of the platelet, which is approximately 10 days. Dose-dependent inhibition of platelet aggregation is seen 2 hours after a single oral dose. With repeated daily doses, maximal inhibition of platelet aggregation (up to 60%) occurs in 3 to 7 days (Clinical Pharmacology Database, 2004). Bleeding time gradually returns to normal approximately 5 days after the drug is discontinued.

Clopidogrel is indicated in the treatment of unstable angina and non-STEMI. It is also routinely prescribed after elective percutaneous coronary interventional procedures. After ACSs and percutaneous coronary interventional procedures, patients stay on clopidogrel for up to 9 months. Some clinical trial data suggest an increased benefit in extending clopidogrel beyond the 2002 American College of Cardiology/American Heart Association guideline recommendations of 1 to 9 months (Clinical Pharmacology Database, 2004). The maintenance dose of clopidogrel is 75 mg per day. Clopidogrel is administered in conjunction with aspirin after discharge.

Clinical Application

Clopidogrel is substantially more expensive than aspirin. Because both medications interfere with platelet function, it is important for patients to understand the added benefit of clopidogrel in order to assure compliance. It is also important prior to discharge to assess for any financial barriers that may limit the patient's ability to comply with treatment. Financial assistance may be available through Partnership for Prescription Assistance (www.pparx.org)

Aspirin

Aspirin was first introduced in medicine in 1899 (Clinical Pharmacology Database, 2004). Since then, it has been widely used for its many therapeutic benefits including its anti-inflammatory, analgesic, antipyretic, and antithrombotic effects. Aspirin 75 mg to 325 mg is prescribed routinely in all patients with acute and chronic ischemic heart disease. Aspirin therapy should be prescribed regardless of symptoms. Aspirin reduces risk in both primary and secondary prevention of cardiovascular disease and reduces adverse cardiovascular events by an average of 33% (Braunwald et al., 2002). In patients with unstable angina, aspirin decreases short-term and long-term risks of fatal and nonfatal MI (Gibbons et al., 2002).

Aspirin works by inhibiting cyclooxygenase and inhibiting the synthesis of thromboxane A_2. Thromboxane A_2 is a potent vasoconstrictor and platelet agonist that is released as a result of vascular injury. Aspirin produces a rapid antiplatelet and vasodilative effect by the immediate inhibition of thromboxane A_2 production. Aspirin also inhibits endothelial production of prostaglandin I_2. Prostaglandin I_2 produces vasodilatation and inhibits platelet aggregation. However, the effects inhibiting thromboxane A_2 dominate over the effects of prostaglandin I_2 inhibition. Aspirin appears to affect platelet function for the life of the platelet and results in prolonged bleeding time. Aspirin may also protect LDL-C from the oxidation process and improve endothelial dysfunction.

Chewing of aspirin can accelerate absorption into the blood during an acute cardiac event. Contraindications to aspirin administration include allergy, history of GI bleeding, and coagulation disorders. Clopidogrel is used in patients who are allergic to aspirin.

Aspirin is specifically indicated after coronary artery bypass graft surgery for multiple reasons. It prevents early saphenous vein graft closure and is also effective in reducing postoperative MI, stroke, renal failure, and bowel infarction. Aspirin also reduces subsequent mortality. To achieve the maximal benefit of postoperative aspirin use, aspirin must be given within 48 hours of surgery. Aspirin is continued indefinitely postoperatively.

Decreased prostaglandin synthesis with aspirin is responsible for the GI side effects. Aspirin also causes direct irritation of the GI tract. Enteric-coated aspirin can help minimize this common side effect.

CONCLUSION

Many of the medications discussed in this chapter are administered indefinitely and, therefore, patients throughout the continuum of health care are actively taking them. Nurses in all settings play an important role in patient education and assessment of therapeutic and adverse effects. Nurses in the cardiovascular setting play a critical role in the accurate administration of potentially dangerous medications, such as IV anticoagulant and antiplatelet therapies. Nurses in the emergency department setting may also play a role in administration of potentially life-saving therapies involving thrombolytic and fibrinolytic agents. The agents that increase myocardial oxygen supply play a major role in the reduction of risk for cardiovascular disease and the mortality associated with it.

EXAM QUESTIONS

CHAPTER 3
Questions 20-25

20. The class of medications most effective in lowering LDL-C is

    a. bile acid sequestrants.

    b. nicotinic acid.

    c. fibrates.

    d. HMG-CoA reductase inhibitors.

21. The two classes of medications most effective in lowering triglycerides are

    a. nicotinic acid and fibrates.

    b. fibrates and bile acid sequestrants.

    c. HMG-CoA reductase inhibitors and bile acid sequestrants.

    d. nicotinic acid and HMG-CoA reductase inhibitors.

22. Patients taking HMG-CoA reductase inhibitors should receive which of the following instructions?

    a. Do not take the medication if you are also taking beta-blockers or angiotensin-converting enzyme (ACE) inhibitors.

    b. Immediately report any muscle weakness to a physician.

    c. Always take the medication with grapefruit juice.

    d. Have a cholesterol level drawn after the second day of therapy so that the dose can be adjusted, if necessary.

23. Patients who receive thrombolytics or fibrinolytics as reperfusion therapy should have the medication administered within what time frame from initial presentation?

    a. 90 minutes

    b. 60 minutes

    c. 30 minutes

    d. 15 minutes

24. Advantages to the use of LMWH include

    a. ability for the patient to self-administer subcutaneously at home if needed.

    b. use of bedside activated clotting time monitoring to measure drug effectiveness.

    c. ability to take the oral form after initial IV loading.

    d. shorter half-life than UFH so it can be continued until right before surgery or another invasive procedure.

25. Patients with cardiovascular disease may be treated with various types of antiplatelet therapy, including

    a. streptokinase, GP IIb/IIIa inhibitors, and aspirin.

    b. aspirin, GP IIb/IIIa inhibitors, and clopidogrel.

    c. warfarin, clopidogrel, and aspirin.

    d. LMWH, UFH, and hirudin.

CHAPTER 4

RISK FACTORS FOR AND PREVENTION OF CORONARY HEART DISEASE

CHAPTER OBJECTIVE

After completing this chapter, the reader will be able to discuss the impact of risk factors on the development of coronary heart disease.

LEARNING OBJECTIVES

After studying this chapter, the reader will be able to

1. describe the difference between primary and secondary prevention.

2. define a risk equivalent for coronary artery disease.

3. list the nonmodifiable risk factors for coronary artery disease.

4. list the modifiable risk factors for coronary artery disease.

5. define the five A's all health care practitioners can use in providing smoking-cessation counseling.

6. define blood pressure goals for healthy people and people with hypertension and diabetes or renal disease as established by the Joint National Committee on Prevention, Detection, Evaluation, and Treatment of High Blood Pressure.

7. describe the two lifestyle modifications most effective in lowering blood pressure.

8. describe the steps of lifestyle modification used in the reduction of cholesterol for primary prevention.

9. define the current low-density lipoprotein treatment goals for those with a coronary heart disease risk equivalent.

10. describe the difference between type II diabetes and metabolic syndrome.

11. describe differences between women and men in heart disease risk and presentation.

INTRODUCTION

A *risk factor* is a characteristic found in a healthy person that is independently related to the future development of a disease, such as coronary heart disease (CHD). A risk factor can be a lifestyle habit, an environmental factor, or an inherited characteristic. Risk factors are classified as modifiable (can be changed) or nonmodifiable (cannot be changed).

Knowledge of risk factors can sometimes aid disease prevention. Prevention has historically been differentiated as *primary* or *secondary*. For CHD, primary prevention is defined as reducing risk in people without known CHD to prevent the development of the disease in the future. Secondary prevention is defined as reducing risk in people with known CHD to prevent a future cardiac event. However, with the increased understanding of the development and progression of coronary atherosclerosis, the lines between primary and secondary prevention are merging. Atherosclerosis, the underlying cause of most heart attacks, begins early in life, often before the age of 20. There is strong evidence that CHD is largely preventable and, therefore, the topics of risk assessment and reduction are vitally important in cardiovascular nursing.

Those at greatest risk for developing CHD are people with a history of CHD. Those with a *risk equivalent* for CHD have the same risk for having a cardiac event as someone with a history of CHD.

There are three CHD risk equivalent groups:

1. people with other forms of atherosclerotic vascular disease (peripheral vascular disease, abdominal aortic aneurysm, or symptomatic carotid disease)

2. people with type II diabetes

3. people with two or more CHD risk factors who score at the equivalent risk on the Framingham risk tool (a mathematical health risk appraisal model in which points are assigned to each risk factor in order to calculate the probability of developing CHD in a 2-year period).

NONMODIFIABLE RISK FACTORS

Previous Cardiac Event

History of past CHD is the most powerful risk factor for a future event. People with known CHD, or a CHD risk equivalent, have a 20% risk of having a cardiac event within the next 10 years (Levine, 2002).

Family History

Family history refers to the presence of CHD in a first-degree relative. A first-degree relative is defined as a mother, father, brother, or sister. Development of CHD in people younger than age 55 for men and younger than age 65 for women is considered premature. A history of myocardial infarction (MI) in a first-degree relative doubles the risk for CHD (Newton &

Froelicher, 2005). The risk is greater when the MI occurs at a premature age.

Age

Cardiovascular disease is a disease of the aged. Eighty-five percent of people who die from CHD are older than age 65. The lifetime risk of developing CHD after age 40 is almost 50% for men and approximately 30% for women (Levine, 2002). Women generally lag behind men in the initial presentation of heart disease by about 10 years (Newton & Froelicher, 2005).

Gender

Men are generally considered to be at a higher risk for CHD than women until women reach menopause. After this time, the risk begins to equalize. In general, men between ages 35 and 65 have a higher risk of CHD than women. For this reason, historically, many women have not believed that they are vulnerable to heart disease.

In addition, women commonly present with different symptoms (more nausea and fatigue) and have less documented disease on cardiac catheterization (angiography) than men. For these reasons, women have historically been misdiagnosed and undertreated. In recent years, however, a major initiative has been underway to educate health care providers and women about the realities of women and heart disease. This educational movement is getting important messages out to women, including these facts:

*   CHD kills more women than all cancers combined.

*   Of every 2.5 women who die, 1 dies of MI, stroke, or other cardiovascular disease. This rate of death from cardiovascular disease compares to 1 in 30 women who die of breast cancer.

*   Women have a higher mortality rate than men after a heart attack.

(Levine, 2002)

Despite the information known today about women and heart disease, misconceptions still exist, leading people to believe heart disease is not a real problem for women.

Clinical Application

Women commonly exhibit what some providers call "atypical" symptoms of CHD, including nausea, fatigue, shortness of breath, and abdominal discomfort. However, these symptoms are not necessarily atypical for women. Any woman with discomfort from the nose to the navel, especially if she has risk factors for CHD, should be carefully evaluated for CHD.

Socioeconomic Status

In developed countries, CHD is concentrated in the lower socioeconomic, less educated portion of society. In less developed countries, CHD is a disease of the middle and upper classes. Coronary disease is virtually nonexistent in traditional tribal villages (Levine, 2002).

MODIFIABLE RISK FACTORS

Tobacco Use

Cigarette smoking is the leading avoidable cause of death in the United States and accounts for one out of every five deaths (Levine, 2002).

Smoking is also the single most important modifiable cardiovascular risk factor. A person who smokes more than 20 cigarettes per day has a two- to four-fold increased risk for CHD (Martin & Froelicher, 2005). The risk associated with smoking increases with the number of cigarettes smoked per day, the duration of smoking in years, and the younger the age at onset of smoking. Smoking low-tar, low-nicotine, or filtered cigarettes does not decrease the risk of CHD. In addition to increasing the risk of CHD, smoking also increases the risk of cancer and lung disease.

Cigarettes are the delivery system for nicotine. Nicotine and carbon monoxide are the two most important chemicals in cigarette smoke. Nicotine is the physically addictive substance in tobacco, and therefore smoking cessation can lead to nicotine withdrawal. Nicotine withdrawal can cause irritability, anxiety, depression, anger, inability to focus, insomnia, and increased appetite (Fiore et al., 2000). These symptoms are commonly observed in smokers who are admitted for acute coronary events.

To provide effective patient counseling, it is important to understand the effects of tobacco, nicotine, and carbon monoxide on cardiovascular health. Box 4-1 outlines these effects.

BOX 4-1: CARDIOVASCULAR EFFECTS OF TOBACCO, NICOTINE, AND CARBON MONOXIDE

- Endothelial dysfunction: Increased arterial wall stiffness with increased coronary vasoconstriction
- Increased catecholamine release: Increased incidence of cardiac arrhythmias
- Enhanced oxidation of low-density lipoprotein cholesterol (LDL-C)
- Lowered high-density lipoprotein cholesterol (HDL-C) level
- Enhanced hypercoagulability and thrombosis formation: Increased C-reactive protein and fibrinogen levels and increased platelet aggregation
- Increased blood viscosity: Increased hematocrit
- Decreased oxygen-carrying capacity of the blood

Net effect: Accelerated development of atherosclerosis and increased risk for acute cardiac events

(Fiore et al., 2000; Martin & Froelicher, 2005)

Smoking Cessation Interventions

Due to extensive public health efforts in the 1980s, smoking prevalence decreased substantially until about 1990 (Fiore et al., 2000). Since that time, no further substantial decrease in smoking has occurred. Approximately one in four adult Americans continues to smoke. In the year 2000, there were approximately 46.5 million adult smokers in the United States (Martin & Froelicher, 2005). Smoking cessation is a safe and cost-effective risk factor intervention for all patients. Smoking cessation counseling has also proven effective in reducing tobacco use (Fiore et al., 2000). Although smoking cessation counseling is effective, safe, and cost effective, it is still highly underutilized. Some studies show that up to one half of smokers have not been advised by their health care providers to quit (Fiore et al., 2000).

Patients who have had an acute cardiac event or are experiencing symptoms from CHD are most receptive to smoking cessation counseling. Smoking cessation advice given by physicians and other health care workers increases the likelihood of cessation. Structured programs can be very beneficial to the success of smoking cessation, which is critical in achieving risk reduction for CHD. Types of structured programs include nurse-led cessation counseling beginning in the hospital and continuing after discharge with follow-up telephone calls. They can also be part of a comprehensive cardiac rehabilitation program. Referral to a formal nurse-led smoking cessation program can improve the effectiveness of smoking cessation counseling by up to 61% (Gibbons et al., 2002).

Cessation of smoking after an initial MI reduces CHD mortality rates by 50% (Martin & Froelicher, 2005). Therefore, cessation counseling is an imperative nursing intervention. A rapid and substantial reduction in coronary risk occurs when smoking cessation is achieved. After 15 years of smoking cessation, the CHD risk for a former smoker approaches that of a nonsmoker (Martin & Froelicher, 2005).

Factors critical to achieving smoking cessation are:

- brief counseling sessions by multiple health care providers during every patient encounter, including relapse prevention counseling
- individual or group counseling strategies
- use of pharmacotherapies, including nicotine replacement therapy and antidepressant therapy. (Gibbons et al., 2002)

Although structured group-cessation programs can be very effective, the majority of smokers prefer to quit on their own or with individual counseling. In addition, the majority of people who have achieved cessation have done so on their own. Most smokers who successfully quit have 3 to 4 unsuccessful attempts before achieving success (Fiore et al., 2000). It is crucial for nurses not to underestimate the importance of individualized education and support in the success of smoking cessation.

Because the rate of relapse in smoking cessation efforts is high, especially early in cessation efforts, relapse prevention is an important aspect of smoking cessation counseling and education. Relapse prevention counseling includes helping patients identify high-risk situations and providing coping skills to deal with those high-risk situations. When patients achieve smoking cessation, health care providers should congratulate them and encourage them during each visit to remain nonsmokers.

The use of nicotine-replacement therapy can double smoking cessation success rates (Fiore et al., 2000). However, nicotine replacement therapies are often underutilized in smoking cessation efforts. Historically, there has been concern about the use of nicotine replacement therapy in any patient with cardiovascular disease. Although nicotine replacement therapy should be used with caution in patients with very recent MI (within 2 weeks), worsening angina, or serious arrhythmias, its effects on the cardiovascular system are no worse than cigarette smoking (Martin & Froelicher, 2005).

Nicotine replacement therapy comes in several forms, including a patch, gum, inhaler, or nasal spray. The patch and gum can be purchased over the counter. Nicotine replacement therapy works by supplying the patient with either a bolus or continuous dose of nicotine. Some patients who are highly addicted to nicotine may require two forms of replacement therapy. Nicotine replacement therapy is not recommended for people who smoke less than 10 cigarettes per day.

The other pharmacotherapy used in smoking cessation is the oral agent bupropion, which has been used for many years in the treatment of depression. Bupropion's exact mechanism of action in achieving smoking cessation is not fully understood. Like nicotine replacement therapy, the use of bupropion can double the rate of cessation success (Fiore et al., 2000). Unlike nicotine replacement therapy, bupropion is initiated while the patient is still smoking. Therapeutic blood levels are achieved in approximately 1 week. Patients are usually instructed to pick a quit date during the second week of therapy. Therapy is generally continued for 7 to 12 weeks. If the patient has not stopped smoking by the seventh week, then therapy is discontinued (Martin & Froelicher, 2005).

Issues that negatively affect cessation include depression and weight-management concerns. The average weight gain associated with smoking cessation is 6 to 10 lb (Martin & Froelicher, 2005). Weight gain is caused by the metabolic changes associated with smoking cessation. If depression is associated with smoking cessation, then weight gain can increase. Weight gain is particularly a concern among female smokers. Premenstrual stress can also play a role in the smoking-cessation efforts of women. Planning a smoking cessation date to avoid the peak of premenstrual stress is an important consideration.

Clinical Application
Listed here are practical guidelines for smoking cessation counseling in any setting:

1. *Ask the patient if he or she uses tobacco.*
2. *Assess the patient's interest in quitting.*
3. *Inform the patient about the importance of quitting.*
4. *Assist the patient by helping him or her pick a quit date. Also assist by linking the patient to resources that can provide counseling and pharmacotherapy.*
5. *Arrange a follow-up phone call with the patient.*

(Fiore et al., 2000)

Internet resources available for patients include:

- American Heart Association: www.americanheart.org
- American Cancer Society: www.cancer.org
- American Lung Association: www.lungusa.org
- Agency for Healthcare Research and Quality: www.ahcpr.gov

Hypertension

Hypertension is another major risk factor for CHD, including MI and sudden cardiac death. Those with hypertension have double the risk of developing CHD than those who have normal blood pressure (Cunningham, 2005). Hypertension can cause direct vascular injury and also increases myocardial oxygen demand. Hypertension increases the work of the left ventricle, causing hypertrophy and increased left ventricular wall thickness. Increased wall thickness puts patients at risk for subendocardial ischemia and diastolic dysfunction. Left ventricular hypertrophy can lead to left ventricular dilatation and, eventually, systolic dysfunction and heart failure. Hypertension is also an important risk factor for stroke.

Researchers estimate that nearly 29% of all adults have hypertension. At least 58 million people in the United States alone and approximately 1 billion people worldwide have hypertension (Cunningham, 2005). Among those who have hypertension, these are the sobering statistics:

- Only 69% of those with hypertension are aware of the problem.

- Only 58% are treated with medication.

- Of those being treated, only 53% have blood pressures less than 140 / 90 mm Hg.

(Cunningham, 2005)

The incidence of hypertension rises with age. Seventy-five percent of people over age 75 have hypertension (Levine, 2002). Hypertension is more prevalent in males of all ages, and it is more common and severe in African-Americans. The prevalence of hypertension is also higher in American-Indians (Levine, 2002). Women who take oral contraceptives have a higher prevalence of hypertension than women of childbearing age who do not take oral contraceptives.

For people younger than age 50, diastolic blood pressure is very important. There is a greater than 25% increase in risk for every 7 mm Hg increase in diastolic blood pressure (U.S. Department of Health and Human Services [DHHS], 2003). As a person ages, however, systolic blood pressure becomes a more important indicator of cardiovascular risk. In people older than age 50, a systolic blood pressure greater than 140 mm Hg is a more important indicator of cardiovascular risk than is diastolic hypertension (DHHS, 2003). Although systolic blood pressure continues to rise with age, diastolic blood pressure begins to decline at age 60. Systolic hypertension is more difficult to control than diastolic hypertension.

Isolated systolic hypertension is defined as a systolic blood pressure greater than 160 mm Hg with a normal diastolic blood pressure. Isolated systolic hypertension increases the risk of nonfatal MI and cardiovascular death in low-risk patients and the general population. Isolated systolic hyperten-

sion accounts for 70% of cases of hypertension in the elderly (DHHS, 2003).

In adults, 90% to 95% of hypertension is known as *primary,* or *essential,* hypertension. Essential hypertension is characterized by the existence of hypertension with no known cause. *Secondary hypertension* refers to hypertension with an identifiable cause that can be corrected. The vast majority of hypertension in children is secondary. The exact pathophysiology involved in essential hypertension is not fully understood. Possible contributing factors in essential hypertension include:

- excessive salt and water retention from impaired ability of the kidneys to excrete sodium and water

- dysfunction of the autonomic nervous system with increased sympathetic nervous system stimulation and higher levels of circulating norepinephrine, resulting in increased vasoconstriction

- impaired endothelial dysfunction with decreased production of nitric oxide, causing local vasodilatation

- dysfunction of the renin-angiotensin-aldosterone system (RAAS).

Coexisting risk factors are also associated with essential hypertension including hyperlipidemia, diabetes, and obesity. Although the majority of hypertension in adults is essential, health care providers should always assess for identifiable causes of secondary hypertension. The most common causes of secondary hypertension in adults include:

- chronic renal disease

- renovascular disease

- primary aldosteronism

- oral contraceptive use.

Other possible causes of secondary hypertension include a variety of renal, endocrine, neurologic, and cardiac disorders. For example, coarctation of the aorta is a cardiac cause of secondary hypertension.

Genetic disorders, pregnancy, and exposure to exogenous materials can also cause secondary hypertension. Sleep apnea is increasingly being studied for its role as a cause of secondary hypertension.

Certain clinical findings provide clues to the cause of secondary hypertension:

- Abdominal or renal bruits are associated with renovascular disease.

- Unexplained hypokalemia can be associated with primary aldosteronism. (Aldosterone promotes retention of sodium and water and excretion of potassium.)

- Lower blood pressure in the legs than in the arms is associated with aortic coarctation.

Treatment of Hypertension

The Joint National Committee on Prevention, Detection, Evaluation, and Treatment of High Blood Pressure is a coalition of leaders from 46 health care agencies that establishes guidelines for treating hypertension. The most recent guidelines, released in May 2003, contain seven key points:

1. A systolic blood pressure greater than 140 mm Hg in people over age 50 is a more important cardiovascular risk factor than a high diastolic blood pressure.

2. People with normal blood pressure at age 55 have a 90% lifetime risk of developing hypertension.

3. Blood pressure is considered normal only if it is less than 120 mm Hg systolic and less than 80 mm Hg diastolic. People who are considered prehypertensive (systolic pressure between 120 and 139 mm Hg and diastolic pressure between 80 and 89 mm Hg) require lifestyle modification to prevent cardiovascular disease. There are now two stages of hypertension rather than three:

   Stage 1: Systolic 140 to159 mm Hg or diastolic 90 to 99 mm Hg

   Stage 2: Systolic 160 mm Hg or greater or diastolic of 100 mm Hg or greater.

4. Thiazide diuretics are the first-line treatment in uncomplicated hypertension. Other agents may be used as first-line treatment in patients with preexisting conditions, such as diabetes or coronary artery disease.

5. Two or more medications are usually required to effectively treat hypertension in the majority of patients.

6. When initial blood pressure assessment is more than 20 mm Hg systolic or greater than 10 mm Hg diastolic above the blood pressure goal, then initiation of therapy with two medications should be considered. One of the two medications should be a thiazide diuretic.

7. Patient motivation is critical in the effective treatment of hypertension. Empathy is a powerful motivator, and motivation improves when patients have a positive relationship with their health care providers.

(DHHS, 2003)

Effective antihypertensive therapy reduces CHD risk but it does not reduce the risk back to baseline. Goals of hypertension management include the prevention of target organ damage:

- Heart: Hypertension is associated with the development of left ventricular hypertrophy, coronary artery disease, MI, and heart failure.

- Brain: Hypertension increases the risk of transient ischemic attacks and ischemic or hemorrhagic stroke. Malignant hypertension can also cause cerebral encephalopathy when blood pressure is so high that the brain can no longer maintain autoregulation.

- Kidneys: Hypertension causes nephropathy through the production of atherosclerotic renal lesions. Chronic renal disease causes hypertension, and hypertension accelerates the progression of chronic renal disease to end-stage disease.

- Peripheral arteries: Hypertension produces vascular damage that impairs endothelial vasodilatation and accelerates atherosclerosis in the peripheral arteries as well as in the coronary and cerebral arteries.

• Eyes: Vessel damage to the retina caused by hypertension is called *hypertensive retinopathy*.

Four lifestyle interventions have been shown in clinical trials to delay or prevent the onset of hypertension:

1. weight reduction
2. increased physical activity
3. sodium reduction
4. the DASH diet.
(DHHS, 2003)

Weight reduction is the most effective lifestyle modification. Weight reduction can reduce blood pressure by 5 to 20 mm Hg per 5 lb of weight loss (Levine, 2002). For effective blood pressure management, patients should in engage in physical activity almost every day for 30 to 45 minutes.

Some individuals are salt sensitive and others are not; therefore, sodium reduction impacts blood pressure for some patients and not others. All patients with high blood pressure should evaluate the effects of a sodium-restricted diet.

Clinical Application
It is important for patients with hypertension to understand that 75% of sodium intake comes from processed food, not from added salt.

After weight loss, the DASH diet is the second most effective lifestyle intervention. DASH stands for Dietary Approaches to Stop Hypertension. The DASH diet manipulates potassium, calcium, and magnesium, while holding sodium constant. Low calcium consumption is associated with hypertension and high potassium consumption is associated with lower blood pressure in people with hypertension.

The DASH diet is high in fruits, vegetables, and low-fat dairy products. It is low in both saturated fat and total fat and rich in potassium and calcium. This diet has been found to reduce both systolic and diastolic blood pressure. The DASH diet can reduce

blood pressure by 8 to 14 mm Hg (DHHS, 2003). Unlike weight reduction, smoking cessation has not been shown to decrease blood pressure.

Pharmacological treatment of blood pressure has been shown to protect against stroke, coronary events, heart failure, and progression of renal disease and to reduce all-cause mortality. Thiazides are the first-line treatment option, unless another class of medication is indicated based on a coexisting medical condition. Thiazide diuretics are cost effective and have a low risk of side effects.

If a patient's blood pressure is greater than 20 mm Hg above systolic goal or 10 mm Hg above diastolic goal, then therapy can be started with two medications, one of which is typically a thiazide diuretic. Stage two hypertension treatment is started with two initial medications. All patients with hypertension should have their blood pressure aggressively controlled to less than 140/90 mm Hg. Patients with diabetes or coexisting renal disease have lower blood pressure targets.

Special Considerations for the Elderly

Target blood pressure goals are the same for the elderly as for younger adults. The elderly can show substantial benefits when hypertension is adequately treated. Systolic pressure, rather than diastolic, is a better predictor of events among this group of patients. Pseudohypertension may occur in the elderly due to excessive vascular stiffness. Thiazide diuretics are also the preferred first-line treatment in the elderly. Long-acting dihydropyridine calcium channel blockers can also be used.

Clinical Application
Assessment for orthostatic hypotension is particularly important in elderly patients being treated for hypertension. Their risk of orthostatic hypotension is greater because the percentage of water as body weight declines with age.

Special Considerations for African-Americans

African-Americans have the highest prevalence and severity of hypertension (Levine, 2002). Hypertension also develops earlier in life among this population. African-Americans produce less renin and are therefore not as receptive to beta-blockers or medications that block the RAAS (DHHS, 2003).

Special Considerations for patients with diabetes

An angiotensin-converting enzyme (ACE) inhibitor or angiotensin II receptor blocker is usually the first-line agent in diabetic patients. Medications that interrupt the RAAS reduce microvascular and macrovascular complications in both type I and type II diabetes. ACE inhibitors reduce end-organ damage in diabetic patients, even without the presence of hypertension. The blood pressure goal for effective management of hypertension in diabetic patients is below 130/80 mm Hg. Diabetic patients commonly require two or more medications to keep blood pressure within this limit (DHHS, 2003).

Special Considerations for Patients with Renal Disease

Three or more medications are generally needed to keep blood pressure below 130/80 mm Hg and reduce the decline of renal function (DHHS, 2003). Medications that interrupt the RAAS are effective in decreasing renal disease in patients with diabetic and nondiabetic renal disease. Most patients with renal disease also need to be on a loop diuretic.

Resistant Hypertension

A patient is considered to have resistant hypertension if he or she is on full-dose therapy, including a diuretic. Patients with resistant hypertension should be referred to a hypertension specialist if the cause of resistance cannot be determined or corrected. Reasons for resistant hypertension are listed in Box 4-2.

BOX 4-2: CAUSES OF RESISTANT HYPERTENSION

- Volume overload
- Nonsteroidal anti-inflammatory drugs
- Cocaine or amphetamines
- Decongestants
- Oral contraceptives
- Adrenal steroids
- Erythropoietin
- Cyclosporin and tacrolimus
- Licorice (contained in chewing tobacco)
- Over-the-counter dietary supplements
- Excessive alcohol intake

(DHHS, 2003)

Patient Education and Long-term Management Issues

Patient compliance is an important part of therapy. The costs and side effects of medication should be carefully considered and discussed with the patient. Self-monitoring of blood pressure by patients has been shown to improve compliance because patients receive timely feedback from their therapy.

Patients need to be instructed to avoid over-the-counter medications, such as decongestants. They also need to receive information regarding the risk of untreated hypertension. Aggressive risk-factor modification is also indicated in any patient with coexisting risk factors. Patients should have monthly follow-up blood pressure checks with medication adjustments until target results are achieved. More frequent follow-up is indicated for patients with stage 2 hypertension and for those with cardiovascular disease, renal disease, or diabetes.

After blood pressure goals are achieved, follow-up should continue at 3- to 6-month intervals. Serum potassium and creatinine levels should be evaluated twice annually to assess renal function. Dose reduction of medications should be attempted after 1 year of controlled therapy.

Dyslipidemia

Approximately 50% of the adult population and 10% of teenage children have abnormal lipid profiles (Levine, 2002). Elevated levels of cholesterol impact the function of the endothelium, resulting in impaired vasodilatation, increased platelet aggregation and monocyte adhesion, and increased thrombus formation.

Lipid levels may be affected by preexisting conditions, such as renal disease, hypothyroidism, and genetic lipoprotein disorders. LDL-C, HDL-C, and triglycerides are all independent risk factors for cardiovascular disease. Hyperlipidemia includes elevated total cholesterol (hypercholesterolemia), elevated LDL-C, or elevated triglyceride levels. Dyslipidemia refers to hyperlipidemia or a low HDL-C level.

Hypercholesterolemia

Twenty percent of adults, or approximately 37 million Americans, have cholesterol levels greater than 240 mg/dl, and 50% percent of adults, or 105 million Americans, have cholesterol levels greater than 200 mg/dl (Levine, 2002). There is a 20% to 30% increase in CHD risk for each 10% percent increase in serum cholesterol. There is also a corresponding 2% to 3% risk reduction for each 1% reduction in total cholesterol (Gibbons et al., 2002).

Elevated LDL-C

LDL-C levels should be less than 100 mg/dl for those with known CHD or a risk equivalent, according to the current published guidelines of the third Adult Treatment Panel (ATP-III) from the National Cholesterol Education Program (DHHS, 2001). Since the publication of these guidelines, however, new research has been published showing improved risk reduction when LDL-C goals of less than 70 mg/dl were met (Grundy et al., 2004). The most recent report of the National Cholesterol Education Program (Grundy et al., 2004) defines an LDL-C goal of less than 100 mg/dl as the minimal treatment goal for those with coronary artery disease. Setting an LDL-C goal of less than 70 mg/dl is a therapeutic option for high-risk patients. For primary prevention in healthy people, a LDL-C less than 130 mg/dl is considered optimal. Many experts believe the normal value should be lowered to less than 130 mg/dl for all people.

The size of LDL-C particles is also important. Smaller, denser particles are associated with a higher incidence and accelerated progression of coronary artery disease (Fair & Berra, 2005). Smaller particles might also be better able to enter the subendothelial space and be more prone to oxidation.

Hypertriglyceridemia

Borderline-high or high triglyceride levels are now considered independent risk factors for CHD. Borderline-high to high levels are 150 to 500 mg/dl. Alcohol and estrogen use can contribute to hypertriglyceridemia.

Low HDL-C

HDL-C facilitates the transport of excess cholesterol back to the liver. This role helps explain the protection HDL-C provides against the development of heart disease. The lower the concentration of HDL-C, the higher the risk of CHD:

- HDL-C < 40 mg/dl = low HDL-C
- HDL-C > 60 mg/dl = high HDL-C

High levels of HDL-C are associated with a decreased risk of CHD. A 2% to 3% reduction in risk is associated with a 1 mg/dl increase in HDL-C (Newton & Froelicher, 2005). In general, women typically have higher HDL-C levels than do men. Estrogen tends to raise HDL-C levels and might explain why premenopausal women are usually protected from heart disease.

Treatment of Hyperlipidemia

The ATP-III guidelines of 2001 were the first updated management guidelines since 1993. With these new guidelines, the number of people eligible for cholesterol-lowering medications tripled. These guidelines recommend a screening with a fasting lipid profile once every 5 years beginning at age 20. Table 4-1 defines cholesterol values according to the ATP-III guidelines.

LDL-C Treatment Goals

In the Lipid Treatment Assessment Project, only 38% of participants were at target goals after treatment, and only 18% of patients with CHD were at LDL treatment goals (DHHS, 2001). For healthy people with high total cholesterol and high LDL-C, the following therapeutic lifestyle changes within the ATP-III guidelines are recommended:

• Reduce intake of saturated fats: less than 7% calories from saturated fat and less than 200 mg/day of cholesterol.

• Allow monounsaturated fats to be up to 20% of calories. Choose fats and oils with less than 2 g of saturated fat per tablespoon. Use canola oil or olive oil. Avoid tropical oils and hydrogenated vegetable oils.

• Increase soluble fiber to 20 to 30 g per day by eating oats, legumes, grains, vegetables, and fruits.

• Follow a healthy eating plan. Obtain carbohydrates primarily from whole grains, fruits, and vegetables. Include five servings of fruits and vegetables daily with six servings of whole grains. Low-fat dairy products should be included and proteins should come from fish, legumes, skinless poultry, and lean meats. Foods high in calories and low in nutrition should be limited. These include candy and soft drinks containing high amounts of sugar. Limit sodium intake and alcohol intake to a moderate amount. These guidelines do not need to be applied to every meal but rather to an overall eating pattern over several days.

• Achieve a caloric balance between intake and expenditure, and increase physical activity to achieve weight loss if needed. To balance the number of calories consumed with the number expended each day, multiply the patient's weight by 15 calories. This is the typical number of calories used per day by a person who is moderately active. People who are less active require fewer calories.

• Increase physical activity and exercise.

• Use 2 grams of plant sterols or stanols per day. Sterols are a group of compounds found in the cell membranes of plants and animals. Cholesterol is a sterol found in animal cells. Plant

TABLE 4-1: CHOLESTEROL VALUES

Total Cholesterol	LDL-C	HDL-C	Triglycerides
< 200 desirable	< 100 optimal and minimal goal for those with CHD *new research*	< 40 low	< 150 normal
	< 70 optimal		
200-239 borderline	100-129 above optimal	≥ 60 desirable	150-499 borderline-high to high
≥ 240 high	130-159 borderline-high		≥ 500 very high
	160-189 high		
	≥ 190 very high		

(DHHS, 2001; Grundy et al., 2004)

sterols however, are poorly absorbed and not synthesized by the human body and can be used to help lower cholesterol levels. Some sterols are saturated to form a stanol derivative. Spreads fortified with plant sterols or stanols are available commercially. Soybeans and sesame and sunflower seeds also contain plant sterols. Sterols or stanols are added to the diet after 6 weeks if total cholesterol and LDL-C goals are not met.

• Pharmacological agents are added to the treatment plan if target levels not met at 12 weeks.

• Follow an interdisciplinary approach to lowering lipids involving physicians, dieticians, nurse experts, exercise specialists, and pharmacists.

(DHHS, 2001)

If a person has CHD or a risk equivalent, then secondary prevention guidelines are used. These include obtaining a lipid profile within 24 hours of admission for hospital inpatients and initiating lipid-lowering therapy prior to discharge. Patients should continue lifestyle interventions while on medication therapy. In addition, the American College of Cardiology/American Heart Association (ACC/AHA) guidelines for secondary prevention recommend an increased consumption of omega-3 fatty acids.

Clinical trials have shown that reducing cholesterol reduces the risk of MI, stroke, and death for people with and without a history of CHD. A large meta-analysis evaluating 38 cholesterol-lowering trials demonstrated that for every 10% reduction in total cholesterol, there was a 15% reduction in death related to CHD (DHHS, 2001). Results have been shown to be effective regardless of age, sex, or diabetes status. Newer trials have shown that high-risk groups benefit from statins even when they have normal LDL-C levels and outcomes are improved when LDL-C levels are taken below the currently recommended guidelines (Grundy et al., 2004). For most patients with existing coronary artery disease, treatment is indicated (Gibbons et al., 2002). Diabetics are considered to have the same risk as those with known CHD and therefore should have the same target LDL-C goals as those patients with coronary artery disease. Most diabetic patients are prescribed lipid-lowering drugs to achieve an LDL-C reduction of 30% to 40%, regardless of baseline LDL-C levels (Fonseca et al., 2005). As with all high-risk cardiovascular patients, an LDL-C goal of less than 70 mg/dl is a therapeutic option. The LDL-C goal is a primary treatment goal in secondary prevention. Table 4-2 outlines the effects of cholesterol-lowering medications on LDL-C levels.

Decreasing triglycerides and normalizing insulin sensitivity can reduce small, dense LDL-C particles. Certain lipid-lowering medications also have a favorable impact on LDL-C particle size. These medications include bile acid sequestrants, nicotinic acid, and fibrates (Fair & Berra, 2005).

TABLE 4-2: EFFECTS OF LIPID-LOWERING DRUGS ON LDL-C LEVELS	
Class of Drugs	**% Reduction**
HMG-CoA reductase inhibitors	↓ 18-60%
Bile acid resins	↓ 15-30%
Nicotinic acid	↓ 15-30%
Fibrates	↓ 5-20%
Intestinal absorption inhibitors	↓ 18%
(DHHS, 2001; Fair & Berra, 2005)	

Secondary Treatment Goals

Treatment for triglycerides and HDL-C levels are considered secondary to treatment for LDL-C levels. The exception is when a patient's triglycerides are greater than 500 mg/dl; then triglyceride reduction may be considered before LDL-C reduction. Table 4-3 outlines the effects of cholesterol-lowering medications on triglycerides and HDL-C.

Diabetes Mellitus

The American Diabetes Association has established the criteria for diagnosis of diabetes mellitus as a random glucose of > 200 mg/dl or a fasting glucose of > 126 mg/dl (Newton & Froelicher, 2005). Both types I and II diabetes mellitus increase a person's risk for CHD because of the accelerated atheromatous process associated with diabetes. Approximately 17 million people in the United States have diabetes mellitus (Wallhagen & Nolte, 2005), with an increasing number of cases being diagnosed each year. Type II diabetes, or adult onset diabetes, accounts for 90% to 95% percent of all diabetes and therefore is considered a modifiable risk factor. Diabetes increases the risk of all forms of cardiovascular disease, including stroke and peripheral vascular disease. Diabetes doubles the CHD risk for men and increases it five to seven times for women (Newton & Froelicher, 2005).

Underlying causes of type II diabetes include obesity, physical inactivity, and genetics. The onset of diabetes can be postponed or prevented with aggressive lifestyle modification, including weight loss and increased levels of physical activity. Long-term diabetes control is an important measurement of risk and is assessed using hemoglobin (Hb) A_{1C} level. An Hb A_{1C} level greater than 6% indicates uncontrolled diabetes.

Diabetes is associated with both microvascular and macrovascular complications. Microvascular complications include vision loss, nephropathy, neuropathy, and amputation. Macrovascular complications include CHD and stroke. Tight glycemic control reduces the risk of microvascular complications of diabetes (Gibbons et al., 2002). To reduce the risk of macrovascular complications, diabetic patients need a comprehensive plan for risk reduction in addition to tight glycemic control.

Eighty percent of all diabetes-related deaths result from atherosclerotic disease, with CHD accounting for 75% of those deaths (Gibbons et al., 2002). In addition to being at higher risk for developing cardiovascular disease, diabetic patients who suffer MIs are also at risk for developing higher complications, including heart failure, postinfarction angina, and mortality (Newton & Froelicher, 2005).

Many of the modifiable risk factors for coronary artery disease are also risk factors for the development of type II diabetes, including obesity, physical inactivity, hypertension, HDL-C level less than

TABLE 4-3: EFFECT OF LIPID LOWERING DRUGS ON HDL-C AND TRIGLYCERIDE LEVELS		
Class of Drugs	**HDL-C % Increase**	**Triglyceride % Reduction**
Nicotinic acid	↑ 15-35%	↓ 20-50%
Fibrates	↑ 10-20%	↓ 20-50%
HMG-CoA reductase inhibitors	↑ 5-15%	↓ 7-37%
Bile acid sequestrants	↑ 3-5%	does not decrease, may even increase
Intestinal absorption inhibitors	↑ 1%	↓ 8%
(DHHS, 2001; Fair & Berra, 2005)		

35 mg/dl, and triglyceride levels more than 250 mg/dl. Low HDL-C and high triglyceride levels are the common pattern of dyslipidemia in people with type II diabetes. Weight loss and increased physical activity improve these parameters and also modestly lower LDL-C. The Heart Protection Study showed a 22% reduction in major cardiovascular events in diabetics taking simvastatin (a statin lipid-lowering medication). This study also showed that diabetics over age 40 with total cholesterol levels greater than or equal to 135 mg/dl may benefit from statin therapy regardless of baseline LDL-C (Fonseca et al., 2005; Grundy et al., 2004).

Clinical Application:

Diabetic patients without coronary artery disease may need special instructions regarding their goals for LDL-C and blood pressure. Diabetes is considered a risk equivalent for CHD; therefore, patients with diabetes should have an LDL-C level less than 100 mg/dl (or less than 70 mg/dl based on newest research) and blood pressure less than 130/80 mm Hg.

Obesity

Obesity adversely affects most other risk factors for CHD, including hypertension and type II diabetes mellitus. It also increases myocardial oxygen demand in patients with CHD. Obesity is also independently associated with left ventricular hypertrophy. Abdominal obesity (determined by waist-to-hip ratio) is an independent risk factor for vascular disease in women and older men (Levine, 2002). Body mass index (BMI) is commonly used to define overweight and obesity. Box 4-3 defines a method for estimating BMI and for evaluating the results.

BMI measurement is limited because it does not take into account distribution of body fat. Distribution of fat tissue around the abdomen increases CHD risk more than the distribution of fat tissue around the hip and pelvic area. Waist-to-hip ratio provides information about the distribution of fat tissue. A waist-to-hip

---

BOX 4-3: BODY MASS INDEX

Estimated BMI calculation:

$$\frac{\text{Weight in lbs.}}{\text{Height in inches}^2} \times 703$$

BMI measurements

Healthy = 18.5 to 24.9

Overweight = 25.0 to 29.9

Obese = > 30

BMI goal: < 25

(Centers for Disease Control and Prevention, 2005)

---

ratio less than 0.8 for women and less than 1.0 for men is considered normal.

Waist circumference is another way to evaluate body fat distribution around the abdomen. Waist circumferences greater than 35 inches for women and greater than 40 inches for men are considered criteria for abdominal obesity (Levine, 2002).

BMI less than 25 is considered healthy for all adults, regardless of age. A BMI of 25 relates to approximately 110% of ideal body weight. A healthy diet and an exercise program designed for weight loss are recommended for people with BMIs of 25 to 30. A healthy diet and exercise program should strive for 1 lb per week of weight loss. A negative caloric balance of 400 calories per day produces a weight loss of 1 lb per week. Pharmacological agents may be considered in high-risk patients with BMIs greater than 30. The achievement of weight loss is especially important for people with hyperlipidemia, hypertension, or elevated blood glucose levels. Achievement of weight loss has the following beneficial effects:

- improved lipid levels

- improved insulin resistance

- lowered blood pressure.

Obesity is associated not only with the risk of cardiovascular disease but also with many other comorbidities. Although the benefits of weight loss are clear and significant, weight loss goals are difficult to achieve. Both hereditary and environmental factors play a role in weight management.

Clinical Application
Prevention of obesity needs to be a high priority of health care providers because long-term weight loss is difficult to achieve once obesity occurs.

Metabolic Syndrome

Metabolic syndrome represents a grouping of lipid and nonlipid risk factors of metabolic origin. Metabolic syndrome is present in 20% to 25% of the population (Levine, 2002). This represents approximately 48 million people. Metabolic syndrome is closely linked to the generalized disorder of insulin resistance. Excess body fat and physical inactivity promote the development of insulin resistance. Metabolic syndrome abnormalities include:

- defective glucose uptake by skeletal muscle
- increased release of free fatty acids by adipose tissue
- overproduction of glucose by the liver
- hypersecretion of insulin by beta cells in the pancreas.

A diagnosis of metabolic syndrome is made when three or more of the following indicators are present:

- waist circumference greater than 40 inches for men and greater than 35 inches for women
- triglyceride level greater than 150 mg/dl
- HDL-C level less than 40 mg/dl for men and less than 45 mg/dl for women
- blood pressure greater than 135 mm Hg systolic or greater than 85 mm Hg diastolic
- elevated fasting glucose level greater than 100 to 125 mg/dl.

(Levine, 2002)

Physical Inactivity

Like obesity, physical inactivity is associated with other cardiovascular risk factors. Modest amounts of exercise can result in important health benefits. Higher levels of activity and fitness are associated with decreased risk of CHD (Newton & Froelicher, 2005). People who are overweight but fit have risk similar to those without CHD risk factors. Exercise is recommended for primary and secondary prevention of cardiovascular disease. Benefits of exercise include:

- lowered blood pressure
- decreased platelet aggregation
- increased HDL-C
- improved glucose metabolism
- decreased depression and anxiety.

For primary prevention, healthy people should exercise at a moderate level for 30 minutes per day, on most, if not all, days of the week. Walking, as a component of secondary prevention, has been shown to increase survival, decrease reoccurrence rates, and also slow progression of CHD (Gibbons et al., 2002). In addition, walking improves quality of life and decreases hospitalization. For detailed information about cardiac rehabilitation and activity progression after an acute event see chapter 5.

Stress and Other Psychosocial Risk Factors

The body has a physiologic response to psychological stress. Stress can cause coronary vasoconstriction. A release of catecholamines in response to stress also promotes alterations in thrombosis and coagulation to favor clot formation. The number of MIs in the early morning hours are higher than during other times of the day due to morning increases in levels of circulating catecholamines. Exposure to acute stress or highly stressful life events can also increase the risk of an acute cardiac event (Maden & Froelicher, 2005).

Depression, anxiety, anger, and hostility are other psychosocial risk factors associated with the development of CHD. Hostility is the most powerful of these risk factors (Gibbons et al., 2002). There are two theories used to explain the increased risk of CHD related to psychosocial factors. The first theory is based on the physiological neuroendocrine response to psychosocial stress. The second theory is related to poor health behaviors of people with these psychosocial risk factors (Maden & Froelicher, 2005).

Alcohol

Moderate alcohol intake can produce protective cardiovascular effects by increasing HDL-C, lowering platelets, and enhancing fibrinolysis. Light drinkers have lower blood pressures than both nondrinkers and those who drink in excess. Excessive alcohol intake can lead to hypertension and increase the risk of sudden cardiac death, in addition to other adverse effects associated with high alcohol consumption.

The AHA recommends moderate alcohol consumption for appropriate individuals, including those with no contraindications to moderate alcohol consumption and those with no cultural or religious beliefs against alcohol use. Moderate alcohol consumption is defined as no more than one alcoholic beverage per day for women and no more than two alcoholic beverages per day for men.

EMERGING RISK FACTORS

In recent years, much information has developed on what have been termed "emerging risk factors." Some of these emerging risk factors are discussed here.

Hyperhomocysteinemia

Increased homocysteine levels are independently associated with increased risk of cardiovascular disease. Elevated homocysteine levels are responsible for producing endothelial toxicity, accelerating the oxidation of LDL-C, impairing endothelial-derived relaxation factor, and impairing arterial vasodilatation (Levine, 2002; Newton & Froelicher, 2005). Deficiencies in folate and vitamins B_6 and B_{12} lead to elevated serum levels of homocysteine. Supplementation with folic acid and B vitamins

decreases homocysteine levels. However, there is currently no evidence that lowering homocysteine levels decreases cardiovascular mortality and morbidity. Research to evaluate the relationship between homocysteine, vitamin therapy, and cardiovascular outcomes is ongoing (Newton & Froelicher, 2005).

Hypercoagulability

Increased concentrations of fibrinogen are associated with:

- increased age
- obesity
- smoking
- diabetes
- elevated LDL-C and triglyceride levels.

Fibrinogen concentration is inversely associated with:

- high levels of HDL-C
- high alcohol intake
- increased levels of physical activity and exercise.
(Levine, 2002)

Smoking cessation can also favorably alter fibrinogen levels. People in the top one third of baseline fibrinogen concentrations have almost two times the relative risk of cardiovascular events (Levine, 2002). Although antiplatelet and anticoagulant therapy do not directly alter fibrinogen levels, they are prescribed to reduce the risk of cardiac events in patients with elevated levels.

Lipoprotein a Level

Lipoprotein (a) (Lp[a]) has been shown to be an independent factor in cardiovascular risk (Fair & Berra, 2005). Lp(a) is similar to LDL-C. There is currently a lack of standardization for Lp(a) testing, and more research is needed to fully understand its role. In clinical practice, reduction in LDL-C markedly reduces any adverse hazard associated with Lp(a) (Levine, 2002).

Oxidative Stress

Although much has been written about the harmful effects of oxidative stress, the AHA discourages the use of antioxidant vitamin supplements, such as vitamin E, vitamin C, and selenium, and recommends dietary changes instead to increase antioxidant intake. Increased consumption of fruits and vegetables increases antioxidant levels. Cruciferous vegetables and blueberries are particularly high in antioxidants.

Left Ventricular Hypertrophy

Left ventricular hypertrophy increases with age, obesity, and hypertension and is independently associated with an increased risk of cardiovascular disease, including an increased risk for the development of MI, heart failure, and sudden cardiac death (Gibbons et al., 2002). When associated with a reduction in blood pressure, a decrease in left ventricular mass can reduce a person's risk of cardiovascular disease. Reduction of left ventricular mass can be achieved with effective treatment of hypertension.

Inflammation

Atherosclerosis is a diffuse inflammatory process. Extravascular sources of chronic infection such as the gingivae, bronchi, urinary tract, prostate, and diverticula are thought to be possible culprits. Infectious agents being evaluated as contributors to vascular inflammation and injury include cytomegalovirus, *Chlamydia pneumoniae*, *Helicobacter pylori*, and herpes simplex virus (Levine, 2002).

The following inflammatory markers are released during the acute phase of a coronary event:

- high-sensitivity C-reactive protein (hs-CRP)

- intercellular adhesion molecule

- interleukin-6 (cytokine)

- tumor necrosis factor (cytokine).

hs-CRP is a marker of cardiovascular risk. Elevated hs-CRP level increases the relative risk for vascular events by three to four times (Levine, 2002). Elevated levels are found in smokers and in healthy men with other cardiovascular risk factors.

Hormone Replacement Therapy

Hormone replacement therapy was once thought to protect women from heart disease after menopause. Early observational studies and smaller clinical trials suggested that hormone replacement therapy would decrease the risk of cardiovascular disease in women taking therapy. However, the landmark Heart and Estrogen/Progestin Replacement Study concluded that hormone replacement therapy should not be initiated in women with heart disease (Stuenkel & Wenger, 1999).

In addition, the Women's Health Initiative clinical trial arm that examined the effects of continuous combined hormone replacement therapy (estrogen-progestin [Prempro]) was stopped in July 2002, when the risks associated with this therapy were shown to outweigh the benefits (Newton & Froelicher, 2005). This large study demonstrated a substantial increase in cardiovascular risk among women taking this form of hormone replacement therapy. The study showed an increased risk of heart disease, stroke, breast cancer, and dementia in women older than age 65. It also showed a relative risk reduction for hip fracture and colorectal cancer (Newton & Froelicher, 2005).

The estrogen alone arm of the Women's Health Initiative was stopped in March 2004. Again, the risks of therapy were felt to exceed the benefits. The study showed a neutral impact on heart disease and breast cancer but an increased risk of stroke and dementia in women over age 65. There was also a decreased risk of hip fracture with this therapy (Newton & Froelicher, 2005). The Women's Health Initiative demonstrated that hormone replacement therapy should not be used for the primary prevention of CHD in women. Evidence-based guidelines for cardiovascular disease prevention in women recommend combined estrogen plus progestin hormone therapy should not be initiated to prevent

CHD in postmenopausal women, and combined estrogen plus progestin hormone therapy should not be continued to prevent CHD in postmenopausal women (Mosca et al., 2004).

CONCLUSION

The burden of cardiovascular disease is great and, thus, the opportunity for prevention is also great. Risk factors associated with CHD are on the increase in the United States. However, the majority of cardiovascular risk factors are considered modifiable and even small changes in risk factors can have significant results. Risk factor reduction, including smoking cessation, reduction of LDL-C, and effective treatment of hypertension, has been proven to reduce the risk of cardiac events. It is also likely that control and reduction of other risk factors, including diabetes mellitus, HDL-C, triglycerides, obesity, depression, and physical inactivity, will also reduce the risk of cardiac events (Gibbons et al., 2002). Cardiovascular nurses must see risk factor modification as a primary goal for all patients, even healthy ones, in all settings. Through education, motivation, support, and referral, nurses can use their knowledge of cardiovascular risk and risk reduction to make an impact on this devastating disease.

EXAM QUESTIONS

CHAPTER 4
Questions 26-35

26. Secondary prevention of CHD is best described as prevention of

    a. obesity in adolescents.

    b. subsequent cardiac events in people who have already had a cardiac event.

    c. disability from secondhand smoke.

    d. hypertension and hyperlipidemia.

27. One group of people considered to have a risk equivalent for CHD are those with

    a. type II diabetes.

    b. family history and prior symptoms.

    c. hypertension.

    d. type A personality and job stress.

28. Examples of nonmodifiable cardiac risk factors include

    a. smoking and hypertension.

    b. hyperlipidemia and type II diabetes.

    c. family history and obesity.

    d. age and socioeconomic status.

29. One true statement concerning women and heart disease is

    a. women have better survival rates than men after a heart attack.

    b. heart disease is the second leading cause of death in women, after cancer.

    c. women commonly present with different symptoms of heart disease than do men.

    d. hormone replacement therapy has been shown to significantly reduce the risk of heart disease in women after menopause.

30. The single most important modifiable cardiovascular risk factor is

    a. smoking.

    b. physical inactivity.

    c. elevated homocysteine level.

    d. low HDL-C.

31. When providing smoking cessation counseling, it is important to

    a. inform the patient of the minimal risk reduction associated with smoking.

    b. instruct all patients with a cardiac history to avoid nicotine replacement therapy.

    c. include information about relapse prevention.

    d. only provide counseling one time to avoid offending the patient.

32. A true statement concerning lifestyle modifications and blood pressure is

    a. smoking cessation is the most effective lifestyle change for lowering blood pressure.

    b. weight loss and the DASH diet are the two most effective lifestyle interventions for lowering blood pressure.

    c. no lifestyle intervention has proven effective in reducing blood pressure.

    d. lowering cholesterol is the most effective lifestyle change for lowering blood pressure.

33. The ATP-III guidelines for lifestyle changes in cholesterol reduction include

    a. consuming less than 1% of all calories from fat.

    b. using herbal supplements before each meal.

    c. eating 20 to 30 g of fiber daily.

    d. avoiding the use of all monounsaturated fats.

34. The LDL-C goal for patients with coronary artery disease is

    a. less than 100 mg/dl according to the ATP-III guidelines, and even lower according to recent research.

    b. less than one half of total cholesterol.

    c. less than 160 mg/dl if HDL-C is normal.

    d. dependent on the patient's triglyceride and total cholesterol levels.

35. Characteristics associated with metabolic syndrome include

    a. smoking, high circulating hormone levels, and hypertension.

    b. type II hypertension and type II diabetes.

    c. elevated catecholamines, severe obesity, and sleep apnea.

    d. high triglycerides, low HDL-C, and abdominal obesity.

CHAPTER 5

CORONARY HEART DISEASE AND ACUTE CORONARY SYNDROMES

CHAPTER OBJECTIVE

After completing this chapter, the reader will be able to verbalize a comprehensive understanding of the scope of coronary heart disease management throughout the continuum of presentation, from stable angina through acute myocardial infarction.

LEARNING OBJECTIVES

After studying this chapter, the reader will be able to

1. define the difference between stable and unstable angina.

2. describe the pathophysiology associated with vulnerable plaque and acute coronary syndromes.

3. explain the goals of medical treatment of coronary heart disease (CHD).

4. describe the importance of aggressive risk factor management in the treatment of CHD.

5. define the criteria for immediate reperfusion therapy in the presence of an acute myocardial infarction.

6. explain the benefits of participation in a formal cardiac rehabilitation program.

INTRODUCTION

Cardiovascular disease is a leading cause of death in the United States for both genders and all ethnic groups. In this country, approximately 1 million cardiovascular deaths occur per year (Deedy, 2002). Coronary heart disease (CHD) is the most common cause of cardiovascular disease. In 2000, more than 16 million Americans suffered from a myocardial infarction (MI) or angina. Someone dies approximately each minute from a coronary event in the United States (Bene & Vaughan, 2005).

CHD is the presence of atherosclerosis or atherosclerotic plaque in the epicardial coronary arteries. As atherosclerotic plaque progresses, the lumen of the coronary artery can become narrowed and blood flow can be impaired. Reduced blood flow can lead to ischemia, a lack of oxygen to the myocardium. Prolonged ischemia can result in injury, and ultimately necrosis of myocardial tissue. The presentation of CHD ranges from stable angina to acute MI. The term *acute coronary syndrome* (ACS) is used to describe the presentation of CHD in the form of unstable angina, non-ST-segment elevation MI (non-STEMI), or ST-segment elevation MI (STEMI).

PATHOPHYSIOLOGY OF CORONARY HEART DISEASE

The development of CHD begins in adolescence and continues throughout life (Deedy, 2002). CHD is considered a chronic condition. Cardiovascular risk factors (discussed in chapter 4) accelerate the process. Atherosclerosis involves the deposit of lipids, calcium, fibrin, and other cellular substances within the lining of the arteries (Aouizerat, 2005). This deposit initiates a progressive inflammatory response in an effort to heal the endothelium. The end result of this inflammatory process is the production of a fibrous atherosclerotic plaque that can partially or totally occlude blood flow.

Atherosclerosis begins early in life and may not produce clinical symptoms for several decades. The first step in the development of atherosclerotic plaque is the accumulation of intimal macrophage foam cells that are rich in lipids. As time progresses, smooth muscle cells become more involved as they accumulate intracellular lipids, and fatty streaks form between the endothelium and the intima of the artery (Aouizerat, 2005; Deedy, 2002). In this early developmental phase, the inflammatory process is activated and immune cells, such as T lymphocytes and mast cells, begin to invade the lesion (Aouizerat, 2005). As progression continues, extracellular lipids are deposited among the layers of smooth muscle cells. These deposits begin to destroy the integrity of intimal smooth muscle cells.

As the lesion matures into one of clinical significance, an extracellular lipid core develops (Deedy, 2002). This core is sometimes called an *atheroma*. Calcium deposits may be contained within the lipid core. At this stage, foam cells also die and contribute their necrotic components to the growth of the lipid core. The lipid core thickens the artery wall, usually at the external edge, but does not greatly narrow the lumen. Eventually, fibrous tissue, mainly collagen, forms a fibrous cap that covers the lipid core (Aouizerat, 2005; Deedy, 2002). This lesion is sometimes referred to as a *fibrous atheroma* due to the accumulation of the fibrous connective tissue within the intima. These lesions cause more noticeable vessel narrowing and are clinically significant because they are prone to ulcerations and sudden rupture. Microscopic ulcerations of the vulnerable plaque initiate plaque rupture in most coronary events. Both mechanical and inflammatory vascular changes impact the vulnerability of plaque (Gardner & Altman, 2005).

The release of enzymes from immune response cells contributes to the vulnerability of rupture by weakening the collagen matrix of the fibrous cap. When a plaque ruptures, the core of the lipid is exposed to circulating blood (Deedy, 2002). This exposure results in platelet adherence, activation, and aggregation and activation of the coagulation pathway, with resultant thrombus formation. After rupture, reparative cells respond, incorporating existing thrombi into the expanding lesion, as new fibrous tissue is formed to repair the lesion (Aouizerat, 2005). The lumen of the vessel is thus further narrowed. At this stage in the atherosclerosis process, the tunica media and tunica adventitia are also affected by the inflammatory response.

Stable plaques have thick fibrous caps that separate the lipid core from the endothelium. Stable plaques are less complicated than vulnerable plaques and tend to have smooth outlines. More vulnerable plaques have thinner caps. The edge of the fibrous cap, called the *shoulder*, is a particularly vulnerable area and is commonly the location of ruptured plaque (Deedy, 2002). Both mechanical features and inflammatory responses impact the vulnerability of a lesion. The role of the inflammatory response in ACSs has been the focus of new emerging risk factors that measure levels and risk of vascular inflammation. Biomarkers for this inflammation include high-sensitivity C-reactive protein, fibrinogen, homocysteine, lipoprotein A, serum amyloid A, and interleukin-6 (Gardner & Altman, 2005).

Rupture of a coronary plaque produces an acute coronary event and increases the short-term risk of cardiac death or nonfatal MI (Braunwald et al., 2002). It is important to know that most vulnerable plaques identified during cardiac catheterization (angiography) are not found in tightly stenotic vessels. Patients can have plaque in the coronary arteries that does not cause lumen stenosis. This plaque can be visualized using intracoronary ultrasound. It is this plaque that is usually most vulnerable and the cause of ACSs. In most patients, MI results from atheromas that produce less than 50% narrowing of the vessel lumen (Gardner & Altman, 2005). Plaques that cause greater than 75% stenosis, and therefore angina, are usually more stable plaques and less likely to rupture. Figure 5-1 compares features of vulnerable and stable plaque.

FIGURE 5-1: VULNERABLE PLAQUE COMPARED TO STABLE PLAQUE

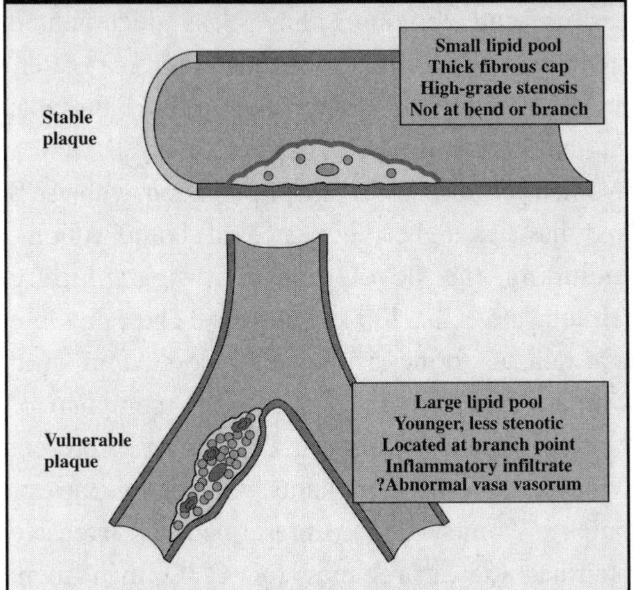

Stable plaque

Small lipid pool
Thick fibrous cap
High-grade stenosis
Not at bend or branch

Vulnerable plaque

Large lipid pool
Younger, less stenotic
Located at branch point
Inflammatory infiltrate
?Abnormal vasa vasorum

Note. From *Atlas of heart ddiseases: Acute myocardial infarction and other acute ischemic syndromes*, by R. Califf. Edited by E. Braunwald (series editor) and R.M. Califf. Copyright 2001, Current Medicine, Inc. Used with permission from Images.MD.

Because vulnerable plaque typically does not produce symptomatic stenotic disease, stress testing has a limited ability to detect vulnerable plaque. Vulnerable plaque may not be visible as a stenotic lesion but may be visualized using intracoronary ultrasound cardiac catheterization.

Clinical Application
When a patient with CHD risk factors has a cardiac catheterization that shows minimal stenotic disease, it is important to understand that this patient may still have a substantial plaque burden and may be at high risk for vulnerable plaque rupture. Aggressive risk factor modification is key in such patients as well as for patients with stenotic disease. Patients with significant risk factors are at the highest risk for progressive atherosclerosis. For this reason, all patients with risk factors should be aggressively treated with risk-reduction strategies regardless of the results of diagnostic tests.

CLINICAL SIGNS AND SYMPTOMS OF CORONARY HEART DISEASE

Angina pectoris is the clinical symptom that results from decreased blood flow to the myocardium. It usually occurs in patients with CHD involving 70% or more stenosis that also involves at least one major epicardial artery (Gibbons et al., 2002). Decreased blood flow results in ischemia, or a temporary lack of oxygen to the heart muscle. Although typically caused by CHD, angina can also be caused by other cardiac conditions, such as coronary artery spasm, valvular heart disease, uncontrolled hypertension, and hypertrophic cardiomyopathy (HCM).

Most patients describe angina as a sensation of pressure, tightness, heaviness, burning, or squeezing. This sensation can be felt behind the sternum and in the upper back, shoulder, arm, jaw, or epigastric area. Angina is rarely described as a sharp or stabbing pain, and it should not worsen with changes in position or respiration. Anginal pain does not usually occur in the middle to lower abdomen and does not usually radiate to the lower extremities. The duration of angina is typically defined in minutes, as opposed to seconds or hours.

Some patients do not experience any of the typical symptoms. Rather they may experience dyspnea, nausea, palpitations, or diaphoresis, alone or in combination. These additional symptoms may also be accompanied by discomfort of the chest, back, shoulder, arm, or jaw. Approximately one half of patients with acute MI have had preceding angina (Gibbons et al., 2002).

When assessing a patient with angina, ask the following questions regarding symptoms:

- What is the quality of discomfort (pressure, squeezing, heaviness)?

- Where is the discomfort located? Does it radiate? If so, where?

- When did the discomfort start, and how long did it last?

- What came before the discomfort?

- What lessens or relieves the discomfort? What makes it worse?

Clinical Application

It is important to use the word "discomfort" when assessing patients with potential angina. Many patients with dyspnea or chest pressure deny the presence of pain.

FEATURES OF ANGINA

Angina pectoris can be classified as stable or unstable.

Stable Angina

Stable angina pectoris typically occurs with physical exertion or emotional stress and is relieved by rest or sublingual nitroglycerin. Angina is considered stable when its pattern is predictable over several weeks. To be considered predictable, angina should be triggered by the same amount of physical or emotional stress and should be easily relieved by rest or sublingual nitroglycerin.

Unstable Angina

Angina is considered unstable when it occurs with minimal exertion or when an increased dose of nitroglycerin is required to achieve relief. Rest angina is also considered unstable angina. Any angina that increases in severity or is very severe on first presentation is considered unstable. Unstable angina is caused by unstable or ruptured plaque that causes abrupt closure of a coronary artery. It is treated very differently than stable angina. This treatment will be discussed later in this chapter, in the section on non-STEMIs.

Angina in Women

The presentation of angina in women is often different than in men. Coronary spasm, mitral valve prolapse, and microvascular disease are more likely to be the cause of symptoms in women. Women presenting with anginal symptoms who proceed to cardiac catheterization have less documented stenotic disease of major epicardial coronary arteries. Women are also more likely to have unstable angina than acute MIs (Braunwald et al., 2002). Women are also older on presentation with ACS and have a higher incidence of complications, including the development of heart failure (Braunwald et al., 2002). Substernal chest pressure that radiates to the arm or jaw is less common in women than in men. Women may complain of more generalized epigastric discomfort or present with less specific complaints, such as dyspnea or fatigue. Women are also prescribed less intensive pharmacological regimes for CHD than men, including less frequent prescription of aspirin (Braunwald et al., 2002).

Many women, and even some health care providers, do not consider heart disease a major health risk for women. For this reason, many women delay presenting with symptoms and may attribute their symptoms to other noncardiac causes. Although heart disease kills more women than all cancers combined, many women still consider breast cancer and other forms of cancer as their primary health risk.

Clinical Application

Women presenting with symptoms of discomfort from their nose to their navel should be evaluated for the presence of CHD. Women should be educated about the risk and specific manifestation of CHD in their gender.

Before menopause, women appear to have a protective mechanism in place against CHD. However, after menopause, the risk of CHD in women begins to approach that of men. However, women lag behind men in their presentation of CHD by about 10 years. The protective effect of the premenopausal state has led to testing and use of hormone replacement therapy as a strategy to reduce the risk of heart disease in women. However, based on the results of the Women's Health Initiative, hormone replacement therapy is no longer a recommended strategy to reduce the risk of heart disease in postmenopausal women (Newton & Froelicher, 2005).

Angina in the Elderly

Among elderly people, angina is commonly described as more generalized symptoms, such as weakness, dyspnea, and confusion. These symptoms are often attributed to the aging process, and the possibility of angina is overlooked.

The elderly also face special challenges in the medical management of angina. In many cases, these patients have multiple factors that impact the effects of cardiovascular drugs. In addition, many medications need to be started at lower doses. The elderly are particularly sensitive to drugs with a hypotensive response. This population is also more likely to have coexisting conditions that complicate treatment.

Angina in Diabetics

Autonomic dysfunction occurs in about one third of patients with diabetes and can affect the symptoms they experience with angina and ACSs.

Diabetic patients may be less likely to experience pain. Up to 25% of all patients presenting with ACSs are diabetic (Braunwald et al., 2002). Diabetic patients have more severe multivessel disease and also have higher rates of complications after acute cardiac events.

DIAGNOSIS OF CORONARY HEART DISEASE

Initial diagnosis of coronary heart disease involves a thorough history and physical examination, including a 12-lead electrocardiogram (ECG). Lab studies, cardiac imaging studies, stress testing, and cardiac catheterization may be used as additional diagnostic tools. Assessment information also includes the presence of cardiovascular risk factors, history of CHD, cerebrovascular disease, or peripheral vascular disease. A history of CHD, cerebrovascular disease, or peripheral vascular disease increases the likelihood that the presentation of symptoms is related to myocardial ischemia.

The 12-lead ECG can be normal in up to 50% of patients with chronic stable angina (Gibbons et al., 2002); therefore, a normal ECG does not exclude CHD. However, an abnormal ECG or the presence of a cardiac arrhythmia increases the likelihood that CHD is the cause of the symptoms.

In addition to a 12-lead ECG, initial assessment parameters for evaluating a patient for CHD include blood pressure, ankle-brachial-index, and laboratory testing, including hemoglobin level and hematocrit to rule out anemia, a fasting blood sugar level to rule out diabetes, and a fasting lipid profile to assess for hyperlipidemia.

When a patient presents with potential symptoms of angina, other cardiac and noncardiac conditions should be considered. Pulmonary disorders, gastrointestinal disorders, chest wall pain, and sometimes psychiatric conditions can have symptoms similar to those of angina.

Stress Testing

Stress testing, with or without myocardial imaging, is a common tool used in the diagnosis of CHD. Stress testing can be done using exercise or chemicals. Treadmills or bicycles are used for exercise stress tests. Certain patients are not candidates for exercise stress testing without accompanying myocardial imaging because the ECG alone may not provide adequate diagnostic information. These patients include those with left bundle branch block, greater than 1 mm ST-segment depression at rest, paced ventricular rhythm, or Wolff-Parkinson-White syndrome (Gibbons et al., 2002).

When patients exercise, myocardial oxygen demand increases and coronary arteries dilate in response to this increased demand. In a patient with CHD, the coronary arteries are not able to adequately dilate to meet the needs of the increased myocardial oxygen demand, and abnormalities occur on the 12-lead ECG or associated imaging studies.

Three pharmacological agents are used in chemical stress testing: dobutamine, dipyridamole, and adenosine. Dobutamine works differently than the other two agents. During a dobutamine stress test, high-dose dobutamine is used to increase contractility and heart rate, thereby increasing myocardial oxygen demand.

Both dipyridamole and adenosine cause coronary microvascular dilatation similar to the coronary artery vasodilatation that occurs with exercise. Dipyridamole is an indirect coronary vasodilator, whereas adenosine causes direct coronary vasodilatation. These medications commonly cause chest pain because vasodilatation pulls blood away from compromised areas of the myocardium. Another common side effect of these medications is flushing caused by vasodilatation. Adenosine can also cause brief episodes of heart block due to its ability to slow or stop conduction through the atrioventricular (AV) node. A rare but severe side effect of both medications in patients with asthma or other lung disease is bronchospasm. Any patient with severe lung disease or active wheezing prior to stress testing is not a candidate for use of these medications. Aminophylline can be given as an antidote to both medications but is seldom needed with adenosine due to its short half-life. All pharmacological stress testing is done in conjunction with myocardial imaging.

Clinical Application

Patients scheduled for chemical stress testing involving adenosine or dipyridamole should be assessed for the presence of lung disease and wheezing prior to the test. Patients who are currently taking aminophylline-containing medications should not undergo chemical stress testing because aminophylline counteracts the medications being administered for the stress test.

Dobutamine stress testing more closely mimics exercise stress testing in that high-dose dobutamine is used to increase myocardial oxygen demand by increasing heart rate and contractility. In response to this increased myocardial oxygen demand, the coronary arteries dilate. They do not, however, dilate to the extent they do with agents that produce more direct coronary vasodilatation. A potential side effect of dobutamine that is not present with dipyridamole or adenosine is cardiac tachyarrhythmias.

Exercise or chemical stress testing is combined with pretest cardiac imaging, such as cardiac echocardiography or radionuclide imaging; pretest and posttest cardiac images are compared. When echocardiography is used, CHD is suspected when echocardiography images show a new wall motion abnormality after exercise or after the administration of high-dose dobutamine. Echocardiography is not used as the imaging modality with dipyridamole or adenosine stress testing. When radionuclide imaging is used, the peak stress images are compared to the resting images. An area of relative hypoperfusion on the peak stress images is suspicious for CHD.

The imaging portion of a stress test provides information about the extent, severity, and location of ischemia. The exercise portion of a stress test (excluding dipyridamole and adenosine testing) can provide prognostic information (Gibbons et al., 2002). One example of prognostic information obtained from exercise stress testing is the heart rate recovery score. This score is calculated by taking the heart rate at peak exercise and subtracting the heart rate at 1-minute after exercise. A normal score is a heart rate greater than 12 beats per minute; this is associated with a low risk of death. A low score is considered less than 8 beats per minute and is associated with a high risk of death. A score of 8 to 12 is considered an intermediate risk (Gibbons et al., 2002). When patients are able to exercise on a treadmill for 6 to 12 minutes, exercise stress testing is generally performed instead of chemical stress testing. Patients on beta-blockers who are scheduled to undergo exercise stress testing should have these medications held for approximately 48 hours prior to testing. If these medications are not held, an adequate heart rate may be difficult to achieve . Exercise stress testing is less sensitive in women than in men (Gibbons et al., 2002).

There are certain absolute contraindications to stress testing in high-risk patients. High-risk patients include those with:

- acute MI ≤ 2 days old
- acute myocarditis or pericarditis
- acute pulmonary embolism
- acute aortic dissection
- symptomatic heart failure
- severe aortic stenosis
- symptomatic arrhythmias
- high-risk unstable angina.

(Gibbons et al., 2002)

Cardiac Catheterization

Cardiac catheterization, or angiography, is currently the gold standard for determining the presence, location, and extent of obstructive CHD. Cardiac catheterization is an invasive procedure that has a small but serious risk of serious adverse outcomes, including stroke, MI, and even death. For this reason, patients are carefully chosen and must meet certain criteria. The American Heart Association and American College of Cardiology have very specific guidelines stating indications for cardiac catheterization. Patients for whom cardiac catheterization is an indication include:

- patients with disabling angina despite medical treatment
- patients with high-risk criteria for CHD on noninvasive testing
- patients who have survived sudden cardiac death
- patients with angina and clinical signs of CHD
- patients with low ejection fractions and ischemia on noninvasive testing
- patients with inadequate information obtained from noninvasive testing.

(Bene & Vaughan, 2005)

In addition to determining the location and severity of lesions, cardiac catheterization can evaluate intracardiac pressures and left ventricular function. Cardiac catheterization is also done to evaluate patients with possible vasospastic angina who have chest pain at rest. Provocative testing can be done in the cardiac catheterization laboratory using ergonovine maleate. If needed, intracoronary vasodilators can be given to treat the induced spasm.

Patients can receive diagnostic cardiac catheterization and return home the same day if no further treatment is done. Cardiac catheterization is performed by inserting a catheter through the femoral artery and guiding it to the heart. If femoral artery access cannot be used, then radial or brachial access can be used. Care of the insertion site, usually the groin, after the procedure is a major nursing focus. A period of bed rest in an observation unit is indicated after the procedure. The amount of bed rest required prior to discharge depends on the type of closure used for the femoral artery insertion site. If the traditional method of sheath removal is used, the patient typically remains on bed rest for 4 to 8 hours. If a closure device is used, then a much shorter period of bed rest and an earlier discharge are possible. Nursing care after cardiac catheterization involves frequent assessment of the insertion site for external bleeding and hematoma development. Distal pulses are also assessed to assure adequate circulation.

Clinical Application

The development of bleeding or a hematoma at the insertion site is treated by applying firm manual pressure. Patients and families must be instructed to activate the Emergency Medical Services (EMS) and apply firm manual pressure to the site if bleeding occurs after discharge.

CARDIAC ISCHEMIA

Aggravating Conditions

Patients with CHD develop symptoms due to an imbalance between oxygen supply and demand. Certain conditions can upset the balance between myocardial oxygen supply and demand. Conditions that can increase myocardial oxygen demand include hyperthermia, hypertension, tachycardia, and conditions that produce overstimulation of the sympathetic nervous system, such as cocaine use and hyperthyroidism. Certain coexisting cardiac conditions can also increase myocardial oxygen demand and reduce supply, including aortic stenosis and HCM. Noncardiac conditions that decrease the delivery of oxygen to tissues can also exacerbate angina. These include conditions that decrease hemoglobin or oxygen saturation levels, such as anemia and pulmonary disease.

Complications of Chronic Ischemic Heart Disease

The extent of ischemia and its impact on left ventricular function determine the outcome in patients with angina (Gibbons et al., 2002). Complications of ischemia include the development of mitral regurgitation or left ventricular thrombi. These complications are a result of left ventricular dilatation and dysfunction.

TREATMENT OPTIONS FOR STABLE ANGINA

Stable patients who are diagnosed with greater than 70% stenosis during cardiac catheterization have three primary treatment options: medical treatment, primary (percutaneous) coronary intervention (PCI), or coronary artery bypass grafting (CABG). Lifestyle modification and aggressive risk factor reduction is included in all three treatment arms. The goals of treatment in CHD are to reduce symptoms (improve quality of life) and prevent complications (improve quantity of life). Complications include disease progression, MI, and death. The highest priority of treatment is to reduce death. When treatment decisions are made, first preference is given to those treatments proven to reduce the risk death (Gibbons et al., 2002).

Pharmacological Management

Treatment of angina usually begins with medical therapy. Medical management of patients with CHD includes the use of a combination of medications from the following list:

- antiplatelet therapy
- antianginal therapy
- lipid-lowering therapy (discussed in chapter 3).

Antiplatelet Therapy

Antiplatelet therapy is prescribed for all patients. Aspirin is the primary antiplatelet agent used for patients with known CHD or those with symptoms suggestive of CHD. For patients with known CHD, peripheral vascular disease, or stroke, aspirin in doses from 75 to 325 mg has been shown to reduce the risk of MI, stroke, and vascular death by approximately 33% (Gibbons et al., 2002).

Clopidogrel is more effective than aspirin in reducing the risk of MI, stroke, and death in patients with atherosclerotic vascular disease (Deedy, 2002). However, there is a dramatic cost difference between aspirin and clopidogrel that prevents clopidogrel from being more widely used as a primary antiplatelet agent. Administration of clopidogrel with aspirin adds an additional 20% risk reduction in patients with unstable angina or non-STEMI (Deedy, 2002).

Antianginal Agents

Patients with CHD are also prescribed antianginal agents. These agents include beta-blockers, nitrates, and calcium channel blockers. The goals of antianginal therapy are to reduce symptoms and improve activity tolerance, thereby improving quality of life.

Beta-blockers. Beta-blockers are the first line agents in the treatment of stable angina. Beta-blockers are very effective in controlling angina brought on by physical exertion. The initial target heart rate goal is 55 to 60 beats per minute at rest for patients with stable angina (Gibbons et al., 2002). Resting heart rate may need to be lowered if angina cannot be controlled. Patients can experience side effects that limit dosing. Beta-blockers are not used to treat vasospastic angina. Beta-blockers are the one class of antianginal medications that have survival benefit in certain groups of patients, such as those patients who have had a recent MI (Antman et al., 2004).

Nitrates. Nitrates improve exercise tolerance and prolong the time to onset of angina. For nitrates to remain effective, patients need to have an 8- to 10-hour nitrate-free period each day. Headache is the most common side effect of nitrate use.

Headaches usually subside over time in patients taking long-acting nitrates. Patients with a history of angina should always carry sublingual nitroglycerin.

Clinical Application
Headaches associated with nitroglycerin administration should be treated because pain activates the sympathetic nervous system, which increases myocardial oxygen demand and, potentially, myocardial ischemia.

Calcium channel blockers. Calcium channel blockers or long-acting nitrates are used as first-line agents for vasospastic angina because they are direct coronary vasodilators. These medications can also be added to beta-blocker therapy when angina is not controlled. Calcium channel blockers must be used very cautiously in patients with impaired systolic left ventricular dysfunction. Amlodipine and felodipine, newer dihydropyridine calcium channel blockers, are more selective coronary arterial vasodilators and are better tolerated than other calcium channel blockers in patients with left ventricular dysfunction (Gibbons et al., 2002). For a more detailed discussion of pharmacological agents, see chapters 2 and 3.

Nonpharmacological Treatment Options

PCI and CABG are the two nonpharmacological treatment options for patients with CHD. These two forms of cardiac revascularization are discussed, along with transmyocardial revascularization, in the next chapter.

External counterpulsation is another nonpharmacological treatment option for patients with debilitating angina on maximal medical therapy; this option is used for patients who are not candidates for revascularization. During this therapy, a series of cuffs are wrapped around the patient's legs. Compressed air is used to apply pressure in the cuffs in synchronization with the cardiac cycle. The cuff pressure results in an increased arterial pressure that is used to increase retrograde aortic blood flow into the coronary arteries during diastole. Patients receive 35 hours of treatment over a 4- to 7-week period (Gibbons et al., 2002).

Long-Term Management

For patients with stable angina, it is important to evaluate the effectiveness of risk factor reduction with each follow-up. An assessment of the patient's anginal symptoms, functional capacity, and tolerance to medications is also important. The patient should know to report worsening angina or rest angina. Follow-up office visits are usually scheduled for every 4 to 6 months during the first year after initiation of antianginal therapy. Long-term follow up is generally based on the patient's other existing medical conditions but should occur at least annually. Patients with conditions that exacerbate angina require more frequent follow-up. Follow-up visits can be alternated between the primary care physician and cardiologist.

Clinical Application

Patients who alternate follow-up visits between a cardiologist, a primary care physician, and perhaps another specialist need to be instructed on the importance of always carrying a current medication list to alert all involved physicians of any medication changes between office visits.

ACUTE CORONARY SYNDROME OVERVIEW

CHD presents in a continuum, as seen in Figure 5-2. Patients presenting with an ACS are treated differently than patients presenting with stable angina. During an ACS, there is an urgency for treatment to preserve myocardial function. Acute myocardial ischemia develops when oxygen supply is insufficient to meet the metabolic demands of cardiac cells. When cells are deprived of oxygen, ischemia occurs within 10 seconds. Myocardial function is affected after 1 minute of ischemia, and cells begin to swell after just a few minutes. After 20 minutes of oxygen deprivation, irreversible cellular injury begins to occur (Gardner & Altman, 2005).

Clinical Application

All patients should be taught the importance of immediately seeking medical attention for any symptoms that could suggest a heart attack. Patients need to understand the physiological importance of early treatment in preserving myocardial function.

ACSs include unstable angina, non-STEMI, and STEMI. The rupturing of unstable vulnerable plaques is a frequent cause of ACSs. When vulnerable plaques rupture, thrombi form at the site of injury, blocking blood flow and causing ischemia or injury to myocardial cells. Patients with a longer history of ischemic heart disease may have collateral circulation that provides protection during the occlusion of a coronary vessel. Collateral vessels are those that connect major branches of coronary

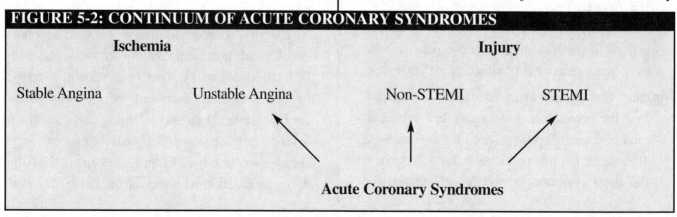

FIGURE 5-2: CONTINUUM OF ACUTE CORONARY SYNDROMES

Ischemia   Injury

Stable Angina   Unstable Angina   Non-STEMI   STEMI

Acute Coronary Syndromes

arteries. As luminal narrowing gradually occurs, pressure changes promote the development and use of these collateral vessels to supply oxygen to ischemic areas. New capillaries can grow in response to ischemia. Younger patients without collateral circulation are more vulnerable to extensive damage from an occluded coronary artery.

When an ACS begins, the endocardial region is the first to become ischemic and is the first area where tissues begin to die. As ischemia continues and the injury extends, the middle myocardium (or subendocardium) is affected. If left untreated and MI continues, the injury can extend toward the epicardium affecting the full thickness of the myocardium. A full-thickness MI is commonly referred to as a *transmural MI*.

Classifications of Myocardial Infarction

MIs are now classified by their initial presentation as either STEMI or non-STEMI. Figure 5-3 compares a normal ST-segment with two examples of ST-segment elevation. Patients presenting with STEMI are candidates for reperfusion therapy.

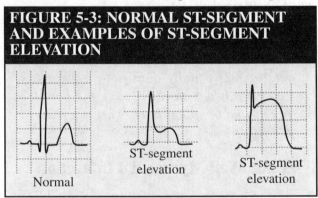

FIGURE 5-3: NORMAL ST-SEGMENT AND EXAMPLES OF ST-SEGMENT ELEVATION

Normal | ST-segment elevation | ST-segment elevation

STEMI and non-STEMI can both produce either a Q-wave or non-Q-wave MI. Non-Q-wave MIs are usually associated with damage that has not extended through the full thickness of the myocardium. A Q-wave MI is diagnosed by the presence of a pathological Q-wave in the leads of infarction on a 12-lead ECG. This type of MI is usually associated with full thickness damage of the myocardium. Q-waves are the first negative deflection of the QRS complex; when they are too large, they represent altered depo-

larization due to necrotic tissue. Figure 5-4 shows an example of a Q-wave that is considered pathological. Q-waves are more common with STEMI.

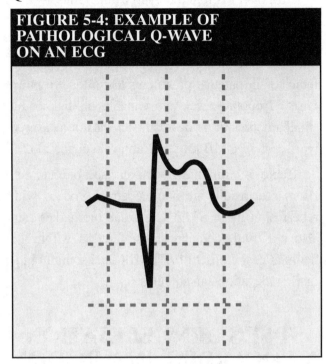

FIGURE 5-4: EXAMPLE OF PATHOLOGICAL Q-WAVE ON AN ECG

A 12-lead ECG is used to differentiate STEMI from non-STEMI. However, a 12-lead ECG cannot distinguish between non-STEMI and unstable angina. Cardiac biomarkers help differentiate between these two conditions.

Cardiac Biomarkers

Cardiac biomarkers are released into the blood when necrosis occurs as a result of membrane rupture of the myocytes. Cardiac biomarkers used in the evaluation of ACSs include myoglobin, creatine kinase (CK), CK-MB, and troponin I and T.

Myoglobin is the biomarker that rises the earliest, within 2 hours after myocardial damage (Braunwald et al., 2002). Although it is a very sensitive biomarker, is it not specific to myocardial damage.

CK is an enzyme present in the heart, brain, and skeletal muscle, so elevations are not specific to myocardial damage. CK-MB is more specific to the heart. Therefore, CK-MB measurements are helpful in identifying more than minor amounts of myocardial damage. CK-MB rapidly rises in the presence of myocardial damage.

Troponin I is found only in cardiac muscle. It is the most sensitive indicator of myocardial damage. Because troponin I remains elevated for a long period, with a gradual return to normal, it is a beneficial indicator in patients presenting late after symptom onset. Troponin levels are capable of diagnosing small amounts of myocardial necrosis not measured by rises in CK-MB levels (Braunwald et al., 2002).

Table 5-1 summarizes the cardiac biomarkers. Biomarker results are not needed to proceed with reperfusion in an STEMI. Cardiac biomarkers are also not used to diagnose reinfarction within 18 hours after the onset of STEMI because initial biomarker elevation can still exist.

ST-SEGMENT ELEVATION MYOCARDIAL INFARCTION

An estimated 500,000 STEMIs occur each year (Antman et al., 2004). Complete occlusion of a vessel by a thrombus produces STEMI. Figure 5-5 shows an occlusive clot responsible for STEMI. Patients with STEMIs are classified more specifically by the portion of the left ventricle suffering injury.

Inferior Wall Myocardial Infarction

On a 12-lead ECG, inferior wall MIs show ST-segment elevation in the inferior leads, leads II, III, and aVF. Figure 5-6 shows a 12-lead ECG representation of an inferior wall MI. The inferior wall of the left ventricle is fed by the right coronary artery (RCA); therefore, an occlusion of the RCA is sus-

pected in patients with inferior wall MI. Inferior wall MIs are sometimes associated with additional involvement of the posterior wall of the left ventricle or the right ventricle. A right-sided ECG using right-sided chest leads should be performed with all patients with inferior wall MIs to assess for involvement of the right ventricle. Patients with right ventricular involvement are treated differently, as discussed later in this chapter. The more proximal the occlusion of the RCA, the greater the amount of myocardium involved in the infarction.

Complications of Inferior Wall MI

Because the RCA also feeds the sinoatrial (SA) and AV nodes in the majority of people, bradycardia and first- and second-degree heart block are common complications of inferior wall MI. Patients with inferior wall MIs have increased parasympathetic activity, which causes nausea and vomiting (Bene & Vaughan, 2005). Patients with inferior-posterior MIs are also at risk for the development of papillary muscle rupture. Papillary muscle rupture results in acute mitral regurgitation and is an emergent situation.

> ### Clinical Application
> *First- and second-degree heart block seen in inferior MI usually does not progress to complete heart block because the bundle of His and bundle branches are not fed by the RCA.*

Anterior Wall Myocardial Infarction

The left anterior descending artery (LAD) supplies blood to the anterior portion of the septum and the anterior wall of the left ventricle. An occlusion of the LAD produces an infarct of the anterior wall

TABLE 5-1: SUMMARY OF CARDIAC BIOMARKERS

Cardiac Biomarker	Specificity Sensitivity	Rise	Peak	Duration
Myoglobin	Sensitive but not specific	Within 2 hours	4 to 10 hours	< 24 hours
CK-MB	Highly specific	4 to 6 hours	18 to 24 hours	2 to 3 days
Troponin I or T	Highly specific and sensitive	4 to 6 hours	18 to 24 hours	10 or more days

FIGURE 5-5: OCCLUSIVE CLOT PRODUCING STEMI

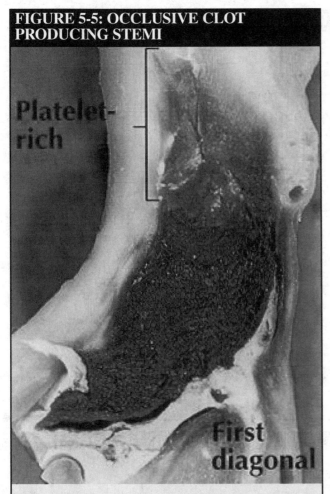

Note. From *Atlas of heart diseases: Acute myocardial infarction and other acute ischemic syndromes* by E. Falk & P. Shah. Edited by E. Braunwald (series editor) and R.M. Califf. Copyright 2001, Current Medicine, Inc. Used with permission from Images.MD.

of the left ventricle, producing ST-segment elevation in leads V_3 and V_4 on a 12-lead ECG. If the lesion is proximal and the septum is involved, ST-segment elevation occurs in leads V_1 through V_4. Figure 5-7 shows a 12-lead ECG representation of an anterior septal MI. Both Figures 5-6 and 5-7 can be compared to the normal ECG in Figure 5-8.

Complications of Anterior Wall MI

Because the bundle branches of the conduction system run through the septum, patients with occlusion of the LAD are at risk for the development of bundle branch blocks and complete heart blocks. Patients with septal infarcts are also at risk for ventricular septal rupture. Patients with anterior wall MIs have a worse prognosis than those with inferior wall MIs (Smith, Zvosec, Sharkey, & Henry, 2002). A large anterior wall MI can result in profound left ventricular dysfunction, leading to heart failure and cardiogenic shock.

Clinical Application

The assessment of a new holosystolic murmur in an unstable patient with an anteroseptal MI can indicate a ventricular septal rupture. This condition is a medical emergency requiring emergency surgery to repair the rupture.

FIGURE 5-6: SUBSTANTIAL ST-SEGMENT ELEVATION OF INFERIOR WALL MI

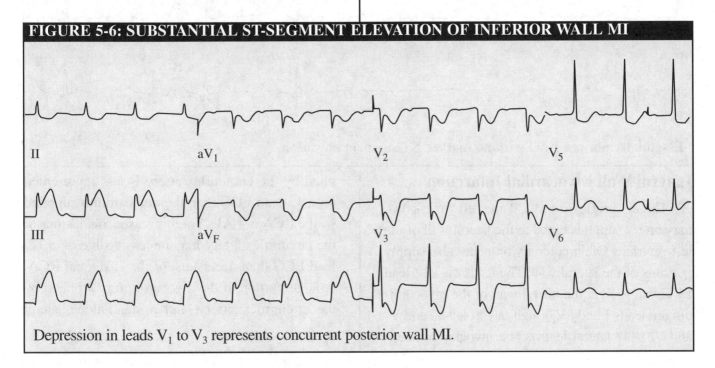

Depression in leads V_1 to V_3 represents concurrent posterior wall MI.

FIGURE 5-7: ST-SEGMENT ELEVATION OF ANTERIOR SEPTAL MI IN LEADS V₁ TO V₄

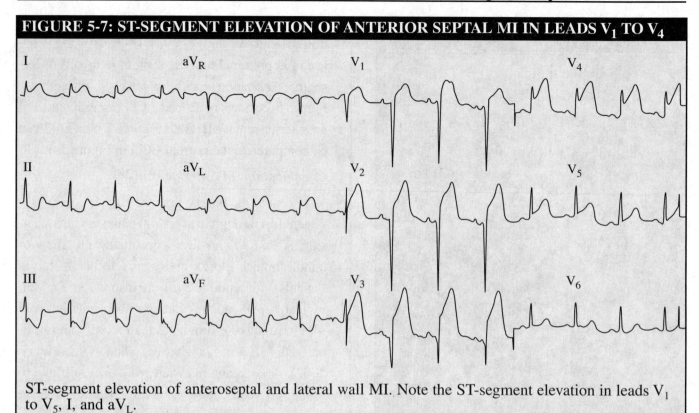

ST-segment elevation of anteroseptal and lateral wall MI. Note the ST-segment elevation in leads V₁ to V₅, I, and aV_L.

FIGURE 5-8: NORMAL ECG

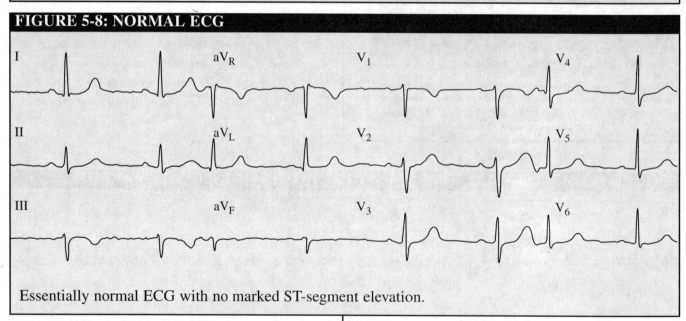

Essentially normal ECG with no marked ST-segment elevation.

Lateral Wall Myocardial Infarction

The circumflex artery off the left main coronary artery supplies blood to the lateral wall of the left ventricle. Other coronary branches also supply portions of the lateral wall. The leads on a 12-lead ECG that look at the lateral wall of the myocardium are leads I and aV_L (high lateral leads) and V₅ and V₆ (low lateral leads). The myocardium sup-

plied by the circumflex artery is less represented on a 12-lead ECG than the myocardium supplied by the RCA or LAD. For this reason, occlusions of the circumflex artery may be less visible on a 12-lead ECG than occlusions of the LAD and RCA. A large portion of the myocardium is supplied by the circumflex artery, and a stand-alone lateral wall MI should be treated as aggressively as other forms of MI.

Complications of Lateral Wall MI

The circumflex artery supplies the AV node, bundle of His, and papillary muscles in about 10% of people. Therefore, conduction abnormalities and papillary muscle dysfunction with resultant mitral regurgitation are potential complications of lateral wall MIs.

Posterior Wall Myocardial Infarction

Posterior wall MIs are caused by obstruction of the posterior descending artery (PDA), usually originating from the RCA. They commonly occur in conjunction with inferior wall MIs. The PDA in some patients can originate from the circumflex artery; in these patients, a posterior MI may occur in conjunction with lateral wall MI. A true isolated posterior MI does not produce ST-segment elevation on a standard 12-lead ECG because no electrodes are placed directly over the posterior wall of the left ventricle. A posterior wall MI may show ST-segment depression in the leads reciprocal to the posterior wall, including leads V_1 to V_3.

Right Ventricular Myocardial Infarction

All of the above types of MIs refer to the location of the infarction of the left ventricle. Infarction of the right ventricle occurs in anywhere from one third to one half of inferior wall MIs (Bene & Vaughan, 2005). The presence of a right ventricular MI is important because mortality is increased when the right ventricle is involved (Bene & Vaughan, 2005). In most people, the marginal branch of the RCA feeds the right ventricle; therefore, an occlusion proximal to this branch infarcts the right ventricle. An ECG with right precordial leads should be done on all patients with inferior MIs to assess for presence of right ventricular infarct. ST-segment elevation can be seen in the right precordial leads if the ECG is performed early during the MI.

Patients with right ventricular infarct with hemodynamic alterations need special treatment. The right ventricle supplies the left ventricle with its preload. When the right ventricle fails, the left side of the heart does not receive adequate preload and, therefore, cardiac output decreases. Patients with right ventricular infarct may show clinical signs of right-sided heart failure, such as increased jugular venous pressure. However, the lungs remain clear because left-sided preload is low. Intravenous (IV) fluids are indicated in the treatment of these patients to help assure adequate preload. Venous vasodilators and diuretics are avoided because they decrease preload. If fluid administration is ineffective in supplying adequate preload to the left side of the heart, inotropic medications, such as dobutamine, may be needed to support the failing right ventricle.

Patients with right ventricular infarctions are at higher risk for development of atrial fibrillation. They also have an increased risk of atrial fibrillation because the right atrium can stretch from volume overload due to right ventricular failure and infarct. The presence of atrial fibrillation can further complicate a right ventricular infarct because the loss of atrial kick further decreases right ventricular preload. Patients who are hemodynamically unstable require emergency cardioversion.

Reperfusion and STEMI

Definition and Options for Reperfusion

Patients with STEMI need to receive reperfusion therapy as quickly as possible. Reperfusion is defined as the restoration of oxygen to ischemic tissue. Two methods of reperfusion are available: administration of fibrinolytics and PCI. If a patient is receiving a fibrinolytic, the drug should be administered within 30 minutes of arrival in the emergency department (ED) or on first contact with the paramedics. If a patient is receiving PCI, balloon inflation should occur within 90 minutes of arrival in the ED or on first contact with the paramedics.

PCI is the preferred method of reperfusion if patients can be promptly treated within the 90-minute time frame by an experienced operator in an experienced cardiac catheterization laboratory. Fibrinolysis is the preferred method of reperfusion when there is a delay to PCI or if PCI is not an option. If any contraindications to fibrinolytic therapy exist, the patient should be transferred directly to a facility capable of performing PCI. PCI is also the preferred option for safety reasons if the onset of symptoms is longer than 3 hours, if there is any question as to the diagnosis of STEMI, and in patients in shock or with severe congestive heart failure (Antman et al., 2004).

Criteria for Reperfusion

In addition to patients with ST-segment elevation on a 12-lead ECG, patients with a new (or presumably new) left bundle branch block and those with evidence of posterior wall MI are also candidates for immediate reperfusion therapy. An initial ECG should be completed within 10 minutes of arrival to the hospital, if not already completed in route by EMS. If the initial ECG is not diagnostic of ST-segment elevation and the patient remains symptomatic, then serial ECGs should be done at 5- to 10-minute intervals until a diagnosis is made or until symptoms resolve (Antman et al., 2004). Imaging studies such as echocardiography can also be done in the ED if the patient's symptoms suggest acute MI but the ECG is not clearly demonstrating ST-segment elevation. An echocardiogram shows wall motion abnormality of the affected wall during an acute MI.

ST-segment elevation may be difficult to determine in the presence of left bundle branch block because a normal degree of ST-segment elevation exists with left bundle branch block. In posterior wall MI, ST-segment elevation does not show on a standard 12-lead ECG, but an echocardiogram may show poor function of the posterior wall, helping to confirm the diagnosis. Reperfusion with PCI is discussed in detail in chapter 6.

Myocardial Mimics

The pain of aortic dissection can mimic the pain of MI. ECG changes associated with pericarditis can also mimic the ECG changes seen in acute MI. It is key in both of these circumstances to differentiate these diagnoses from acute MI because treatment with fibrinolytic therapy could be devastating in either case.

Fibrinolytic Therapy

There are inclusion and exclusion criteria for the administration of fibrinolytics. Criteria necessary to administer fibrinolytics include:

- symptom onset within 12 hours of administration (ideally within 3 hours)

- ST-segment elevation of greater than 1 mm in two leads evaluating the same wall of the myocardium or the presence of a new left bundle branch block

- ECG and other findings consistent with a true isolated posterior wall MI.

Contraindications to the administration of fibrinolytics include:

- prior intracranial hemorrhage

- known structural cerebrovascular lesion

- malignant intracranial neoplasm

- significant closed head injury within last 3 months

- ischemic stroke within last 3 months (unless within last 3 hours)

- suspected aortic dissection

- active bleeding or bleeding diathesis (excluding menses)

- symptoms older than 24 hours

- ST-segment depression (unless indicative of a true posterior wall MI).

(Antman et al., 2004)

Several fibrinolytic agents are available. Some are fibrin selective and, therefore, clot specific, whereas others are nonfibrin selective and, therefore, create more systemic effects. Fibrinolytics are discussed in more detail in chapter 3.

Intracranial hemorrhage is a potential complication of fibrinolytic therapy, and any STEMI patient at substantial risk for intracranial hemorrhage should be treated with PCI rather than fibrinolytic therapy. Any change in neurological status within 24 hours of administration of a fibrinolytic is considered an intracranial hemorrhage until proven otherwise. All fibrinolytic, anticoagulation, and antiplatelet therapy should be immediately discontinued when a change in neurological status occurs until intracranial hemorrhage is ruled out. Signs of successful reperfusion with fibrinolytics include relief of presenting symptoms, reduction of at least 50% of initial ST-segment elevation on repeat ECG, and hemodynamic and electrical stability.

Pharmacological Treatment for Acute STEMI

Aspirin

Initial treatment of all patients presenting with ACSs includes aspirin immediately on arrival, if not already taken at home or given by EMS. Non-enteric-coated aspirin, in the dose range of 162 to 325 mg, should be chewed by the patient. A targeted history and physical should be completed, focusing on the goal of early reperfusion for STEMI patients. Special attention should be paid to contraindications to fibrinolytic therapy and assessment of possible myocardial mimics, such as aortic dissection (pain mimic) and pericarditis (ECG mimic). There is an increasing focus on prehospital care of STEMI patients, including the ability of advanced cardiac life support (ACLS) providers to identify STEMI on a 12-lead ECG and complete a reperfusion checklist prior to arrival in the hospital.

Oxygen

Oxygen is used in patients with an arterial oxygen saturation less than 90%. Oxygen can also be administered to patients with STEMI during the first 6 hours. After the first 6 hours, oxygen is not indicated unless the patient's oxygen saturation is low.

Nitroglycerin

Up to three doses of sublingual nitroglycerin, 0.4 mg, can be given every 5 minutes. If ischemic discomfort continues after sublingual nitroglycerin and beta-blocker administration, an IV nitroglycerin drip can be started at 5 to 10 mcg/min and titrated in increments of 5 to 10 mcg every 5 to 10 minutes. Sublingual nitroglycerin and high-dose intravenous nitroglycerin dilate arteries and veins. In addition to managing ischemic symptoms, IV nitroglycerin can be used in treating patients who are hypertensive or who have signs of pulmonary congestion. Nitroglycerin should not be used in hypotensive patients, patients who are bradycardic or tachycardic, patients who have taken sildenafil (Viagra), or those with right ventricular infarct. If blood pressure is a limiting factor, beta-blockers should be given priority administration over nitrates.

Morphine Sulfate

Morphine sulfate is the pain reliever of choice for ischemic cardiac pain. The initial dose is usually 2 to 4 mg IV. Morphine can be repeated at 5-minute intervals in increments of 2 to 8 mg (Antman et al., 2004). Morphine is a preload reducer and also reduces anxiety and limits activity of the sympathetic nervous system.

Beta-Blockers

Oral beta-blockers should be administered promptly if no contraindications exist. Beta-blockers can be given IV initially, especially if the patient is tachycardic or hypertensive or if pain persists.

ACE Inhibitors

Angiotensin-converting enzyme (ACE) inhibitors are given within the first 24 hours of an acute MI in the following circumstances: anterior wall MI, presence of pulmonary congestion, or left ventricular ejection fraction less than 40% (Antman et al., 2004).

Anticoagulants

Heparin or low-molecular-weight heparin (LMWH) is indicated for 48 hours in STEMI in the following circumstances: large MI or anterior wall MI, presence of atrial fibrillation, previous embolus, known presence of thrombus, or current cardiogenic shock (Antman et al., 2004).

Pathophysiology of Ventricular Remodeling after STEMI

During an MI, cellular edema produces an inflammatory response. This inflammatory response leads to the recruitment of some stem cells and can lead to some tissue regeneration. Catecholamines are also released from myocardial cells during the acute phase of injury, increasing the risk of arrhythmias during this vulnerable time.

Clinical Application
Beta-blockers are particularly important in suppressing cardiac arrhythmias in ischemic tissue because they suppress catecholamine release.

Initially, damaged tissue is bruised and cyanotic. During this period, the cardiac biomarkers are released. By the second to third day, white blood cells invade the necrotic tissue. Scavenger cells release enzymes to break down necrotic tissue. The necrotic wall can become very thin during this phase, and cardiac rupture is most likely to occur at this time (Gardner & Altman, 2005). By the second week, a weak collagen matrix has formed, but the myocardium is still vulnerable to reinjury. By the third week, scar formation has started, and at 6 weeks, the necrotic area is completely replaced with scar tissue (Gardner & Altman, 2005). Although this scar tissue is very strong, it does not contribute to the contractile function of the myocardium.

In addition to postinfarction changes in necrotic tissue, the noninfarcted surrounding areas can also be affected. Surviving myocytes hypertrophy in an attempt to compensate for damaged tissue. Excessive noncontractile collagen is present in the newly hyper-

trophied myocardium, leading to a ventricle that is stiff and noncompliant. A stiff, noncompliant ventricle is unable to fill properly during the cardiac cycle, and cardiac output is impaired.

Hemodynamic Alterations after STEMI

When myocardial function is impaired as a result of MI, stroke volume decreases. To compensate for decreased stroke volume, heart rate increases. If myocardial function is impaired to the point that adequate stroke volume cannot be maintained, diastolic filling pressures increase and pulmonary edema results.

Clinical Application
Tachycardia is a poor prognostic sign in the presence of an acute MI because it is a compensatory mechanism for decreasing stroke volume due to a failing left ventricle.

Hemodynamic alterations depend on the size and location of the infarction. A large MI affecting more than 40% of the myocardium can result in circulatory collapse and cardiogenic shock. The prognosis of patients in cardiac shock remains very poor unless successful revascularization can occur in a timely fashion. Long-term hemodynamic alterations from left ventricular dysfunction result in chronic heart failure. With current reperfusion technology, many patients with MIs are left with no clinical evidence of left ventricular dysfunction.

Ventricular Arrhythmias after STEMI

Ventricular fibrillation is a major cause of preventable death in the early period after MI. Many episodes of prehospital sudden death are caused by untreated ventricular fibrillation. During MI, arrhythmias are caused by ischemia to the electrical conduction system, catecholamine release, and electrolyte imbalances. Hypokalemia and hypomagnesemia increase the risk of ventricular fibrillation. Routine magnesium sulfate is not administered in STEMI; however, any magnesium deficiency should be corrected. Any episodes of torsades de pointes (a special ventricular tachycardia associated with prolonged QT interval) should be treated with IV magnesium sulfate.

Clinical Application

Patients presenting with signs of MI need to be connected to a cardiac monitor immediately and observed in an area with trained personnel who have immediate access to a defibrillator and other emergency cardiac equipment and medications.

Mechanical Complications of STEMI

Septal Rupture

Septal rupture is most common with a large anteroseptal infarction. It most commonly occurs 3 to 7 days after an infarct (Bene & Vaughan, 2005). The patient experiences sudden and severe left ventricular failure. Blood is shunted from the left side of the heart back to the right side through the ruptured area. This shunting of blood results in poor systemic perfusion. The rupture also produces a very loud holosystolic murmur. Emergency measures to reduce afterload are indicated while the patient is prepared for surgical repair.

Papillary Muscle Dysfunction or Rupture

Papillary muscle dysfunction and rupture result in acute mitral valve regurgitation. This complication occurs most frequently with inferior-posterior wall MIs and usually occurs within the first week after infarction (Bene & Vaughan, 2005). As with septal ruptures, emergency measures to reduce afterload are indicated while preparing the patient for emergency surgery.

Other Complications of Myocardial Infarction

Pericarditis

Pericarditis, caused by inflammation of the pericardial sac, can occur immediately after an MI or several weeks later. When pericarditis occurs several weeks after an infarction, it is called *Dressler's syndrome*. When it occurs acutely, it is usually caused by a transmural infarct extending to the epicardium and causing an inflammatory response. Pain associated with pericarditis is sharp and severe. It is worse with inspiration and is relieved by leaning forward. A pericardial friction rub may be heard during auscultation of the heart. As with many complications of MI, the incidence of pericarditis has decreased significantly due to reperfusion therapy (Bene & Vaughan, 2005).

Left Ventricular Aneurysms

Localized dilatation of the left ventricle at the site of infarction can cause a ventricular aneurysm. Aneurysms can be classified as true or false. True aneurysms can be a source of ventricular arrhythmias that originate from the tissue at the junction of the aneurysm. These aneurysms typically do not rupture. False aneurysms, or pseudoaneurysms, are at greater risk for rupture. Rupture of these aneurysms results in death. If identified, these aneurysms require immediate surgical repair (Bene & Vaughan, 2005).

Postreperfusion Care in the Treatment of STEMI

Patients with STEMI are generally admitted to the coronary care unit. Listed here are key coronary care nursing interventions in the care of patients with STEMI:

- Assure aspirin was administered.

- Assess that response to beta-blocker therapy is adequate enough to control heart rate and arrhythmias.

- Assess the need for continued antianginal therapy, including the need for IV nitroglycerin during the first 48 hours. IV nitroglycerin can also be used for patients who are hypertensive or who have pulmonary congestion. Oral or topical agents can be used after 24 hours, if needed. Morphine sulfate can be given for pain that does not respond to antianginal therapy.

Note: If a patient has low blood pressure, life saving treatments such as beta-blocker and ACE inhibitor administration should occur before nitrate administration.

- Initiate ACE inhibitor as ordered within the first 24 hours for patients with anterior STEMIs, heart failure, or ejection fractions less than 40%.

- Reassess oxygen saturation after 6 hours of supplemental oxygen and discontinue if saturation is more than 90%.

- Administer anxiolytics as needed to reduce anxiety.

Clinical Application
Control of pain and anxiety is key not only for patient comfort but also to reduce myocardial oxygen demand. Pain and anxiety activate the sympathetic nervous system and increase myocardial oxygen demand.

- Assess heart sounds for new holosystolic murmurs.

- Restrict activity for at least the first 12 hours, and then begin a step approach to activity progression (phase I cardiac rehabilitation exercises).

- Utilize cardiac monitoring and ST-segment monitoring to assess for recurrent ischemia and the presence of arrhythmias.

- IV insulin may be indicated in first 24 to 48 hours after STEMI to tightly control blood sugars.

- Observe for signs of left ventricular dysfunction, including hypotension or clinical signs of heart failure.

- Include the family. Family visits do not have a negative impact on vital signs or cardiac rhythm.

(Antman et al., 2004)

When hemodynamic stability is achieved, patients can be transferred to a step-down unit. With successful reperfusion, some patients can transfer to a step-down unit within 24 hours. Post-PCI care is discussed in chapter 6.

NON-ST-SEGMENT ELEVATION MYOCARDIAL INFARCTION

Non-STEMI and unstable angina are usually caused by a ruptured plaque that causes a partially occluded vessel. The partial occlusion is generally caused by incomplete thrombosis. A non-STEMI cannot be differentiated from unstable angina at the time of presentation because the 12-lead ECG findings, such as ST-segment depression and T wave inversion, may be similar. In unstable angina, these ECG changes are usually more transient; in non-STEMI, they are usually more persistent. Cardiac biomarkers are used to differentiate between non-STEMI and unstable angina. Approximately 40% of all MIs are non-STEMIs (Bene & Vaughan, 2005). Patients in this category are at an increased risk for recurrent ischemia, MI, and death. The risk is highest during the first 2 months after the acute event (Braunwald et al., 2002).

Pharmacological Treatment of Non-STEMI

All patients with ACSs, including non-STEMI and unstable angina, should initially be treated with aspirin, oxygen, nitroglycerin, and morphine (for pain not relieved by nitroglycerin). Patients should also receive beta-blockers unless contraindicated. ACE inhibitors are given if hypertension is present after nitroglycerin and beta-blocker administration.

Other special pharmacological considerations for this group of patients are listed here.

Clopidogrel

- As soon as possible in patients receiving non-interventional treatment strategies (continued for 1 month)

- Also used in patients with planned interventional treatment strategies (continued for 1 to 9 months)

- Held for 5 to 7 days in patients undergoing CABG surgery

Unfractionated heparin (UFH) or LMWH

- UFH preferred in patients likely to have CABG surgery within 24 hours

Glycoprotein IIb/IIIa inhibitor

- In addition to aspirin and heparin when an interventional treatment strategy is planned

- May also be used in patients with continuing ischemia or elevated troponin levels when an interventional procedure is not planned

(Braunwald et al., 2002)

Additional Treatment Considerations

The two treatment arms for patients with unstable angina and non-STEMI include the early conservative arm and the early invasive arm. The early invasive treatment arm involves cardiac catheterization and revascularization within 24 hours. Early invasive treatment is recommended for high-risk patients, including those with:

- recent PCI or history of CABG

- recurrent ischemia

- depressed left ventricular function or clinical signs of heart failure

- sustained ventricular arrhythmias or hemodynamic instability

- significant ST-segment changes on a 12-lead ECG or high-risk findings on other noninvasive testing

- positive troponins.

(Braunwald et al., 2002)

In other patients presenting with ACSs, either early conservative or early invasive strategies may be used. When patients are treated conservatively, noninvasive testing is indicated to assess for areas of ischemia and the need for revascularization. Approximately 50% of patients presenting with unstable angina or non-STEMI have three vessel disease or left main disease and are therefore candidates for revascularization (Braunwald et al, 2002).

SPECIAL CONSIDERATIONS

Treatment of Cocaine-Induced Chest Pain

Cocaine use leads to sympathetic nervous system activation and direct stimulation of vascular smooth muscle, resulting in vasoconstriction. Cocaine also promotes platelet aggregation and thrombus formation. Chronic cocaine use accelerates the process of atherosclerosis. Cocaine-induced ischemic chest discomfort cannot be distinguished from unstable angina and non-STEMI caused by CHD. Nitroglycerin or calcium channel blockers are used to treat cocaine-induced chest pain. If ST-segment elevation is present, then calcium channel blockers are administered IV. A small percentage of cocaine users develop MIs as a result of cocaine use.

Variant (Vasospastic or Prinzmetal's) Angina)

Variant angina is caused by spasm of the coronary arteries. This type of angina usually occurs spontaneously but can be triggered by exercise, hyperventilation, and cold. The only associated risk factor for variant angina is smoking. Patients can have long asymptomatic periods between episodes. The pathophysiology of variant angina is not fully understood. One possible explanation is that endothelial dysfunction causes an imbalance between local vasodilative and local vasoconstrictive factors.

Transient ST-segment elevation usually occurs with variant angina but usually does not result in MI if the spasm occurs in a nonstenotic vessel. However, if the patient has spasms in vessels that are already stenosed, MI can occur. This type of angina is treated with nitroglycerin and calcium channel blockers.

LONG-TERM MANAGEMENT OF ACUTE CORONARY SYNDROMES

After an acute event, most patients resume a medical management course similar to patients with stable angina. Post-acute coronary syndrome (ACS) patients continue a daily dose of aspirin indefinitely. Clopidogrel is used if a patient is unable to take aspirin. Clopidogrel is also continued for a specified period for patients who underwent PCI. Patients with bare metal stents are prescribed clopidogrel for a minimum of 1 month; patients with drug-eluting stents, for a minimum of 3 months (Antman et al., 2004).

Beta-blockers initiated in the acute phase of MI are continued indefinitely after discharge. ACE inhibitors should be given within the first 24 hours to patients with anterior wall MIs, pulmonary congestion, or left ventricular ejection fractions less than 40%. ACE inhibitors are continued indefinitely. An angiotensin II receptor blocker may be used as an alternative for patients unable to tolerate ACE inhibitors.

Aldosterone blockers are given after MI to patients with ejection fractions less than 40%, those who have clinical heart failure, and those who are diabetic. Aldosterone blockers are added to therapy for patients who are already on ACE inhibitor therapy. Aldosterone blockers cannot be added to therapy for patients with renal dysfunction or hyperkalemia. Discharge medications include a lipid-lowering agent that should be initiated 24 to 96 hours after admission (Braunwald et al, 2002). Patients should not take ibuprofen for pain after STEMI because it interferes with healing and can cause thinning of the scarred area.

Discharge medical management includes three main objectives.

- Medications to improve prognosis
  - Aspirin
  - Clopidogrel (if aspirin sensitive or after PCI)
  - Beta-blockers
  - Lipid-lowering drugs (initiated prior to discharge)
  - ACE inhibitors (especially if ejection fraction is less than 40%)
- Medications to control ischemia
  - Beta-blockers
  - Nitrates (all patients should be given sublingual nitroglycerin)
  - Calcium channel blockers
- Secondary prevention through risk factor reduction
  - Smoking cessation
  - Reduction of hyperlipidemia
  - Hypertension control
  - Diabetes control

Patient Education

Medical Follow-Up

Patients should be instructed on the importance of physician follow-up. High-risk patients should be seen within 2 weeks after discharge, and low-risk patients within 6 weeks. The patient should be instructed to notify the physician anytime there is a change in condition, such as a change in activity tolerance or perceived medication side effects.

Risk Factor Reduction

A major focus of patient education for any patient with CHD is secondary prevention by aggressive reduction of cardiac risk factors. The reduction of cardiac risk factors is discussed in detail in chapter 4.

Recognition of Signs and Symptoms and Emergency Response

Another focus is the recognition of and response to symptoms of an acute coronary event. Patients should know how to activate the EMS and should know the location of the nearest hospital with 24-hour cardiac care. Patients should be instructed on the use of sublingual nitroglycerin or nitroglycerin spray and should be instructed to activate the EMS if symptoms do not improve after 5 minutes or after one sublingual nitroglycerin. Patients with signs and symptoms of ACS should also be instructed to take an aspirin (if not already taken) while awaiting the arrival of EMS.

Patients with a history of stable angina should be instructed to rest with the onset of angina and to take up to three sublingual nitroglycerin. Patients should notify the EMS if pain persists after the use of three sublingual nitroglycerin. Family members who are appropriate candidates may be given resources to learn about cardiopulmonary resuscitation and the use of automated external defibrillators.

Medications

Education regarding prescribed medications is also a key nursing intervention prior to discharge and continuing in the office setting. Patients with chronic cardiac disease are commonly prescribed multiple medications and the risk for noncompliance is high. Patients who have had revascularization and are experiencing an improvement in symptoms might not understand the importance of continued medical treatment. Noncompliance with medications is associated with increased adverse outcomes in the cardiac population. Those patients with fixed or low incomes might also have financial concerns regarding their medication regime.

Activity

Patients should be instructed on special post-discharge activity restrictions, including driving restrictions, weight-lifting restrictions, and instructions regarding sexual activity. These decisions are usually individualized based on the patient's clinical condition. Driving regulations may also vary between states. Most patients with an uncomplicated hospital course can drive about 1 week after discharge (Braunwald et al., 2002). Patients may be uncomfortable asking about resuming sexual relationships, so instructions regarding sexual activity should be included as a routine part of all discharge instructions. Patients with a history of angina during

sexual relationships may be instructed by their physician to take nitroglycerin prior to engaging in sexual activities.

Daily walking is the exercise of choice after an acute cardiac event. After the initial recovery period, stable patients should walk a minimum of 30 minutes daily. Patients should walk preferably every day but at least 3 to 4 days per week. The daily walking regime should be supplemented by an increase in activities of daily living (ADLs). Special considerations for the initial recovery period are discussed below. All STEMI patients should be referred to formal comprehensive multidisciplinary cardiac rehabilitation programs. All ACS patients at moderate to high risk, and with multiple risk factors, should also be referred to formal cardiac rehabilitation programs, where supervised exercise and continued patient education can be provided. Additional information about exercise and cardiac rehabilitation is provided in the next section.

Anxiety and Stress

Anxiety is common during and immediately after the acute phase of a cardiac event. Nurses can help reduce anxiety by helping the patient gain accurate perceptions of the recovery process. Teaching the patient about relaxation techniques and methods of worry control can help reduce anxiety. An example of a worry-control technique is to schedule 5-minute times to worry twice a day. At other times of the day, worries are set aside.

Patient and family education is a very important tool in relieving stress when the patient and family are ready to receive information. If the patient and family are not ready, providing information can actually increase stress.

Teaching Principles

The key to effective patient education is to individualize the approach and take advantage of every patient encounter. Nurses should be prepared to utilize all teachable moments. Many patients are afraid or have anxiety or depression after an acute cardiac event. Patients must be allowed to express concerns and have questions answered before they are able to accept new information. Patients should be active participants in the education process. Adult patients need to be in control of their learning; therefore, it is critical to assess the patient's readiness and desire for information.

In many cases, sharing scientific information about the value of the treatment or risk factor plan increases motivation and compliance. Patients who are engaged should be encouraged to seek out additional information and resources from the library or on the internet. Family, as defined by the patient, should be included in education. When providing patient education, it is helpful to individualize the information to the patient. For example, discuss the patient's individual risk factors, type of CHD, area of infarction, and specific ejection fraction. This allows the patient to assimilate and take ownership of the information being provided.

Effective patient education requires a great deal of time and is often neglected. However, the rewards of effective patient education can be tremendous. Patients can benefit from improved physical functioning and quality of life and even improved survival from increased adherence to the medical regime.

Cardiac Rehabilitation

Exercise in the Early Recovery Period

Initiation of activity early in the recovery period after an acute cardiac event is important because 3% of total body muscle mass deconditions per every day of bed rest (Levine, 2002). Patients also develop altered distribution of body fluids with bed rest and can develop orthostatic intolerance. The goal of rehabilitation in the early recovery period is to counteract the negative effects of deconditioning. Complications after an acute event are not increased with early activity progression in stable patients. Phase I cardiac rehabilitation exercises are initiated in a post-MI patient as soon as the patient is med-

ically stable and after evaluation for orthostatic hypotension. Phase I exercises usually begin on day 1 or 2 for an acute MI patient, depending on the size of the MI. Cardiac rehabilitation is typically initiated on postop day 1 for CABG patients. Cardiac contraindications to beginning or continuing exercise include unstable angina, complete heart block, uncontrolled tachyarrhythmias, uncontrolled hypertension, and decompensated heart failure (Myers, 2005). The development of thrombophlebitis or other complicating illness may also restrict the ability to begin exercise.

In the early recovery period, patients should walk 5 to 10 minutes at a time. Only non-resistive range-of-motion (ROM) exercises should be done because resistive exercises increase afterload and, therefore, the workload of the ventricles. The best exercises involve flexion and extension of arms and legs. Internal and external rotation and abduction of legs should be avoided because these exercises can also increase afterload (Levine, 2002).

The majority of patients begin with a 1.5 to 2.0 metabolic equivalent (MET) level of exercise (using bedside commode, transferring to a chair, feeding self, washing face and hands), progressing to 2 to 3 MET of activity (sitting up longer, walking to bathroom, showering). The goal is for patients to be at a rehab level of activity equivalent with ADLs by the time of discharge. With shorter hospital stays, the steps involved in inpatient rehabilitation programs have been modified to allow for more rapid progression. During early recovery, an increase of 20 beats per minute above resting heart rate, or a heart rate more than 110 beats per minute, may be used as a guideline for assessment of activity intolerance (Levine, 2002). These signs demonstrate an inappropriate chronotropic response to activity. Other guidelines for assessing activity intolerance include failure of systolic blood pressure to increase or a decrease in systolic blood pressure of 20 mm Hg (Levine, 2002).

Exercise in the Late Recovery Period

Most patients should be at a 3 to 4 MET level of activity by the time of discharge. Once a steady state of activity is well tolerated at home, the duration may be increased in 5-minute increments each week, up to 30 minutes per session. Activity should be done at least three to four times and may be done up to six times, per week (Levine, 2002). Intensity may also be increased as activity is progressed. Exercises should involve large muscle groups and include a warm-up and cool-down. The warm-up should be active, such as slow walking, and the cool-down should include stretching. Isometric activities should be limited due to their potential to increase afterload. Isometric exercises involve the contraction of a muscle with no movement of the joint. Driving requires only 1.5 to 3.0 METS; however many MI patients do not drive until they return to work.

Patients need to be instructed to balance myocardial oxygen supply and demand by monitoring their response to activity. Shortness of breath means overexertion. Patients should lower activity if breathing and heart rate do not return to normal within 10 minutes of stopping exercise. Activity that is well tolerated is accompanied by no adverse symptoms and no arrhythmias or excessive tachycardia. The same heart rate guidelines are used as with activity progression early in the recovery period.

Walking and secondary prevention have been shown to increase survival, decrease reoccurrence rates, and possibly slow progression of CHD (Gibbons et al., 2002). In addition, a regular walking program after an acute cardiac event improves the patient's perception of quality of life. Exercise as part of cardiac rehabilitation limits disability and improves the physical function of participants (Myers, 2005). The hemodynamic benefits of exercise include reduction of heart rate and blood pressure. Exercise stress testing is recommended before starting an exercise program after an acute cardiac event. Exercise later in recovery should be guided by a symptom-limited stress test.

Low-risk patients can implement an exercise prescription at home or in a community setting. Low-risk patients include those with absence of ischemia or arrhythmias on a stress test. High-risk patients should be in medically supervised exercise programs. High-risk patients are defined as those with ischemia or serious arrhythmias on a stress test. The majority of patients exercising for secondary prevention are classified as low risk. Exercise testing should be done on an annual basis for low-risk patients (Levine, 2002).

Formal Cardiac Rehabilitation

A formal cardiac rehabilitation program involves medically supervised exercise after an acute cardiac event. It usually begins 1 to 2 weeks after discharge and involves exercise three times weekly for a period of 4 to 12 weeks . The program is multidisciplinary and requires physician referral. Patients enrolled in a formal cardiac rehabilitation program must have baseline exercise testing and annual follow-ups. Exercise prescription is guided by exercise physiologists, and the patient's plan of care is directed by a registered nurse. Aerobic exercise and resistive training are components of the exercise program. Risk factor counseling, patient education regarding signs and symptoms and medications, and psychosocial support are also components of a comprehensive program.

Health insurance generally covers formal cardiac rehabilitation programs during the immediate recovery period after admission for MI, percutaneous transluminal coronary angioplasty (PTCA), and CABG for those with chronic stable angina. A patient copayment may be required. Many cardiac rehabilitation programs have sliding-scale fee structures to allow participation of those with financial limitations. Cardiac rehabilitation services have also been expanded to include patients with chronic heart failure, and those who have undergone valve surgery or implantable cardioverter-defibrillator implantation.

Pooled data from a meta-analysis of studies involving cardiac rehabilitation in secondary prevention show a benefit of reduced cardiovascular mortality of approximately 25% at 1 and 3 years (Gibbons et al., 2002; Myers, 2005). Participation in formal exercise training is safe, and patients benefit from increased functional capacity and exercise tolerance (Gibbons et al., 2002). However, exercise training needs to continue to show sustained improvement.

Patients who exercise experience a decrease in low-density lipoprotein cholesterol and triglyceride levels (Gibbons et al., 2002). Some patients experience a reduced need for oral hypoglycemic agents or insulin. Symptom reduction has been demonstrated in patients with angina and heart failure. Patients also experience improved psychosocial well-being and stress reduction. Patients who benefit from cardiac rehabilitation include those with the following cardiovascular conditions: angina, compensated heart failure, and decreased ejection fractions. Those with decreased exercise tolerance at baseline can benefit the most from participation but are often among those not referred. Cardiac rehabilitation exercises are safe and beneficial in clinically stable coronary patients. Unfortunately, only 10% to 20% of appropriate cardiac candidates participate in outpatient cardiac rehabilitation (Levine, 2002).

Psychosocial Issues

During postdischarge follow-up or during cardiac rehabilitation, the patient's psychosocial status should be evaluated. Many patients with left ventricular dysfunction as a result of acute MI will experience role identity crisis after their acute event. Many patients miss large amounts of work and many have to alter their work roles if high levels of physical exertion and stress are involved. Altered work roles may add family and financial stresses. Patients may also experience anxiety and sleep disorders. An assessment of the patient's support system is an important part of the psychosocial assessment. Social isolation is a predictor of worse outcomes after an acute cardiac event, such as MI (Maden & Froelicher, 2005).

Depression is not uncommon after an acute cardiac event. Patients with depression are three to four times more likely to die within the first year following an MI (Maden & Froelicher, 2005). Depression also impacts participation in exercise, medication compliance, seeking attention for symptoms, and return to work. Minor depression may respond to increased accomplishment and association with others. Exercise can also improve minor depressions so patients should be referred to formal cardiac rehabilitation programs for the social support as well as exercise component. Mended Hearts is an organization for those who have survived a cardiac event. Referral to Mended Hearts is another option for social support for those who are depressed and those with limited social support.

Selective serotonin reuptake inhibitors can be useful in treating depression during the first year after an acute MI or in cardiac patients with co-existing depression. This group of medications is generally considered safer than other antidepressant medications for use in the cardiac population (Maden & Froelicher, 2005).

CONCLUSION

Cardiac nurses have made a tremendous impact on patient outcomes, beginning with the introduction of coronary care units in the 1960s. From the original focus of arrhythmia detection and treatment to hemodynamic monitoring and aggressive intervention for all aspects of the disease process, cardiac nurses continue to play an important role in impacting patient outcomes.

CHD is a chronic, progressive, and systemic process. The systemic disease – not just the symptomatic stenosis – must be treated. Medical advances in the treatment of CHD and ACS offer hope in altering the course of disease progression. Nurses in all settings care for patients with cardiovascular disease at some stage on the continuum. Nursing knowledge linked to clinical practice can make a difference in the care of cardiac patients.

EXAM QUESTIONS

CHAPTER 5
Questions 36-45

36. Stable angina is best defined as angina that

    a. increases in severity.

    b. is new.

    c. occurs at rest.

    d. has a predictable pattern over time.

37. The gold standard diagnostic procedure to definitively diagnose the presence, location, and severity of CHD is

    a. stress testing with nuclear imaging.

    b. stress echocardiography.

    c. cardiac catheterization.

    d. spinal computed tomography.

38. Vulnerable plaque and ACSs are related in what way?

    a. The rupture of vulnerable plaque is the most frequent cause of ACSs.

    b. They are not related in any way.

    c. The episode of an ACS causes plaque to become vulnerable.

    d. They are only related in men with ACSs.

39. Goals of medical treatment for CHD include

    a. providing surgical revascularization for all patients.

    b. reducing symptoms, preventing complications, and reducing the risk of death.

    c. placing all patients on antiarrhythmic drugs to prevent sudden cardiac death.

    d. placing all patients on warfarin to reduce the risk of stroke.

40. Risk factor modification is important for all patients with CHD because

    a. risk factor modification can eliminate all possible chance of developing CHD.

    b. CHD only occurs in patients with three or more risk factors.

    c. although it does not benefit patients with CHD, risk factor modification sets a good example for their children.

    d. CHD is a systemic and progressive disease.

41. Which of the following patients is a candidate for reperfusion therapy?

    a. A patient with a 5-year history of stable angina who develops chest pain with extreme exertion.

    b. A patient with a history of CHD who develops shortness of breath with exertion after he stops taking his cardiac medications.

    c. A patient with no history of CHD who presents with STEMI.

    d. A patient who underwent CABG who presents for the second time with a non-STEMI.

42. During an acute MI the medication that is not routinely administered prior to reperfusion is

    a. morphine.

    b. lipid-lowering agent.

    c. aspirin.

    d. nitroglycerin.

43. A potential mechanical complication of acute MI that requires surgical repair is

    a. reinfarction.

    b. death.

    c. pericarditis.

    d. papillary muscle rupture.

44. A non-STEMI is definitively differentiated from unstable angina by

    a. location of chest pain.

    b. cardiac biomarkers.

    c. ECG changes.

    d. extent of cardiac history.

45. Proven benefits of participating in formal exercise training (cardiac rehabilitation) include

    a. increased functional capacity and exercise tolerance.

    b. ability to eliminate all cardiac medications.

    c. increase in earning potential after return to work.

    d. access to a cardiac rehab nurse in the home environment at all times.

CHAPTER 6

CARDIAC REVASCULARIZATION

CHAPTER OBJECTIVE

After completing this chapter, the reader will be able to discuss the indications for, benefits of, and potential complications of cardiac revascularization.

LEARNING OBJECTIVES

After studying this chapter, the reader will be able to

1. define the indications for revascularization with coronary artery bypass graft (CABG) surgery.

2. discuss advances in CABG that make the procedure less invasive.

3. describe complications and related nursing interventions associated with CABG.

4. explain the expected differences in the postoperative course of patients being fast tracked after CABG.

5. define the historical limitations of using primary (percutaneous) intervention (PCI) as a revascularization option in the treatment of coronary artery disease.

6. define advances in PCI in recent years and the impact of those advances on patient outcomes.

7. explain key nursing interventions in the care of a patient receiving PCI.

INTRODUCTION

There are two types of cardiac revascularization: surgical and percutaneous. Surgical revascularization is performed by coronary artery bypass grafting (CABG), and percutaneous revascularization is performed by percutaneous coronary intervention (PCI). CABG involves the use of graft material from the patient's arteries or veins to reroute blood around areas of long stenosis in coronary arteries. PCI is a catheter-based procedure in which mechanical devices are used to open shorter areas of stenosis in the coronary arteries.

CABG was first introduced in 1967; PCI followed 10 years later (Gibbons et al., 2002) with the introduction of percutaneous transluminal coronary angioplasty (PTCA), sometimes referred to today as *plain old balloon angioplasty,* or *POBA*.

Cardiac revascularization is performed to achieve several goals:

• improve survival

• minimize complications of ischemia

• relieve symptoms of ischemia

• improve functional capacity.

(Eagle et al., 2004)

In asymptomatic patients, revascularization is only performed if there is an expected survival advantage. Several factors must be considered in making a decision about cardiac revascularization. These factors include suitable coronary anatomy for the procedure, left ventricular function and amount of viable myocardium, symptoms of disease and impact on functional capacity, and other comorbid conditions and factors influencing life expectancy. Patients who have coronary anatomy unsuitable for revascularization are not candidates. Other conditions that limit the option for revascularization include advanced or metastatic cancer with a life expectancy of less than 1 year, end-stage cirrhosis with severe portal hypertension, and intracranial disorders that limit the ability to anticoagulate or substantially limit cognitive function (Braunwald et al., 2002).

It is difficult to adequately compare CABG and PCI today because there have been so many advances not only with both procedures but also with medical therapy used in conjunction with both revascularization techniques. There has not been sufficient time to evaluate the long-term effects of these many recent advances. Results of previous studies evaluating long-term outcomes do not account for these recent advances. In addition, many early studies that evaluated revascularization did not include large numbers of women, elderly people, or patients presenting for repeat revascularization.

CORONARY ARTERY BYPASS GRAFTING

Indications for Coronary Artery Bypass Grafting

CABG surgery has an average initial hospital cost of $30,000 per patient. When applied to the annual number of patients in the United States, CABG costs approximately 10 billion dollars annually (Eagle et al., 2004). For this reason, CABG is performed only in patients whose survival and symptomatic benefit have been proven. When performed in this group of patients, CABG is considered a cost-effective intervention. With the increasing use of less-invasive strategies for CABG, and with the increasing use of drug-eluting stents,

the initial hospital cost difference between CABG and PCI is narrowing.

Patients with left main disease or multivessel disease with decreased left ventricular function have a survival advantage with CABG (Antman et al., 2004; Braunwald et al., 2002; Eagle et al., 2004; Gibbons et al., 2002). Other indications for CABG include:

- left main equivalent disease with a significant left anterior descending (LAD) and left circumflex blockage.

- proximal LAD disease with greater than 75% occlusion, plus another vessel, plus a very positive stress test and an abnormal ECG

- coronary heart disease (CHD) in patients who have survived sudden cardiac death.

(Eagle et al., 2004)

CABG increases the chance of survival in patients with reduced left ventricular function, severe ischemia, or potential for severe ischemia (Braunwald et al., 2002). The poorer the left ventricular function, the greater the potential mortality benefit with CABG (Eagle et al., 2004). Reduced left ventricular function can be a result of chronic hypoperfusion in addition to past myocardial infarction (MI). Areas with chronic hypoperfusion can be assessed for viability using noninvasive cardiac testing. Patients with large areas of viable myocardium can benefit from revascularization. There is also some evidence that CABG is the preferred method of revascularization in diabetic patients with multivessel disease (Eagle et al., 2004).

Compared to high-risk patients, lower-risk patients receive only a modest survival benefit with CABG. Low-risk patients are generally only considered for CABG when their symptoms have been unresponsive to medical treatment and are limiting their quality of life or functional capacity. CABG has the greatest survival benefit for patients who are at greatest risk of death without surgery (Gibbons et al., 2002).

In addition to increasing survival, CABG is indicated to relieve symptoms and improve other outcomes. Angina is initially relieved in more than 90% of patients who undergo CABG (LeDoux & Luikart, 2005); however, angina can gradually reoccur over time due to either graft stenosis or progression of the patient's underlying CHD. Approximately 80% of patients remain free from angina at 5 years (Gibbons et al., 2002). These results are superior to medical treatment alone. The indications for CABG are very similar for patients with stable angina and unstable angina. However, there is a greater sense of urgency for those with unstable angina.

Myocardial Protection during CABG

The traditional approach to CABG involves a median sternotomy and the use of a cardiopulmonary (heart and lung) bypass machine (see Figure 6-1). The distal aorta is clamped during surgery to prevent coronary blood flow. Myocardial protection is required when the aorta is clamped to prevent myocardial ischemia and injury. Myocardial protection is accomplished by the use of cardioplegia to arrest the heart. A cardioplegia solution is infused either antegrade through the coronary arteries or retrograde through the coronary veins. Solutions for cardioplegia can be either crystalloid or crystalloid and blood mixtures and can be infused at normal or hypothermic temperatures. Cardioplegia involving the use of blood is commonly used and is definitely recommended in emergent and urgent cases as well as in patients with depressed left ventricular function. Cardioplegia solutions containing blood provide additional cardiac protection because of the increased oxygen-carrying capacity of blood (LeDoux & Luikart, 2005). The optimal type and delivery of cardioplegia remains the subject of current research. Cardioplegia solutions contain a variety of substances to aid in cardiac protection, such as potassium, and magnesium and procainamide to produce cardiac arrest (LeDoux & Luikart, 2005).

FIGURE 6-1: HEART AND LUNG BYPASS MACHINE

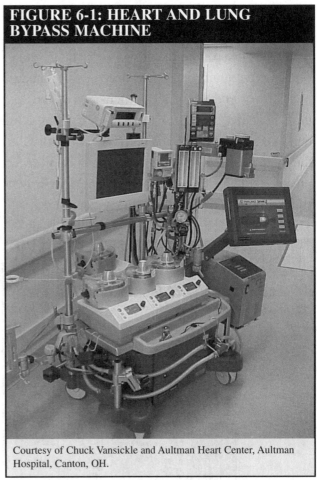

Courtesy of Chuck Vansickle and Aultman Heart Center, Aultman Hospital, Canton, OH.

Prophylactic use of an intra-aortic balloon pump 2 or more hours before cardiopulmonary bypass can also increase myocardial protection in high-risk patients. Intra-aortic balloon counterpulsation involves the placement of a balloon catheter in the descending aorta. The balloon is inflated during diastole and deflated during systole, delivering counterpulsation therapy. During balloon inflation during diastole, myocardial perfusion is increased. During balloon deflation, just before systole, a vacuum is created to reduce afterload, thereby reducing the work of the left ventricle.

Graft Material

One of the limiting factors of CABG has been the failure of saphenous vein grafts. Up to one half of all vein grafts close within 10 years after surgery (Eagle et al., 2004). Antiplatelet therapy with aspirin reduces short-term vein graft occlusion, and lipid-lowering therapy reduces long-term occlusion.

Initially, all CABG surgeries were done using solely saphenous vein grafts. The most common vein graft material is taken from the greater saphenous vein of the leg. Vein grafts can be harvested using standard incisions or endoscopically. After harvest, the vein graft is attached at one end to the ascending aorta and at the other end to the coronary artery distal to the blockage. Flow through vein grafts depends on pressure. Figure 6-2 shows a saphenous vein graft sutured both to the aorta and to the coronary artery. The saphenous vein graft is the graft on the left.

FIGURE 6-2: SAPHENOUS VEIN GRAFT AND INTERNAL MAMMARY ARTERY GRAFT

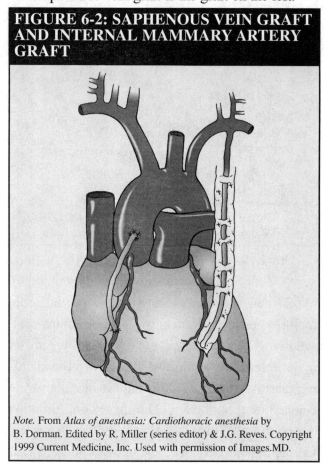

Note. From *Atlas of anesthesia: Cardiothoracic anesthesia* by B. Dorman. Edited by R. Miller (series editor) & J.G. Reves. Copyright 1999 Current Medicine, Inc. Used with permission of Images.MD.

Clinical Application
Patients with hypotension or poor left ventricular function are at increased risk for acute vein graft closure due to low pressures and resultant poor flow through the vein graft.

A very important surgical advancement is the success of internal mammary artery grafts. These grafts have shown major improvement in late patency rates, with more than 90% patency at 10 years (Eagle et al., 2004). Internal mammary artery grafts have also improved long-term survival rates and reduced postoperative mortality (Eagle et al., 2004). Harvesting of the internal mammary arteries is technically more difficult than harvesting of saphenous vein grafts (LeDoux & Luikart, 2005). The left internal mammary artery is most commonly used to bypass the LAD. When the LAD is bypassed using an internal mammary artery, patients have improved long-term outcomes (Antman et al., 2004; Eagle et al., 2004).

When used as a pedicle graft, a graft left attached to the original site, the proximal end of the internal mammary artery is left intact and the distal end is sutured beyond the site of stenosis. Figure 6-2 shows an internal mammary artery graft on the right. Most CABG surgeries involve a combination of a left internal mammary artery graft and a saphenous vein graft. Both internal mammary arteries can also be used.

In some young patients, revascularization with all-arterial grafts may be considered, with the hope of achieving longer-term patency and avoiding the need for reoperation. The need for one or more reoperations is a concern in younger patients because reoperation carries a higher risk. Lack of an acceptable conduit is also a concern if reoperation must be performed more than once. The radial artery can be used as conduit; however, it is prone to spasm because of its thick muscular nature. The risk of spasm can be decreased with the use of nitrates and calcium channel blockers, both intraoperatively and postoperatively. The advantage of the radial artery is its length, which enables it to be used to reach most distal targets. The radial artery is not used unless the patient has adequate patency of the ulnar artery. The radial artery is most often harvested from the patient's nondominant hand.

Clinical Application
Ulnar pulse and distal circulation should be checked postoperatively if the radial artery was harvested for graft material during surgery.

The right gastroepiploic artery supplies blood to the greater curvature of the stomach. When this artery is used as graft material in CABG, a more extensive surgery results because abdominal entry is also required (LeDoux & Luikart, 2005). This artery can be used as a pedicle graft or a free graft.

When patients have no available arterial or venous conduit, cryopreserved saphenous vein grafts or umbilical vein grafts that have been treated with glutaraldehyde can be used. Unfortunately, these grafts have poor long-term patency, so they are used only when no other options are available. Other nonhomologous grafts have been used but also have poor patency. These grafts include bovine internal mammary arteries and synthetic grafts (Eagle et al., 2004).

Advantages

CABG has proven mortality benefits in certain high-risk patient groups, as previously discussed. CABG also has proven long-term success, with graft patency rates at more than 90% at 10 years with the use of arterial conduits (Smith, et al., 2001). CABG allows revascularization to some occlusions that are not accessible using catheter-based techniques.

Contraindications

Patients who have inadequate conduits are not ideal candidates for CABG. Very small coronary arteries distal to the site of stenosis are also a limiting factor in performing CABG. Patients with severe atherosclerosis of the aorta are at very high risk for intraoperative neurological complications and may not be able to undergo CABG.

Minimally Invasive Techniques

MIDCAB

Minimally invasive CABG (MIDCAB) is performed on a beating heart without cardiopulmonary bypass and without the use of a median sternotomy to gain access. Due to limited access through an anterolateral thoracotomy, this procedure is typical-ly done to the easily accessible proximal LAD. This approach is cosmetically appealing for patients because the incision from a small thoracotomy is less noticeable than an incision from a median sternotomy. However, this procedure is technically challenging because visibility is not the same as with a sternotomy. In addition, the intercostal nerves can be irritated, producing increased postoperative pain (Niinami, Ogasawara, Suda, & Takeuchi, 2005). Another approach being used for MIDCAB is the ministernotomy. In this approach, the LAD and right coronary artery (RCA) can be bypassed using the same incision (Niinami, Ogasawara, Suda, & Takeuchi, 2005). Internal mammary artery grafts can be used during MIDCAB with both approaches; however, access to the internal mammary arteries is improved with the ministernotomy approach.

To allow for suturing, medications such as beta-blockers or adenosine can be given to slow or temporarily stop the heart. Mechanical stabilizers are also used to hold the coronary artery still while suturing occurs. The advantages of MIDCAB are associated with its avoidance of the sternotomy and cardiopulmonary bypass. Some patients experience less pain with no sternotomy and require less blood transfusions by avoiding cardiopulmonary bypass. Both of these factors can lead to shorter hospital stays.

OPCAB

Off-pump CABG (OPCAB) is another less-invasive form of CABG. This surgery is done without cardiopulmonary bypass but involves a median sternotomy. A full sternotomy offers better access to bypass the vessels that supply the lateral and posterior walls. Intraoperative techniques are used to stabilize the coronary arteries and to clear the operative field of blood. The avoidance of cardiopulmonary bypass eliminates the need to clamp the aorta in patients with high-risk aortic atherosclerosis. Other potential advantages include a decreased need for blood transfusions and shorter hospital stays. The number of OPCAB procedures performed each year has increased since the late 1990s. In the state of New York, 27% of CABG procedures in the year 2000 were done off pump (Racz et al., 2004). Today, some cardiovascular surgical programs do a substantial portion of their procedures as OPCABs. Both MIDCAB and OPCAB are relatively new procedures, and the results of these techniques are expected to improve over time.

Other Techniques

Other advances in cardiac surgery include port-access and video-assisted CABG with a closed chest. During this procedure, the aorta can be occluded and cardioplegia delivered via endovascular techniques. Cardiopulmonary bypass is used during this procedure and access occurs through the femoral artery and vein. One advantage of this technique is the avoidance of a median sternotomy. However, this procedure has not yet been evaluated through large controlled trials (Eagle et al., 2004). Additional techniques for CABG using robotics are also being investigated.

Potential Complications

The use of cardiopulmonary bypass causes a diffuse inflammatory response. This response results in transient multiorgan dysfunction and can also delay recovery after surgery. Various strategies are used to limit the immune response associated with cardiopulmonary bypass:

- Preoperative corticosteroids block complement activation and reduce the levels of proinflammatory cytokines. (Steroids may not be indicated in diabetic patients.)

- Aprotinin, a serine protease inhibitor and hemostatic agent used in high-risk patients to prevent bleeding, also has a role as an anti-inflammatory agent because it blocks complement activation and cytokine release. Aprotinin is an expensive medication and is not widely used for this purpose.

- The administration of leukocyte-poor blood and leukocyte depletion via filtration during the perioperative period has been shown to be beneficial in improving myocardial performance during acute or chronic ischemia.

(Eagle et al., 2004)

Patients undergoing CABG today are older and have more comorbidities than patients of the past. However, advances in CABG continue to allow for improved outcomes even for high-risk patients.

Low Cardiac Output State

The most common cause of mortality after CABG is a low cardiac output state (Eagle et al., 2004). Myocardial damage from a perioperative MI can occur as a complication of CABG and is a common cause of a low cardiac output state. Perioperative MI can occur due to graft spasm or embolization into the graft. Perioperative MI can also occur as a complication of cardiopulmonary bypass if myocardial protection is not adequate. Patients with perioperative MI are at increased risk for increased adverse outcomes. These patients are treated with maximal medical therapy, including antiplatelet agents, beta-blockers, and angiotensin-converting enzyme inhibitors. Low cardiac output after CABG can be caused by reversible conditions after surgery, including acidosis and hypoxemia.

Neurological Complications

The second most common cause of postoperative mortality is postoperative stroke (Eagle et al., 2004). Neurological complications after CABG are classified as type I or type II. Type I deficits include major focal deficits and coma. Type II deficits include various degrees of intellectual deterioration and memory loss. Neurological complications can be caused by intraoperative or postoperative hypoxia, emboli from cardiopulmonary bypass, hemorrhage, or metabolic abnormalities (Eagle et al., 2004). Risk factors for type I and II neurological complications include advanced age and hypertension. Additional risk factors for type I complications include atherosclerosis of the proximal aorta, previous history of neurological disease, unstable angina or diabetes, and intraoperative use of an intra-aortic balloon pump. Additional risk factors for type II complications include prior CABG, alcohol consumption, arrhythmias, heart failure, and history of peripheral vascular disease (Eagle et al., 2004).

Type II complications may be related to the brain's own microcirculation in addition to microemboli during cardiopulmonary bypass. Sophisticated arterial line filters within the cardiopulmonary bypass circuit help protect against microemboli. Type II complications have been associated with periods of hypotension or hypoperfusion and may be reversible. Minimizing type I complications is critical because stroke is the second leading cause of mortality. A type I neurological injury can produce a 21% mortality rate (Eagle et al., 2004). The use of ultrasound via transesophageal echocardiography or epiaortic imaging to assess the aorta for the presence of atherosclerotic plaque is a technique to help minimize type I complications.

When atherosclerotic plaque is identified in the ascending aorta, the patient is at high risk for an adverse neurovascular outcome. Embolization of atherosclerotic plaque is the most common cause of perioperative stroke (LeDoux & Luikart, 2005). Atherosclerotic emboli can be dislodged from the aortic arch during cannulation for cardiopulmonary bypass or during clamping of the aorta. In very high-risk patients, a no-clamp strategy may be used (Eagle et al., 2004).

Other factors that contribute to postoperative stroke are recent anterior wall MI with left ventricular thrombus and recent stroke. Patients with recent stroke should not have CABG for at least 4 weeks. If CABG is done within 4 weeks of a stroke, then the patient is at high risk for hemorrhagic complications of stroke. Patients who also have symptomatic or severe carotid stenosis should be treated with carotid endarterectomy prior to CABG. Patients routinely have carotid ultrasound exams prior to surgery to assess for significant carotid stenosis. Carotid endarterectomy is generally not performed in asymptomatic carotid disease unless stenosis is 80% or greater (Eagle et al., 2004).

The risk of neurovascular complications also increases with the time spent on cardiopulmonary bypass. Hyperglycemia can also worsen neurological impairment.

Peripheral neurovascular complications, including brachial plexus injury and ulnar nerve injury, can also occur as complications of surgery.

Atrial Fibrillation

Another complication of CABG is the development of atrial fibrillation postoperatively. Atrial fibrillation occurs in 20% to 40% of postoperative patients and is most commonly seen on the second to third hospital day (LeDoux & Luikart, 2005). If atrial fibrillation persists more than 24 hours, warfarin can be initiated to prevent clot formation and future stroke. Several patient factors increase the likelihood of developing atrial fibrillation postoperatively:

- chronic obstructive pulmonary disease (COPD) or proximal RCA disease (can cause right ventricular and right atrial enlargement)

- cessation of beta-blockers prior to surgery

- increased cross-clamp time, producing atrial ischemia

- advanced age.

(Eagle et al., 2004)

Increased circulating catecholamines, volume overload, hypoxia, and electrolyte disturbances in the postoperative state can also contribute to the development of atrial fibrillation (LeDoux & Luikart, 2005). Atrial fibrillation not only extends length of stay but also greatly increases the risk of postoperative stroke.

The standard therapy for the reduction of postoperative atrial fibrillation is the initiation of beta-blockers preoperatively or very early postoperatively. Patients who were on beta-blockers preoperatively and have them withdrawn perioperatively are at increased risk for developing atrial fibrillation as a complication of CABG. Amiodarone can be used if beta-blockers are contraindicated.

Wound Infection

Preoperative antibiotic administration is routinely used to help prevent postoperative infection. Cephalosporins are the class of choice. Because an adequate tissue level of antibiotics is required at the time of incision, timing of preoperative antibiotics is important. Preoperative antibiotics should be administered within 30 minutes of incision time (Eagle et al., 2004). Additional antibiotic dosing may be required for longer surgeries. Postoperative intravenous (IV) antibiotics are continued for 1 to 2 days.

Mediastinitis, or deep sternal wound infection, is a serious complication of CABG that results in a mortality rate as high as 25% (Eagle et al., 2004). Sternal wound infections typically manifest several days to 2 weeks after surgery (LeDoux & Luikart, 2005). Skin and nasopharyngeal gram-positive organisms are the leading cause of postoperative deep sternal wound infections (Eagle et al., 2004). Obesity, diabetes, reoperation, and excessive use of electrocautery are risk factors. In addition, the use of both internal mammary arteries increases the risk because the sternum receives less blood flow. Superficial wounds are treated with antibiotics and drainage, whereas deep sternal wounds require surgical debridement and closure with a muscle flap (LeDoux & Luikart, 2005).

Several strategies are used during surgery to decrease the risk of mediastinitis and sternal wound infection (See Box 6-1.)

Renal Dysfunction

Renal dysfunction is another potential complication after CABG because cardiopulmonary bypass decreases glomerular filtration rate. The following characteristics place a patient at risk for developing renal dysfunction after bypass: advanced age, heart failure, type I diabetes, preexisting renal dysfunction,

---

BOX 6-1: STRATEGIES TO DECREASE STERNAL WOUND INFECTIONS

1. Meticulous aseptic technique
    a) Double gloving of operating room (OR) team
    b) Reduced OR traffic
2. Clipping, rather than shaving, hair and avoidance of hair removal
3. Shorter perfusion times
4. Avoidance of unnecessary electrocautery
5. Proper timing of preoperative and perioperative antibiotics
6. Strict control of blood sugars during and after surgery

(Eagle et al., 2004)

---

and prior CABG (Eagle et al., 2004). Mortality is high for those who develop renal dysfunction perioperatively and is especially high for those who require dialysis. Early recognition of renal insufficiency and assurance of adequate volume administration are key nursing interventions in preventing postoperative renal failure.

Clinical Application

Nephrotoxic medications, including nonsteroidal anti-inflammatory drugs (NSAIDs) and aminoglycoside antibiotics, should be avoided in high-risk patients.

Patients with end-stage renal disease are at very high risk for mortality and morbidity if they undergo CABG. However, their risk for mortality may be even higher if they do not undergo revascularization; therefore, CABG may be considered for some of these patients. Patients with end-stage renal disease have a particularly high risk of developing postoperative infection and sepsis (Eagle et al., 2004).

Pulmonary Complications

Mild pulmonary complications can occur simply as a result of cardiopulmonary bypass. During cardiopulmonary bypass, capillary permeability and pulmonary vascular resistance increase and noncardiac pulmonary edema can occur (LeDoux

& Luikart, 2005). Acute respiratory distress syndrome (ARDS) is a serious potential complication. Patients undergoing reoperation and those requiring blood transfusions are at higher risk for developing ARDS. Preoperative pulmonary edema should be resolved prior to surgery because pulmonary edema increases with cardiopulmonary bypass.

Most patients experience postoperative atelectasis. Postoperative thoracic and abdominal surgery patients are prone to hypoventilation due to postoperative pain.

Clinical Application
Postoperative pain control is an effective intervention in preventing atelectasis by promoting adequate ventilation.

The most common preoperative pulmonary problem is COPD. Those with moderate to severe COPD, including those with elevated partial pressure of carbon dioxide levels and those who use home oxygen, are at increased risk for postoperative complications. These patients are likely to remain on ventilators longer, which places them at risk for the development of nosocomial pneumonia. In addition to their risk of pulmonary complications, these patients also experience an increased risk of ventricular arrhythmias postoperatively (Eagle et al., 2004).

Clinical Application
Smoking cessation is an important intervention to decrease the risk of pulmonary complications in patients electively undergoing CABG.

All pulmonary infectious processes should also be resolved prior to surgery. Before surgery, it is important for patients to receive incentive spirometry and to perform coughing and deep breathing exercises. This preoperative treatment also provides the instruction for postoperative exercises. If time allows, weight loss should be achieved in obese patients electively undergoing CABG; this can help to decrease the risk of adverse pulmonary effects and other complications.

Clinical Application
It is important to accomplish preoperative respiratory teaching (incentive spirometry and coughing and deep breathing) even in patients without pre-existing lung disease because postoperative sedation and pain interfere with the patient's ability to learn during the early postoperative period.

Patients who are unable to be extubated in a timely fashion due to pulmonary complications are usually ventilated using low tidal volume. The use of low tidal volume is one lung-protective strategy to limit damage to pulmonary tissue caused by mechanical ventilation. Pneumothorax can also occur as a postoperative complication and can happen at the time of removal of pleural chest tubes.

Postoperative Bleeding

Postoperative bleeding is usually venous in nature and originates from the site of sutures. Bleeding can also occur from pericardial adhesions during a reoperation. Blood loss should be less than 300 ml/hr during the first several hours and then should begin to taper. Average total blood loss is approximately 1 L (Ferraris et al., 2003). Patients who experience prolonged cardiopulmonary bypass are at risk for developing coagulapathies postoperatively. Coagulation profiles are drawn postoperatively to determine any deficiencies in clotting factors. Recognized deficiencies are replaced with administration of the appropriate clotting factors. Platelet count should be kept above $100,000/mm^3$.

Patients who are at high risk for bleeding preoperatively, including those undergoing reoperation and those with expected long cardiopulmonary bypass, may receive aprotinin to inhibit plasmin. Aprotinin can help preserve platelet function during cardiopulmonary bypass. If bleeding cannot be adequately controlled; then mediastinal re-exploration may be needed to reduce the risk of cardiac tamponade, a life-threatening postoperative emergency.

Transfusion

CABG patients account for 10% of blood transfusions in the United States. However, only 20% of the CABG patients are the recipients of the vast majority of blood transfusions in this patient population (Eagle et al., 2004). Blood transfusions produce an immunosuppressive effect and increase the risk of nosocomial infection, particularly nosocomial pneumonia. Therefore, the goal is to avoid the need for perioperative transfusion whenever possible. The risk of complications from transfusion increases when the transfused blood is older than 1 month old (Raghavan & Marik, 2005). In CABG patients, the proinflammatory substances that accumulate during the storage of blood can increase pulmonary complications postoperatively (Raghavan & Marik, 2005).

There is some evidence that many of the detrimental effects of blood transfusions are related to donor white blood cells and how they react with stored red blood cells (RBCs) (Raghavan & Marik, 2005). Depletion of leukocytes can be helpful in blunting this immunosuppressive response. This procedure can occur in the blood bank or at the bedside at the time of transfusion using a filter. Several factors increase the patient's risk of needing a blood transfusion during or after surgery. These risk factors are listed in Box 6-2.

BOX 6-2: RISK FACTORS FOR PERIOPERATIVE BLOOD TRANSFUSION

- Increased age
- Increased time on cardiopulmonary bypass
- Reoperation
- Emergent or urgent operation
- Low RBC volume preoperatively
- Preoperative fibrinolytic, anticoagulant, or antiplatelet therapy

(Eagle et al., 2004)

Anticoagulation and Antiplatelet Therapy Prior to Surgery

If a patient is expected to need CABG within 24 hours, then low-molecular-weight heparin (LMWH) is not used; unfractionated heparin (UFH) is used instead. LMWH should be stopped 18 to 24 hours before surgery and replaced with UFH (Ferraris et al., 2003). UFH can be continued until a short time before incision (Ferraris et al., 2003). In addition, a direct thrombin inhibitor, such as hirudin, can be continued until immediately before surgery (Ferraris et al., 2003).

Aspirin and clopidogrel should also be held prior to elective CABG to reduce the risk of postoperative bleeding. Aspirin is recommended to be held for 3 to 10 days prior to surgery (Eagle et al., 2004; Ferraris et al., 2003). Clopidogrel is recommended to be held for 5 to 7 days before surgery (Eagle et al., 2004). The American College of Cardiology (ACC)/American Heart Association (AHA) guidelines for ST-segment elevation MI (STEMI) say aspirin should not be held prior to elective or nonelective CABG in patients with STEMI (Antman et al., 2004). The benefits of continuing aspirin therapy in patients with acute coronary syndromes (ACSs) need to be weighed against the risks of postoperative bleeding.

The glycoprotein (GP) IIb/IIIa inhibitors tirofiban and eptifibatide need to be discontinued 4 to 6 hours before CABG, and abciximab needs to be stopped 12 to 24 hours before surgery (Ferraris et al., 2003). In patients who proceed to CABG after receiving abciximab, platelet aggregation does not return to normal for 48 hours. These patients receive special precautions during CABG to minimize the risk of bleeding. Such precautions include:

- lower doses of intraoperative heparin
- minimal hemodilution
- platelet transfusion
- possible use of antifibrinolytics, such as aprotinin.

(Eagle et al., 2004)

Aprotinin acts as a hemostatic drug. It is effective in decreasing postoperative blood loss and transfusion requirements in high-risk patients, including those who have remained on aspirin therapy because their condition did not permit discontinuation of aspirin.

Patients can donate their own blood during the 30 days prior to surgery to be used as an autologous transfusion if needed during or after surgery. Patients who have adequate hemoglobin levels and do not have unstable or potentially unstable ischemic disease may be candidates. In another technique, blood is taken from the patient prior to cardiopulmonary bypass and then reinfused in the patient immediately after bypass. Autotransfusion from mediastinal-shed blood has also been used to decrease the number of blood transfusions. However, some researchers express concern that autotransfusion can stimulate fibrinolysis (Eagle et al., 2004).

Late Postoperative Complications

Weeks to months after CABG, some patients experience an autoimmune response of the pericardial tissue. This response causes inflammation of the pericardium and is termed *postpericardiotomy syndrome*. The pleural space can also be involved. Patients are treated with NSAIDs. Steroids can also be used, if needed.

Cardiac tamponade can also occur late in the postoperative period. It can occur alone or as a complication of postpericardiotomy syndrome. Late tamponade is most typically seen in patients on warfarin (LeDoux & Luikart, 2005).

Special Populations

Emergency CABG Patients

Any emergent or urgent surgery carries an increased risk of mortality and morbidity. Whenever possible, PCI, an intra-aortic balloon pump (IABP), and medical treatment should be used to stabilize the patient prior to surgery. Failed PCI procedures in patients who are ischemic or who have hemodynamic instability may warrant emergency CABG.

Emergency CABG may also be performed at the time of a repair of a mechanical complication of acute MI, such as septal or mechanical rupture. Emergency CABG is not performed in patients with only a small area of myocardium at risk who are hemodynamically stable (Antman et al., 2004).

Acute MI Patients

Patients who have had acute MIs have higher mortality with CABG for the first several days after the infarction. For patients with large MIs who are stabilized, surgery should be delayed to allow the myocardium to recover. However, some patients with acute MIs are unable to wait to have CABG, including those with left main or triple vessel disease and those with symptomatic valve disease. CABG mortality is elevated for the first 3 to 7 days after an MI (Antman et al., 2004).

Right Ventricular MI Patients

Patients with large right ventricular MIs are at particularly high risk and may need surgery delayed for up to 4 weeks to allow for recovery of the right ventricle. During surgery, the pericardium is no longer able to contain the acutely injured right ventricle and it dilates. This dilatation may even prevent the chest from closing (Eagle et al., 2004).

Elderly Patients

The greatest increase in CABG is among patients over age 85. The elderly have an increased risk of mortality and morbidity; however, improvement in functional capacity and quality of life can be achieved in most patients in this age-group (Eagle et al., 2004).

Women

Some studies have found differences in CABG mortality and morbidity rates when comparing women to men, with women having higher complication rates. However, the evidence is conflicting as to whether gender is the determining factor. General consensus is that risk factors and patient comorbidities are more important than gender, and CABG should not be delayed as a treatment option for women (Eagle et al., 2004).

Diabetics

Patients with diabetes have an increased risk of mortality with CABG compared to nondiabetic patients (Woods, Smith, Sohail, Sarah, & Engle, 2004). However, in the Bypass Angioplasty Revascularization Investigation (BARI) trial, CABG was shown to provide a greater survival benefit to appropriate patients with diabetes than does PCI (Woods et al., 2004). In addition to diabetes, any hyperglycemia during the perioperative period increases risk, especially for sternal wound infections. Hyperglycemia can occur in nondiabetic patients due to surgical stress, hypothermia, commonly used postoperative medications, and other complex metabolic changes that occur during CABG (Lorenz, Lorenz, & Codd, 2005). Tight glycemic control, with the use of IV insulin to keep blood sugar levels below 200 mg/dl, is recommended in CABG patients (Lorenz, Lorenz, & Codd, 2005).

Patients with Peripheral Vascular Disease

Patients with peripheral vascular disease commonly have coexisting CHD. Patients with peripheral vascular disease who undergo CABG have an increased short- and long-term risk of mortality.

Patients with Low Ejection Fractions

Patients with low ejection fractions or clinical heart failure also have an increased risk of operative mortality. However, this group of patients, when treated with CABG, also have the greatest survival benefit when compared to treatment with medical therapy. In addition, this population can benefit from symptom relief and improvement in functional capacity (Gibbons et al., 2002).

Patients with Valve Disease

Patients with coexisting moderate to severe aortic stenosis commonly undergo aortic valve replacement at the time of CABG. In addition, patients who have clinically symptomatic mitral regurgitation with structural abnormalities undergo mitral valve repair

at the time of CABG (Bonow et al., 1998; Eagle et al., 2004). If the mitral valve is structurally normal and regurgitation is not severe, the regurgitation may be caused by reversible ischemia that will be corrected with the revascularization procedure. Combined procedures increase the operative risk of complications and mortality. When a valve procedure is added to CABG, the risk of stroke substantially increases (Bonow et al., 1998; Eagle et al., 2004).

Postoperative Nursing Care

All patients who have undergone open heart surgery are cared for in a similar fashion, regardless of the exact operation performed. They receive care in an intensive care unit for the immediate postoperative period. During this period, patients are on mechanical ventilation for a minimum of 2 to 4 hours (LeDoux & Luikart, 2005) and are monitored via a cardiac monitor. In addition, patients have an arterial line and pulmonary artery catheter in place for invasive monitoring of systemic and intracardiac pressures. The arterial line allows for continuous monitoring of blood pressure, which can be unstable during the early postoperative period. Hypertension or hypotension can occur after surgery. Hypotension frequently occurs in the early postoperative period as the patient warms up. The patient can also experience hypovolemia due to fluid volume alterations associated with cardiopulmonary bypass.

The pulmonary artery catheter allows for assessment of preload, afterload, and contractility. Pulmonary artery catheters with the capability of continuous cardiac output and venous oxygen saturation monitoring are commonly used. Poor cardiac output can occur due to problems with heart rate, preload, afterload, and contractility. Venous oxygen saturation levels provide a good assessment of the delivery and consumption of oxygen by measuring the patient's venous reserve. Postoperative patients also have epicardial temporary pacing wires in place.

Bradycardic arrhythmias can occur postoperatively, especially in patients who have received valve repair or replacement. The suture lines from valve surgery are close to the conduction system, and postoperative edema can cause temporary heart block.

Pleural and mediastinal chest tubes connected to water-seal chambers and 20 cm of suction are also used. Stripping of chest tubes postoperatively should be avoided because of the risk of damaging bypass grafts. Mediastinal chest tubes can recover blood during the immediate postoperative period to be used for autotransfusion. Packed RBCs generally are not given unless hemoglobin falls below 8 g/dl (LeDoux & Luikart, 2005). Control of hypertension is important during the postoperative period to reduce the risk of bleeding.

Early postoperative aspirin administration, initiated at least within the first 48 hours, is important to prevent saphenous vein graft closure. Aspirin also reduces many other postoperative complications and decreases postoperative mortality (Eagle et al., 2004; Ferraris et al., 2003).

Fast Tracking

Low-risk patients can be selected for fast tracking after CABG. These patients are targeted for early extubation, early ambulation, and early discharge. Special pathways are used to guide care in patients being fast tracked. Patients who are fast tracked are sedated postoperatively with short-acting agents and receive lower doses of opioids to allow for earlier extubation. Patients can be extubated postoperatively when they are awake, respond appropriately, and are able to have pain controlled without using medications that interfere with extubation. Prior to extubation, patients must also have no serious postoperative bleeding and have stable vital signs. Pharmacological strategies to prevent atrial fibrillation are also a key component of fast tracking.

Early ambulation and phase I cardiac rehabilitation exercises are also a part of the fast track program. Patients who are fast tracked are generally discharged 3 to 5 days postoperatively. Older patients are commonly more difficult to fast track because of higher numbers of preoperative comorbidities.

Postdischarge Care

Administration of postoperative aspirin is continued indefinitely. All patients also receive statin therapy to reduce the progression of vein graft disease. CABG patients are placed on a 20- to 25-lb lifting restriction, with no more than 10 lbs over the head for 6 to 8 weeks after discharge. Bypass patients generally wait to drive, even after their restrictions are over, due to chest soreness and fear of injury.

A formal cardiac rehabilitation program referral should be made for all patients prior to discharge. Patients usually begin participation in outpatient cardiac rehabilitation 4 to 8 weeks after surgery. In one long-term study of CABG patients who participated in cardiac rehabilitation, outcomes at 5 years included increased physical mobility, perception of better health, and perception of better overall life situation. Compared to those who do not participate in cardiac rehabilitation, a larger percentage of those who complete the program are working at 3 years (Eagle et al., 2004).

Assessment of depression and presence of psychosocial support are important nursing interventions in the postdischarge period. Depression occurs in up to 33% of patients after CABG (Eagle et al., 2004). Psychosocial interventions for CABG patients are similar to those for patients with CHD. These interventions were discussed in detail in chapter 5.

Clinical Application
Facilitating participation in cardiac rehabilitation is a key nursing intervention in the prevention and treatment of postoperative depression and social isolation.

Many patients and their caregivers experience major psychosocial adjustments after discharge. Adapting to postoperative pain, changes in body image, activity limitations, and financial burdens are a few of the areas for which nurses need to provide support during the discharge transition

(Theobald & McMurray, 2004). Telephone follow-up programs are one method of providing postoperative support, especially to assure a smooth home transition in patients who are fast tracked.

Presentation with Angina after CABG

Up to 20% of patients presenting with unstable angina have undergone CABG. These patients are at higher risk for mortality and morbidity than patients who have never received revascularization (Braunwald et al., 2002). Patients who present with ACSs or other symptoms suggestive of ischemia after having CABG are generally candidates for cardiac catheterization. It is difficult to distinguish between graft closure and progression of native vessel disease using only noninvasive testing. Most patients who present with ischemia within 30 days of surgery have graft failure due to thrombosis. This acute graft closure can occur in vein grafts and arterial conduits. These patients are usually candidates for PCI to treat the focal stenosis. If multiple vein grafts are stenosed or if the stenotic graft is supplying the LAD, then repeat CABG is often indicated.

Reoperation

Mortality and morbidity risks are higher for patients who undergo repeat CABG. These patients may also have limited available graft options. Long-term results are not as successful with repeat operations as with initial operations.

PERCUTANEOUS CORONARY INTERVENTION

PCI refers to a group of catheter-based technologies used to treat coronary stenosis. PTCA was the first of these catheter-based techniques. Intracoronary stents are now used in the vast majority of PCI procedures. In addition, a variety of other techniques and therapies are used in PCI.

Prior to the use of intracoronary stenting, coronary interventional technique was primarily limited to PTCA. Sometimes referred to as *plain old balloon angioplasty,* PTCA is a catheter-based procedure in which a balloon is inflated at the site of coronary stenosis to increase the vessel lumen diameter. Balloon inflation causes plaque rupture and disruption of the endothelium (see Figure 6-3). PTCA has two primary limitations: acute vessel closure and restenosis. Prior to stents, the acute closure rate during PTCA was approximately 5%, and the 6-month restenosis rate was 35% to 45% (Braunwald et al., 2002). The risk for acute vessel closure made it necessary for standby of a CABG team in case emergency CABG was needed.

Interventional Devices and Adjunct Therapy

Cutting Balloons

Special cutting balloons are now available that can be used to make incisions into the plaque prior to dilatation. This technique allows for greater plaque compression in lesions resistant to balloon dilatation (Deelstra, 2005).

Intracoronary Stenting

The first U.S. Food and Drug Administration (FDA) approval for an intracoronary stent occurred in 1993 (Deelstra, 2005). Both stent design and the associated pharmacology with stent use have improved significantly since that time. Stenting and the use of GP IIb/IIIa antiplatelet therapy have made PCI a safer procedure and have also contributed to substantially improved outcomes. Stenting involves the placement of a metal scaffold-type structure to help prevent elastic recoil and to keep open the lumen of the vessel. Stents can be made from various metals and have different structural designs. Most stents are delivered and expanded with the use of a balloon system (see Figure 6-4). Self-expanding stents are also available. After a stent is deployed and expanded, a high-pressure balloon is typically used to assure that the stent is fully deployed.

FIGURE 6-3: BALLOON INFLATION CAUSING PLAQUE DISRUPTION DURING PTCA

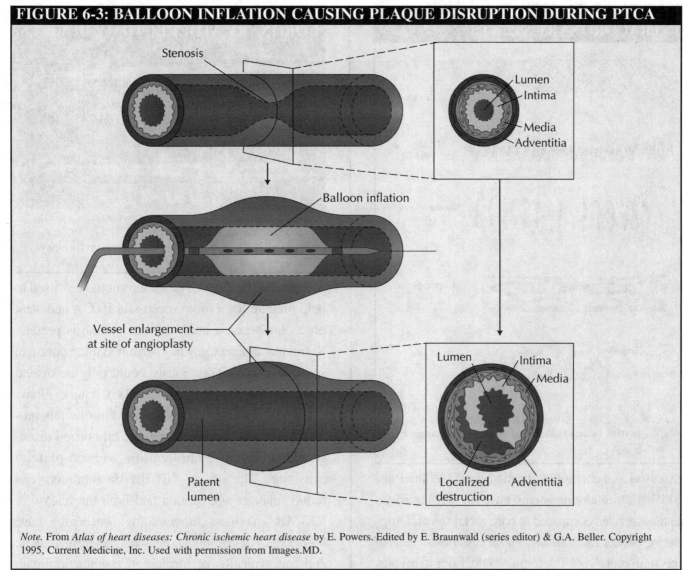

Note. From *Atlas of heart diseases: Chronic ischemic heart disease* by E. Powers. Edited by E. Braunwald (series editor) & G.A. Beller. Copyright 1995, Current Medicine, Inc. Used with permission from Images.MD.

Stenting reduces the risk of acute vessel closure, which can lead to STEMI. Intracoronary stents have also reduced the need for emergency CABG by preventing and treating dissections caused by balloon inflation. Stenting also reduces the percentage of late vessel restenosis. Stents impact restenosis by decreasing the elastic recoil of the vessel and also by decreasing the remodeling that occurs after vessel injury associated with PTCA. Stenting with bare metal stents reduces restenosis rates to approximately 20% to 30% (Deelstra, 2005). With the use of intracoronary stenting, results in patients older than age 75 are similar to those of younger patients (Smith et al., 2001).

Drug-Eluting Stents

Stents coated with pharmacological agents aimed at decreasing restenosis have been FDA-approved since 2003 (Deelstra, 2005). Two pharmacological agents are currently used with drug eluting stents: sirolimus and paclitaxel. Currently, two stents are approved to deliver these agents. Only one agent is coated per stent. Both agents are used to specifically prevent in-stent restenosis. Sirolimus is an immunosuppressive agent that is also used to prevent organ rejection during kidney transplantation (MedlinePlus, 2005a). This drug reduces cytokine production and inflammation and also inhibits proliferation of smooth cells (Deelstra, 2005). Paclitaxel is an antiproliferative, or antineoplastic agent, that is

FIGURE 6-4: TYPES OF INTRACORONARY STENTS

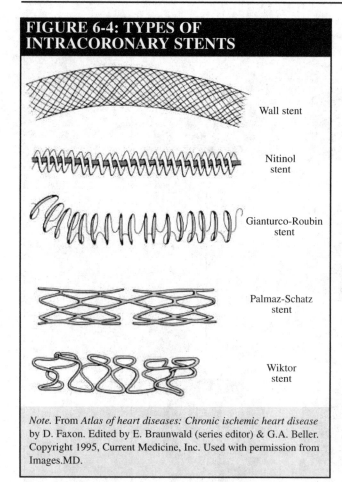

Wall stent

Nitinol stent

Gianturco-Roubin stent

Palmaz-Schatz stent

Wiktor stent

Note. From *Atlas of heart diseases: Chronic ischemic heart disease* by D. Faxon. Edited by E. Braunwald (series editor) & G.A. Beller. Copyright 1995, Current Medicine, Inc. Used with permission from Images.MD.

FIGURE 6-5: DIRECTIONAL CORONARY ATHERECTOMY DEVICES

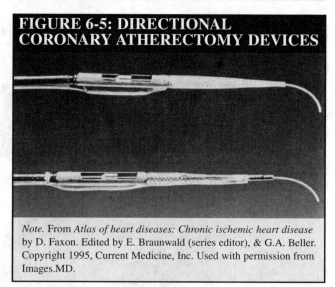

Note. From *Atlas of heart diseases: Chronic ischemic heart disease* by D. Faxon. Edited by E. Braunwald (series editor), & G.A. Beller. Copyright 1995, Current Medicine, Inc. Used with permission from Images.MD.

also used as a chemotherapeutic agent (MedlinePlus, 2005b). Drug-eluting stents have shown improved restenosis rates compared to bare metal stents. Drug-eluting stents have shown initial restenosis rates of approximately 10% (Deelstra, 2005). Long-term outcome data are still needed.

Directional Atherectomy

Directional atherectomy can be used to cut and remove plaque in native vessels or in saphenous vein grafts. A rotating cutter is directed toward the plaque to be removed. Both directional and rotational atherectomy "debulk" coronary arteries containing a large amount of atherosclerotic plaque. Directional atherectomy can be used in calcified lesions. Figure 6-5 displays pictures of devices used for directional coronary atherectomy.

Rotational Atherectomy

Rotational atherectomy involves the use of high-speed rotating blades or burs to remove components of the atherosclerotic plaque. This technique is not used in the presence of acute thrombus. It is used to help prepare for a more successful PTCA and stent procedure when a hard, calcified lesion is present. Rotational atherectomy has permitted intervention in some lesions that previously could only be treated with CABG (Eagle et al., 2004). Creatine kinase (CK)-MB enzymes can be released during this procedure because microparticles are embolized distally. This distal embolization causes platelet activation. The use of GP IIb/IIIa inhibitors can reduce platelet aggregation and limit the release of CK-MB enzymes. Atherectomy procedures have higher rates of complications when performed alone and are typically performed in conjunction with intracoronary stent placement (Smith et al., 2001).

Extraction Techniques

Other atherectomy techniques, such as angiojet thrombectomy and transluminal extraction atherectomy, are used for the extraction of visible thrombi within the coronary artery. An angiojet thrombectomy device works by delivering high-velocity saline jets. The jets are also given retrograde to assist in removal of thrombotic material (Deelstra, 2005). When thrombi are removed prior to intervention, the risk of postprocedure complications may be decreased. These techniques are also proposed to remove degenerative graft material and thrombi commonly seen with saphenous vein graft stenosis.

Laser

With laser techniques, tissue is ablated using a combination of photochemical, thermal, and mechanical effects. These techniques are not widely used. Early results demonstrated increased dissection and perforation with ablative techniques (Deelstra, 2005).

Radiation

Ionizing radiation has also been used to treat in-stent restenosis. Radiation decreases the intimal hyperplasia associated with in-stent restenosis by interfering with smooth cell proliferation. Both gamma and beta radiation have been used. Patients who have undergone radiation treatment need to be on clopidogrel for an extended period because a reduction in neointimal hyperplasia increases the risk of contact between blood and stent material as well as thrombus formation.

Intravascular Ultrasound

With intravascular ultrasound, a miniature ultrasound transducer on the end of catheter provides a cross-sectional image of the coronary artery that can be used to evaluate results in high-risk procedures. This technology can guide assessment of lesions that are difficult to visualize with angiography. Intravascular ultrasound can also be used to assess the quality of lesions, including those that are calcific. It can also be used to guide atherectomy procedures and to assure that intracoronary stents are optimally deployed.

Advantages

Advantages of PCI include low rates of procedure mortality and morbidity. These procedures also take less time to perform and are easier to repeat if needed than is CABG. No general anesthesia, thoracotomy, or cardiopulmonary bypass is required. Patients experience much shorter hospital stays and are able to return to work sooner. Central nervous system complications are also decreased. However, patients must have suitable anatomy to be candidates for PCI. Not all lesions can be reached by a catheter-based technique.

Indications

PCI is performed in a wide range of patients, from stable to unstable and with a varying amounts of myocardium at risk. PCI is more effective than medical treatment in relieving angina (Deedy, 2002). PCI was historically limited to single vessel proximal CHD; however, with newer techniques, the scope of interventional cardiology has expanded. For patients with two vessel disease, PCI is routinely considered an acceptable alternative to surgery. PCI may even be considered in three vessel disease if left ventricular function is normal and the patient is not diabetic.

There is insufficient evidence regarding the mortality benefits of PCI in high-risk patients. Elective PCI is an option for revascularization in patients with normal left ventricular function. However, CABG is recommended for severely symptomatic patients with abnormal left ventricular function (Gibbons et al., 2002). Some evidence shows that CABG improves survival in diabetic patients with three vessel disease (Eagle et al., 2004; Gibbons et al., 2002). However, abciximab, a GP IIb/IIIa inhibitor, has been shown to improve the outcomes of PCI in diabetic patients (Braunwald et al., 2002). Continued advances in PCI may open the door for more PCI procedures in groups of patients who are currently only recommended for CABG.

PCI is not indicated in non-LAD disease except if ischemia is found on noninvasive testing. PCI is also not performed on lesions with less than 60% stenosis unless ischemia is found on noninvasive testing. Many patients with chronic angina undergo PCI for control of symptoms, even though there may be no associated survival benefit. As with all medical decisions, physician judgment and, often, patient preferences play an important role in treatment decisions.

Success Rates

Success of PCI procedures is typically defined in four different ways: angiographic success, procedural success, clinical success, and long-term success. These definitions are listed in Table 6-1.

With the use of stents and GP IIb/IIIa inhibitors, angiographic success rates with PCI are as high as 99% (Smith et al., 2001). Results of PCI are similar in patients presenting with either stable or unstable angina. The limiting factor for long-term success with PCI continues to be restenosis. The majority of restenosis occurs during the 3- to 6-month period after the procedure. It is unusual for restenosis to occur after 12 months (Smith et al., 2001). Bare metal stents help eliminate the elastic recoil associated with restenosis, and drug-eluting stents show promise of greatly impacting the neointimal hyperplasia that still limits long-term success. However, the use of drug-eluting stents is new, and long-term outcomes have not yet been evaluated. Other patient factors that affect long-term success include age, left ventricular function, diabetes, and the presence of diffuse, small, or multivessel disease. Many patients with these factors are referred for CABG.

Complications

Major hospital complications from PCI include death, periprocedural MI, the need for emergency CABG, stroke, renal failure, significant bleeding, and major vascular complications. Significant bleeding is defined as a greater than 3.0 g/dl decrease in hemoglobin level or bleeding that results in transfusion or extended length of stay (Smith, et al., 2001). Nurses play an important role in assessing for vascular complications after the procedure. Vascular complications can include:

- occlusion of the artery at the site of access

- vessel dissection (splitting and separation of arterial layers) at the site of entry

- arteriovenous fistula (connection between artery and vein) at the site of entry

- pseudoaneurysm (dilatation of the artery) at the site of entry.

A retroperitoneal bleed resulting from a large hematoma in the retroperitoneum can be potentially life-threatening. Patients typically experience lumbar pain, hypotension, and a drop in hematocrit. A computed tomography (CT) scan is performed to confirm the diagnosis. The patient is treated with IV fluids and blood transfusion, and surgical repair of the artery may also be needed.

Interventional patients are at increased risk for hemorrhagic and ischemic embolic stroke. Hemorrhagic stroke results from the anticoagulation therapy used during the procedure. A more common complication, however, is ischemic stroke, which is caused by plaque embolization during the procedure.

The use of contrast agents during PCI increases the risk of renal insufficiency and renal failure after the procedure. Patients with existing renal insuffi-

TABLE 6-1: PCI SUCCESS

Term	Definition
Angiographic success	Substantial enlargement of the vessel lumen at the site of intervention; less than 20% residual stenosis
Procedural success	Angiographic success + Freedom from major hospital complications
Clinical success	Angiographic success + Procedural success + Relief from signs and symptoms of ischemia
Long-term success	Clinical success for longer than 6 months

(Smith et al. 2001)

ciency, the elderly, and those with diabetes are at highest risk for renal complications with PCI. It is important that high-risk patients are well hydrated with normal saline solution prior to, during, and after PCI. Careful use of contrast agents to avoid any over-use during the procedure is also important in pre-venting renal complications. Diabetic patients who are taking metformin need to have the agent held prior to and after the procedure. Contrast-induced nephropathy can produce temporary or permanent renal dysfunction. The definition of post-PCI renal failure includes creatinine greater than 2.0 mg/dl, a greater than 50% increase in baseline creatinine, or the need for dialysis (Smith et al., 2001).

Distal microembolization during an interven-tion can result in postprocedure chest pain and a small rise in cardiac enzymes. Chest pain from embolization of microparticles is usually transient and lessens with time. There is an increased risk for embolization from larger debris during PCI with acute thrombus, saphenous vein graft PCI, and rota-tional atherectomy (Deelstra, 2005). The risk of acute and subacute (1 to 2 days postprocedure) stent thrombosis has been reduced with improved tech-niques for stent deployment and aggressive use of antiplatelet therapy. Although these remain very serious complications, they occur in only approxi-mately 1% of patients (Deelstra, 2005).

Additional complications that can occur during the procedure include spasm and vessel perforation. Spasm is most common during rotational atherecto-my and is treated with intracoronary nitroglycerin. Vessel perforation is rare but can be a very serious complication. When perforation occurs, a balloon is inflated in an attempt to stop blood leakage from the perforated site. Specially coated stents are also used to tack up the vessel wall. If too much blood is lost, tam-ponade can occur. Pericardiocentsis may be indicated.

Special Circumstances

Emergency PCI

Emergency PCI can usually be performed with-out additional cardiac assistive devices. If a patient shows signs of hemodynamic instability, has ongoing ischemia, or is in cardiogenic shock, an intra-aortic balloon pump is inserted to provide cardiac support and improve outcomes. Patients who are in cardio-genic shock and have severely depressed left ventric-ular function may be placed on full cardiopulmonary support during emergency PCI. Emergency PCI is ideally performed in a setting with onsite surgical backup. If performed in a facility with no onsite sur-gical backup, there should be the ability to transfer the patient to a cardiac OR within 1 hour (Smith et al., 2001). Emergency PCI as a reperfusion strategy dur-ing an acute MI should be done within 90 minutes from contact with Emergency Medical Services (Antman et al., 2004). Primary PCI is superior to fib-rinolytic therapy when reperfusion can be achieved within 90 minutes by an experienced operator. If a fibrinolytic is given and is not successful, then PCI is indicated. PCI is termed *rescue* or *salvage* when it is performed after failed fibrinolytic therapy in a patient who is actively ischemic.

Emergency PCI is also beneficial in reducing mortality in patients who develop cardiogenic shock as an early complication of acute MI. PCI is not beneficial when cardiogenic shock is the result of a mechanical complication, such as papillary muscle or septal rupture.

Vein Graft Stenosis after CABG

Patients with acute graft closure (vein graft or arterial conduit) within 30 days of surgery usually have successful PCI to the focal area of stenosis. PCI across suture lines has been accomplished safely within 10 days of surgery (Smith et al., 2001).

Vein graft disease can produce very serious and unstable lesions. It can be caused by hyperplasia or atherosclerosis. Vein grafts are at a particularly high risk for developing brittle plaques and thrombotic occlusions. These lesions are very complex.

Patients with late vein graft stenosis (longer than 5 years after surgery) in a graft supplying the LAD and patients with more than one stenotic vein graft generally need reoperation (Eagle et al., 2004; Smith et al., 2001). Vein graft stenosis that occurs within 5 years from the time of surgery may be able to be effectively treated with PCI. Unfortunately, the use GP IIb/IIIa inhibitors has failed to substantially improve results of PCI for vein graft stenosis (Smith et al., 2001). Ischemia that occurs more than 1 year after CABG can represent new stenosis within the graft or new native vessel disease.

One of the challenges of PCI for vein graft stenosis is the unique brittle nature of the plaques, which can cause embolization of graft material. Extraction devices to remove thrombi prior to intervention have been helpful in preventing distal embolization. In addition, devices have been developed to catch this debris and protect the patient from distal embolization. Distal protection devices include balloons or filters that are deployed distal to the site of intervention to collect debris that dislodges during the procedure. The goal is to prevent small amounts of myocardial damage that can occur due to distal embolization.

Medications Before, During, and After PCI

Aspirin should be given prior to PCI. Patients coming in for elective procedures should be instructed to take aspirin at home. Oral hypoglycemic agents are usually withheld the morning of the procedure because of the patient's nothing-by-mouth (NPO) status. Metformin should be held for 24 to 38 hours prior to the procedure and should continue to be held after the procedure because of the potential for renal toxicity.

LMWH can be used in patients undergoing PCI if it is held the morning of the procedure. If the patient is going to have the procedure done more

than 8 hours from the holding of the dose, UFH can be started to maintain adequate anticoagulation before the procedure. UFH is the anticoagulant of choice during PCI. A GP IIb/IIIa inhibitor is also typically initiated during the procedure and continued for several hours after the procedure. If a GP IIb/IIIa is used during the procedure, then UFH dosages are lowered.

Additional antiplatelet therapy is initiated during and continued after the procedure as well. Typically, 300 mg or higher of clopidogrel are given as a loading dose, during or immediately after the procedure. Clopidogrel is continued at 75 mg per day for 1 to 12 months, or longer, after the procedure. Clopidogrel is continued for a minimum of 1 month in patients with bare metal stents and for a period of 3 to 6 months in patients with drug-eluting stents (Smith et al., 2001). Folic acid is also commonly prescribed after stenting to help reduce restenosis (Deedy, 2002).

Before the procedure, it is important to assess for allergy to iodine-based contrast agents. If a patient has never been exposed to an iodine-based contrast agent, assess for allergy to shellfish because many contain organic iodine. If a patient has an iodine allergy, he or she will be premedicated with steroids and antihistamines to avoid an anaphylactic reaction.

Intraprocedure Care

Patients normally receive conscious sedation. Arterial access is achieved with sheath insertion, most typically via the femoral artery. If the femoral artery cannot be accessed, then the radial or brachial artery can be used. Common procedure technique involves the threading of a guidewire across the lesion, followed by the advancement of the interventional device over the guidewire. Heparin is typically the anticoagulant used during the procedure to avoid thrombotic complications associated with the insertion of foreign devices. Bedside activated clotting times are monitored during the procedure to assure the appropriate level of anticoagulation.

Ischemia from balloon inflation may cause or increase arrhythmias during the procedure.

Postprocedure Nursing Care

A major focus of postprocedure nursing care is the prevention of complications related to the vascular access site. The arterial sheath is generally removed 4 to 6 hours after the procedure if a vascular closure device is not used. Upon return to the nursing unit, bedside activated clotting times are drawn until they return to acceptable levels and the arterial sheath can be safely removed. After the arterial access sheath is removed, hemostasis is a priority. Hemostasis can be achieved with manual pressure, the use of a C-clamp, or the use of a commercial compression device. Pressure is applied for a minimum of 20 minutes to achieve hemostasis.

Vasovagal response is a potential complication of arterial sheath removal. Hypotension, bradycardia, diaphoresis, nausea, and vomiting can also occur. This response is triggered by pain and anxiety associated with the sheath removal process. If the patient is hypovolemic, the response is exaggerated. Treatment involves fluids, atropine and, whenever possible, the elimination of pain and anxiety.

If a vascular closure device is used, the arterial sheath is removed in the interventional laboratory. The most common vascular closure devices in use are VasoSeal or AngioSeal, Duett, and Perclose. The VasoSeal and AngioSeal devices work by injecting collagen and inducing thrombus formation. The Duett works by using a combination of both collagen and thrombin. Perclose is a different type of closure device that uses absorbable sutures to close the access site (Deelstra, 2005). The benefits of vascular closure devices include improved patient comfort and earlier ambulation. Associated risks of these devices include infection, bleeding from the site, and leg ischemia, which can potentially result in the need for vascular surgery (Deelstra, 2005).

After arterial sheath removal, the access site should be frequently assessed for external bleeding or development of a hematoma.

Clinical Application
Patients should be instructed to immediately report any feeling of warmth or moisture, which may indicate bleeding, and any new burning at the insertion site, which commonly accompanies the development of a hematoma.

Pressure is applied to treat bleeding or hematoma formation that occurs after arterial sheath removal. Most hematomas are self-limiting and resolve without further treatment. In addition, nurses must frequently assess for other potential vascular complications, such as thrombosis at the access site. Access site thrombosis can cause vessel occlusion. Nursing assessment includes frequent pulse, pain, and sensation checks to the area distal from the insertion site. After sheath removal, these assessments are typically done every 15 minutes for the first hour and then with decreasing frequency if the patient remains free from complications.

The clinical trial Standards of Angioplasty Nursing Techniques to Diminish Bleeding Around the Groin (SANDBAG) found the following nursing interventions effective in preventing postprocedure groin bleeding:

* nurse-to-patient ratio of 1:1.5 or less during the sheath removal process

* prompt removal of the sheath within 4 to 6 hours of the procedure

* patient comfort measures, including pain medication and head of bed elevation to 30 degrees

* avoidance of a sandbag, which has been shown not to decrease bleeding but to increase discomfort

* patient ambulation 8 hours after sheath removal. (Deelstra, 2005)

Adequate hydration both preprocedure and postprocedure is an important component to preventing renal complications related to contrast administration. NPO status prior to the procedure increases the importance of IV hydration. Assessment of blood urea nitrogen and creatinine levels is important in the postprocedure evaluation. Whenever possible, nephrotoxic drugs should be held for 48 hours prior to and after PCI. Examples of common nephrotoxic drugs include metformin, NSAIDs, and some antibiotics. Metformin is important because diabetic patients have an increased risk of developing postprocedure nephropathy.

Post-PCI patients should also be monitored for recurrent ischemia. The ST-segment should be monitored in the leads evaluating the vessel receiving intervention. Many patients are cared for in specialized postinterventional units. Uncomplicated patients who undergo elective procedures are discharged within 24 hours. Patients with PCI during an acute MI have extended stays that vary based on the amount of myocardial damage.

Postdischarge Instructions

Elective PCI patients are generally discharged the day after the procedure, limiting time during the inpatient hospital stay for patient education regarding risk factor reduction. Patients should be encouraged to participate in outpatient cardiac rehabilitation programs so they can receive the same education and support for risk factor modification as those who have had surgery. Place special emphasis on the importance of risk reduction to manage disease progression in these patients.

Clinical Application

PCI has a shorter recovery period and does not provide the long-term reminder of a midsternal scar. For this reason, PCI patients may minimize the importance of their CHD and their future risk. It is important that they fully understand that PCI does not treat the underlying disease process and that aggressive risk reduction is critical in managing the underlying disease.

TRANSMYOCARDIAL LASER REVASCULARIZATION

Transmyocardial laser revascularization (TMLR) is limited to patients who have angina refractory to maximal medical treatment and who are not candidates for other forms of revascularization. Patients who are candidates for this surgery but not other forms of revascularization usually have very diffuse small vessel disease. During this procedure, a series of transmural endomyocardial channels are created with lasers to improve myocardial blood supply. These channels are created on the epicardial surface and go through to the endocardium. The typical number of channels ranges from 20 to 40, with the size of the channels approximately 1 mm wide. The physiology behind the treatment is more complex than simply creating channels for oxygenated blood to flow from the endocardium up through the myocardium to the epicardium. Two theories are proposed regarding the mechanism of action: 1) The laser treatment stimulates angiogenesis and causes improvement in regional blood flow to the ischemic area of myocardium, and 2) The laser treatment creates denervation of the myocardium and an improvement of symptoms (Bridges et al., 2004).

TMLR has been effective in improving anginal symptoms, functional capacity, and quality of life. This procedure is typically done in the cardiac surgery suite as a standalone surgery, or it can be done with CABG when not all ischemic areas can be reached by grafting. Percutaneous options are currently being investigated.

CONCLUSION

Advancements continue to improve the safety and outcomes associated with CABG and PCI revascularization options. These advancements improve treatment options and outcomes for patients with CHD.

Interventional cardiologists and thoracic surgeons are also coming together in some situations to complement each other and perform hybrid revascularization procedures. An example of a hybrid revascularization procedure is a left internal mamary artery to the LAD via a MIDCAB, and additional interventional techniques to the RCA and circumflex arteries. The major challenge to hybrid procedures is timing. Antiplatelet therapy, including clopidogrel, which is a standard part of post-PCI treatment for at least 30 days is also held for several days prior to elective CABG procedures.

With the increasing elderly population, the number of revascularization procedures continues to increase. The impact of nursing on the care of these patients before, during, and after these procedures is important. Revascularization does not alter the underlying disease process; therefore, patient education and risk factor reduction remain key nursing elements in all settings.

EXAM QUESTIONS

CHAPTER 6
Questions 46-53

46. The patient who would be a good candidate for CABG is

    a. a patient with 90% left main occlusion.

    b. a patient with less than 50% LAD occlusion and less than 50% circumflex occlusion.

    c. a patient with an RCA lesion with normal left ventricular function.

    d. a patient with very diffuse and very small vessel disease.

47. The term OPCAB refers to

    a. the use of thoracotomy instead of sternotomy.

    b. patients who are fast tracked to be discharged in less than 5 days.

    c. CABG surgery without the use of cardiopulmonary bypass.

    d. combination open heart surgery and percutaneous procedure.

48. Which patient in the following list is at high risk for an adverse neurovascular complication after CABG?

    a. A previously healthy 50-year-old woman undergoing cardiopulmonary bypass.

    b. A patient with an atherosclerotic aorta undergoing cardiopulmonary bypass.

    c. A patient undergoing OPCAB.

    d. A 67-year-old man having a MIDCAB to the LAD with no known history of hypertension.

49. A characteristic of a fast-track pathway after CABG would include

    a. extubation by the third postop day.

    b. anticipated discharge between postop days 7 and 8.

    c. liberal use of opioid medications to increase patient comfort during the ventilator weaning process.

    d. a defined medication strategy to prevent postoperative atrial fibrillation.

50. The primary limitation of PCI as a revascularization option in the treatment of coronary heart disease (CHD) is

    a. restenosis.

    b. cost.

    c. lack of trained physicians.

    d. patient preference.

51. Recent advances in PCI that have improved safety and long-term outcomes include

    a. beta-blocker and calcium channel blocker administration to relax coronary arteries and improve blood flow immediately after the procedure.

    b. permanent implantable radiation to prevent stents from developing initial restenosis.

    c. the use of an IABP prior to all procedures.

    d. intracoronary stents and GP IIb/IIIa inhibitors.

52. Key nursing interventions immediately after PCI include

    a. assessing for vascular complications and assuring adequate hydration.

    b. monitoring blood sugar level every hour for 4 hours.

    c. limiting fluids and holding all medications for 6 hours after the procedure.

    d. performing range-of-motion on the affected extremity to avoid vascular complications.

53. Key patient education and discharge planning principles after revascularization include

    a. assuring patients that there will be no activity restrictions after discharge.

    b. assuring patients that they no longer have CHD.

    c. informing patients that aggressive risk factor modification is necessary to manage their underlying CHD.

    d. informing patients that it is normal to continue to have angina after revascularization.

CHAPTER 7

HEART FAILURE

CHAPTER OBJECTIVE

After reading this chapter, the reader will be able to describe current strategies for the management of heart failure.

LEARNING OBJECTIVES

After studying this chapter, the reader will be able to

1. define the clinical syndrome of heart failure and the hallmark manifestations of the syndrome.

2. describe the difference in pathophysiology between systolic and diastolic dysfunction.

3. explain the most common cause of heart failure.

4. describe two neurohormonal responses to heart failure that produce negative end results over time.

5. describe the one positive neurohormonal response in heart failure.

6. define the two classifications of medications used to slow progression of left ventricular remodeling and heart failure disease progression.

7. describe two nonpharmacologic treatments for heart failure.

8. describe key nursing considerations regarding patient education in heart failure patients.

INTRODUCTION

Understanding heart failure and its management is very important in cardiovascular nursing. Approximately 5 million Americans live with heart failure today, and 550,000 new cases are diagnosed annually. Moreover, 300,000 patients die each year of heart-failure related causes. Once diagnosed with heart failure, approximately 50% of patients die within 5 years (Hunt et al., 2005). Heart failure is the single most common cause of hospitalization in the United States for people older than age 65, and one third of hospitalized patients are readmitted within 90 days due to further decompensation (Hobbs & Boyle, 2004). In addition, another 20 million people with asymptomatic cardiac impairment are likely to develop heart failure symptoms within a 5-year period (Laurent, 2005).

The increasing number of people with heart failure is attributed to several factors, including the aging population, improved short-term survival of myocardial infarction (MI) patients (placing this group in the high-risk category for development of heart failure in the future), and an increased awareness of heart failure and established guidelines, resulting in increased diagnosis and management of the syndrome (Hunt et al., 2005).

Definition

Heart failure is a complex clinical syndrome that can result from any cardiac disorder that impairs the ability of the ventricle to either fill properly or eject optimally. This syndrome results in a pathologic state in which the heart is unable to pump enough oxygenated blood to meet the metabolic needs of the body.

Patients with heart failure present with one or both of the hallmark manifestations:

1. dyspnea and fatigue, which may impact exercise tolerance

2. extracellular fluid (ECF) retention, which can cause peripheral edema and pulmonary congestion.

(Hunt et al., 2005)

Patients may have only one of the two manifestations of heart failure at any given time. For this reason, the term "heart failure" is more accurate than "congestive heart failure." With either dyspnea and fatigue or ECF retention, the patient's functional capacity and quality of life are affected.

CLINICAL PRESENTATION

Most patients with heart failure present with decreased exercise tolerance due to dyspnea or fatigue. Because these presenting symptoms are non-specific, many patients are not readily diagnosed with heart failure. These symptoms are sometimes attributed to deconditioning associated with the aging process. Many heart failure patients also have coexisting conditions, such as pulmonary disease, that contribute to exercise intolerance. These coexisting conditions make differential diagnosis challenging.

Symptom assessment is more difficult in elderly patients. Many elderly do not experience exertional dyspnea because they have developed more sedentary lifestyles to accommodate their decreased functional capacity.

Clinical Application

When assessing for exertional dyspnea, remember to do so within the context of the patient's activity level. The nurse must not only ask the patient about dyspnea with exertion but must also assess the degree to which the patient has been exerting himself or herself. A patient who sits in chair for the majority of the day may not present with the same complaint of dyspnea on exertion as a patient attempting to complete activities of daily living (ADLs).

Patients may also present with ECF overload, manifested as peripheral edema or abdominal swelling. Anorexia commonly accompanies abdominal swelling. Additional findings during a physical exam that indicate fluid overload are the presence of a third heart sound (S_3) and jugular venous distention. Patients with pulmonary congestion present with dyspnea on exertion, orthopnea, and paroxysmal nocturnal dyspnea. Pulmonary congestion usually occurs when the ventricle rapidly fails. Many patients with left ventricular end-stage heart failure have no signs of pulmonary congestion. Regardless of initial presentation, progressive changes in symptoms over time are common to most heart failure patients.

ETIOLOGY

A variety of cardiac disorders can cause heart failure, but the most common cause is left ventricular dysfunction (Hobbs & Boyle, 2004; Hunt et al., 2005). The most common cause of left ventricular dysfunction is ischemic coronary heart disease (CHD), followed by hypertension. The American Heart Association (AHA) reports that up to 75% of patients with heart failure have hypertension (Hunt et al., 2005). Because coronary heart disease (CHD) and hypertension increase the risk of heart failure, strategies to reduce risk and control disease progression in these disorders are also key in reducing heart failure risk.

Other causes of left ventricular dysfunction include:

- valvular disease

- thyroid disease

- viral infection

- alcohol abuse

- idiopathic (no known cause).

When a patient presents with heart failure syndrome and left ventricular dysfunction is suspected or identified, the following questions can help determine the cause:

- Does the patient have a history of ischemic CHD or associated risk factors, including diabetes, hypertension, hyperlipidemia, or peripheral vascular disease?

- Does the patient have a history or evidence of valvular heart disease?

- Has the patient been exposed to chest irradiation or had any exposure to cardiotoxic agents?

- Does the patient's lifestyle involve any illicit drug or excessive alcohol use?

- Does the patient have a family history of idiopathic cardiomyopathy or unexplained, sudden cardiac death?

- Is there any suspicion for noncardiac causes, such as:
    - hyperthyroidism
    - infectious process
    - collagen vascular disorder
    - pheochromocytoma?

(Hunt et al., 2005)

INITIAL EVALUATION OF HEART FAILURE PATIENTS

Recommendations from the American College of Cardiology (ACC) and AHA Guidelines for the Management of Heart Failure include:

1. thorough history and physical examination to identify cardiac and noncardiac conditions that contribute to the development and acceleration of heart failure

2. initial and ongoing assessment of functional capacity based on the patient's ability to perform routine ADLs

3. initial and ongoing assessment of fluid volume status

4. initial electrocardiogram (ECG) and chest radiogram

5. initial two-dimensional echocardiogram with Doppler to assess the function of the left ventricle

6. initial lab work evaluation, including complete blood count, electrolytes, blood urea nitrogen, creatinine, blood glucose, thyroid-stimulating hormone, liver function studies, and urinalysis.

Because of the high association between ischemic CHD and heart failure, most patients with chest pain of unknown etiology, presenting with the clinical syndrome of heart failure also undergo cardiac catheterization (Hobbs & Boyle, 2004; Hunt et al., 2005).

PATHOPHYSIOLOGY

The AHA/ACC staging system (see Table 7-1) classifies heart failure as a progressive disorder. In this model of progression, left ventricular dysfunction begins with an initial insult to the myocardium. Even without further identifiable insults, left ventricular dysfunction continues to progress.

Left ventricular dysfunction can range from predominantly diastolic dysfunction to predominantly systolic dysfunction. Patients with heart failure can also have a combination of both systolic and diastolic dysfunction. Patients with combined systolic and diastolic dysfunction have a worse prognosis than those with isolated systolic or diastolic dysfunction (Hobbs & Boyle, 2004).

TABLE 7-1: STAGES OF HEART FAILURE

Stage A	Stage B	Stage C	Stage D
• High risk of developing heart failure • No identified structural or functional abnormalities • No signs or symptoms of heart failure	• Presence of structural heart disease strongly associated with development of heart failure • No signs or symptoms of heart failure	• Past or present symptoms of heart failure associated with underlying structural heart failure	• Advanced structural heart disease **Specialized interventions required** • Marked symptoms of heart failure at rest despite maximal medical therapy

(Hunt et al., 2005)

Systolic Dysfunction

In predominant systolic dysfunction, ejection is a problem. With substantial dilatation of the ventricle, reduced wall motion occurs and the heart is unable to contract effectively (see Figure 7-1). The patient's ejection fraction (percent of blood the ventricle ejects per beat relative to the total amount of blood in the ventricle) decreases. A normal ejection fraction is greater than or equal to 55%. An ejection fraction less than 40% percent generally defines systolic dysfunction (Laurent, 2005). Systolic dysfunction is found in two thirds of patients with heart failure (Hunt et al., 2005). Patients with systolic dysfunction also have low cardiac output. As a result, left ventricular end-diastolic volume (preload) increases, leading to pulmonary congestion.

Dilated cardiomyopathy (ischemic or idiopathic) is a common cause of systolic dysfunction. However, cardiomyopathy should not be used interchangeably with systolic heart failure. Cardiomyopathy is a structural disorder associated with the development of heart failure, but heart failure is a clinical syndrome characterized by the presentation of certain symptoms. Cardiomyopathy is discussed in detail in the next chapter.

FIGURE 7-1: LEFT VENTRICULAR SYSTOLIC DYSFUNCTION

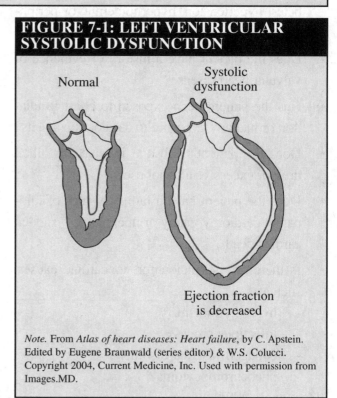

Normal

Systolic dysfunction

Ejection fraction is decreased

Note. From *Atlas of heart diseases: Heart failure*, by C. Apstein. Edited by Eugene Braunwald (series editor) & W.S. Colucci. Copyright 2004, Current Medicine, Inc. Used with permission from Images.MD.

Diastolic Dysfunction

The remaining one third of patients with the clinical syndrome of heart failure have predominant diastolic dysfunction. In predominant diastolic dysfunction the ventricle is not dilated and ejection fraction remains within normal limits. In diastolic dysfunction, however, the ventricle has impaired relaxation and does not fill properly. Diastolic dysfunction is commonly associated with chronic systemic hypertension and left ventricular hypertrophy. The aging process affects the elastic properties of the heart. In particular, elderly women are at high risk for diastolic dysfunction. Ischemic heart disease and restrictive or hypertrophic cardiomyopathy can also cause diastolic dysfunction. In these conditions, the ventricle can become stiff or noncompliant. A noncompliant ventricle is unable to completely relax during diastole, impairing filling (see Figure 7-2).

FIGURE 7-2: LEFT VENTRICULAR DIASTOLIC DYSFUNCTION

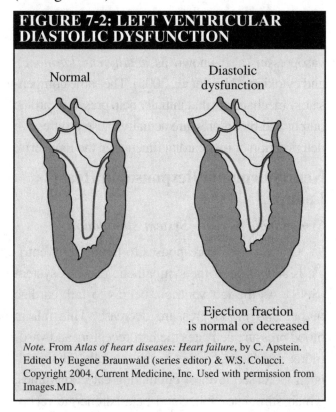

Note. From *Atlas of heart diseases: Heart failure*, by C. Apstein. Edited by Eugene Braunwald (series editor) & W.S. Colucci. Copyright 2004, Current Medicine, Inc. Used with permission from Images.MD.

In diastolic dysfunction, end-diastolic pressures are elevated; however, volumes remain low to normal. To increase diastolic filling, the pressure in the left atria increases. When increased left atrial pressure rises above the pressure in the pulmonary capillaries, pulmonary edema can result. Patients with diastolic dysfunction commonly become symptomatic with exertion when heart rate is increased. When heart rate is increased, ventricular filling time is reduced. Increased levels of circulating catecholamines also increase heart rate and worsen diastolic dysfunction.

Three conditions are required for diagnosis of diastolic dysfunction: 1) signs and symptoms of heart failure, 2) normal or only slightly decreased ejection fraction, 3) increased diastolic filling pressure and abnormal relaxation of the left ventricle (Hunt et al., 2005). For practical purposes, the diagnosis of diastolic heart failure is made in patients presenting with the clinical syndrome of heart failure with no evidence of systolic dysfunction. Table 7-2 summarizes the comparison between systolic and diastolic heart failure. Figure 7-3 compares the concentric hypertrophy of diastolic heart failure with the eccentric hypertrophy of systolic heart failure. Remember that patients can have coexisting systolic and diastolic dysfunction.

Echocardiography

Two-dimensional echocardiography with Doppler flow studies is the most frequently used diagnostic test in evaluating patients with the clinical syndrome of heart failure. A noninvasive, cost-effective diagnostic tool, the echocardiogram can identify systolic and diastolic dysfunction, including a measurement of ejection fraction. When systolic dysfunction is identified, the echocardiogram

TABLE 7-2: SUMMARY COMPARISON OF SYSTOLIC AND DIASTOLIC DYSFUNCTION

Systolic dysfunction	Two thirds of heart failure patients	Decreased left ventricular contractility and ejection fraction	Most common cause is CHD resulting in myocardial infarction or chronic ischemia
Diastolic dysfunction	One third of heart failure patients	Impaired left ventricular relaxation and abnormal filling	Usually related to chronic hypertension or ischemic heart disease

FIGURE 7-3: COMPARISON OF CONCENTRIC HYPERTROPHY OF DIASTOLIC DYSFUNCTION AND ECCENTRIC HYPERTROPHY OF SYSTOLIC DYSFUNCTION

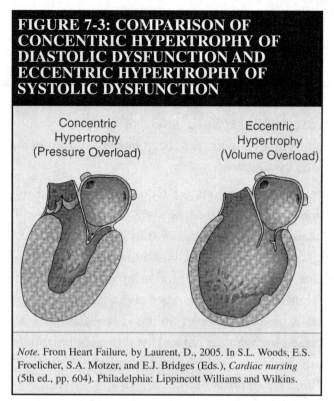

Concentric Hypertrophy (Pressure Overload)

Eccentric Hypertrophy (Volume Overload)

Note. From Heart Failure, by Laurent, D., 2005. In S.L. Woods, E.S. Froelicher, S.A. Motzer, and E.J. Bridges (Eds.), *Cardiac nursing* (5th ed., pp. 604). Philadelphia: Lippincott Williams and Wilkins.

can assist in determining the etiology. Regional wall-motion abnormalities indicate ischemic CHD as the cause, whereas global dysfunction indicates a nonischemic origin. An echocardiogram can also identify other causes of heart failure, such as valvular or pericardial disease. Although an echocardiogram can provide essential information regarding the possible cause of heart failure, it cannot identify the exact cause.

Left and Right Ventricular Failure

The left and right ventricles are part of a closed circulatory system. Right ventricular failure usually results from prolonged left ventricular failure. Isolated right ventricular failure can occur with right ventricular MI, pulmonary hypertension, or chronic severe tricuspid regurgitation. Signs of right ventricular heart failure include weight gain, jugular venous distention, peripheral edema, abdominal swelling, and hepatomegaly.

Neurohormonal Responses to a Failing Heart

Neurohormonal responses are the body's response to decreased cardiac output and poor organ perfusion. Initially, these responses are helpful in improving cardiac output and organ perfusion. Over time, however, these responses actually lead to clinical deterioration. Several neurohormonal responses have been identified in the progression of left ventricular dysfunction. Among the most important and well-understood of these responses are sympathetic nervous system stimulation and activation of the renin-angiotensin-aldosterone system (RAAS).

Other neurohormonal responses to heart failure include increased circulating levels of endothelin, vasopressin (also known as *antidiuretic hormone*), and cytokines (Hunt et al., 2005). The same compensatory mechanisms that initially help preserve cardiac output and blood pressure actually cause progressive deterioration of myocardial function in the long term.

Neurohormonal Responses in Heart Failure

Sympathetic Nervous System Stimulation

One of the first responses to failing left ventricle is activation of the sympathetic nervous system (SNS). As the left ventricle begins to fail, cardiac output and blood pressure decrease. This fall in blood pressure activates the baroreceptors and vasomotor regulatory centers in the medulla. The result is an increased level of circulating catecholamines, which stimulate alpha- and beta-adrenergic receptors to increase heart rate, increase peripheral vasoconstriction (increase afterload), and increase contractility. In chronic heart failure, beta-receptors are less able to respond to circulating catecholamines. This decreased response to circulating catecholamines is called *beta-receptor down regulation* and is an attempt to protect the failing heart from chronic overstimulation of the SNS (Laurent, 2005). Beta-receptor down regulation contributes to the exercise intolerance associated with heart failure. Chronic stimulation of the SNS also accelerates the ventricular remodeling process.

Increased heart rate, afterload, and contractility not only help maintain cardiac output and blood pressure but also have the negative effect of increasing myocardial oxygen demand. Over time, this increased stimulation of the SNS can worsen ischemia and cause cardiac arrhythmias and even sudden cardiac death. In addition, norepinephrine, one of the circulating catecholamines, has direct cardiotoxic properties (Hobbs & Boyle, 2004). These cardiotoxic properties are responsible for the beta-receptor down regulation seen with chronic heart failure.

Renin-angiotensin-aldosterone System

Activation of the RAAS is another compensatory neurohormonal response to a failing heart. The RAAS is activated as the kidneys respond to decreased renal perfusion. It is also activated by an increase in SNS stimulation. When the RAAS is activated, circulating levels of renin, angiotensin II, and aldosterone increase. Angiotensin II is a potent vasoconstrictor, thus systemic vascular resistance and afterload increase. Aldosterone is a mineralocorticoid responsible for sodium and water retention. When sodium is retained by the body, so is water; therefore, preload increases. Enhanced preload increases end-diastolic volume, which further dilates the ventricles and enhances the ventricular remodeling process. If the left ventricle becomes overstretched, contractility is depressed.

Vasopressin and Endothelin

In chronic heart failure, angiotensin II and osmotic stimuli produce an increase in vasopressin release, causing a reabsorption of water and additional vasoconstriction. Levels of endothelin, an endogenous hormonal vasoconstrictor, are elevated in heart failure in response to angiotensin II, vasopressin, and circulating catecholamines (Laurent, 2005). Figure 7-4 summarizes the neurohormonal responses of the SNS and RAAS.

Clinical Application
Current treatment of heart failure involves inhibition of neurohormonal systems with beta-blockers and angiotensin-converting enzyme (ACE) inhibitors. Patients typically do not understand the neurohormonal blockade associated with these medications or the importance they play in stopping disease progression. If patients think these medications are only used to treat hypertension and their blood pressures are normal, they may be less compliant because they do not fully understand the impact of therapy.

FIGURE 7-4: NEUROHORMONAL RESPONSES OF THE RAAS AND SNS IN HEART FAILURE

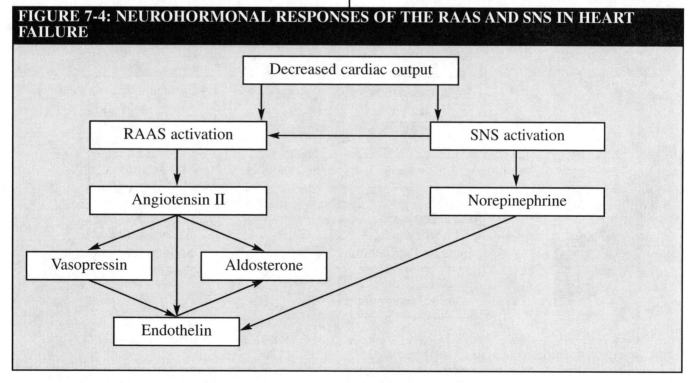

Inflammatory Response

Cytokine levels are also elevated in heart failure, producing both local and systemic inflammatory responses. Local inflammatory responses occur early in the course of the disease; systemic responses occur later in the course. Cytokines promote cell growth (hypertrophy) and cell death (apoptosis) (Laurent, 2005; Opie, 2004). Hypertrophy and apoptosis are seen in the ventricular remodeling process. Figure 7-5 shows the vicious cycle of heart failure caused by uninterrupted neurohormonal responses.

Positive Neurohormonal Response

The release of the hormones atrial natriuretic peptide and brain natriuretic peptide (BNP) from cardiac myocytes is the one beneficial neurohormonal response in heart failure. These hormones have the positive effect of systemic and pulmonary vasodilatation and also enhance sodium and water excretion.

Other neurohormonal responses work to counteract the vasoconstrictive effects of the SNS and RAAS stimulation. However, the vasoconstrictive effects of neurohormonal activation commonly overpower these countereffforts.

Table 7-3 summarizes the results of neurohormonal responses to heart failure.

Left-ventricular Remodeling

Left-ventricular remodeling is another response to the initial left ventricular injury. Remodeling is a process of pathological growth whereby the ventricles hypertrophy and then dilate. Ventricular remodeling occurs due to myocyte hypertrophy in response to either pressure or volume overload in the ventricles. When pressure overload occurs, the myocytes thicken and concentric hypertrophy results. When volume overload occurs, the myocytes elongate and eccentric hypertrophy results (Laurent, 2005; Opie, 2004). Concentric and eccentric hypertrophy are shown in Figure 7-3.

The process of ventricular remodeling is very complex at the cellular level. Concentric hypertrophy causes left-ventricular wall thickening and leads to an increased risk of subendocardial ischemia. Eccentric hypertrophy and eventual

FIGURE 7-5: VICIOUS CYCLE OF NEUROHORMONAL RESPONSES IN HEART FAILURE

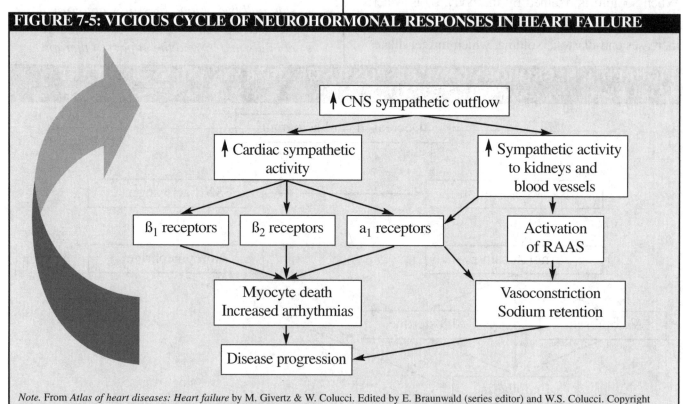

Note. From *Atlas of heart diseases: Heart failure* by M. Givertz & W. Colucci. Edited by E. Braunwald (series editor) and W.S. Colucci. Copyright 2004, Current Medicine, Inc. Used with permission from Images.MD.

TABLE 7-3: SUMMARY OF RESULTS OF NEUROHORMONAL STIMULATION IN HEART FAILURE

SNS	• Stimulation of RAAS and endothelin • Vasoconstriction (increased afterload), increased heart rate, increased contractility • Aggravation of ischemia • Potentiation of arrhythmias • Acceleration of ventricular remodeling • Direct toxicity to cardiac myocytes
RAAS	• Arterial vasoconstriction from angiotensin II • Stimulation of vasopressin and endothelin • Sodium and water retention from increased aldosterone • Endothelial dysfunction from increased aldosterone • Organ fibrosis from increased aldosterone
Vasopressin	• Reabsorption of water • Vasoconstriction
Endothelin	• Vasoconstriction • Fluid retention • Increased contractility • Hypertrophy
Cytokines	• Pro-inflammatory response • Contribution to apoptosis (programmed cell death) • Contribution to cardiac cachexia (systemic inflammatory response)
Natriuretic peptides*	• Systemic and pulmonary vasodilatation • Increased sodium and water excretion • Suppression of other neurohormones
Nitric oxide*, bradykinin*, some prostaglandins*	• Arterial smooth muscle relaxation and vasodilatation

* Neurohormonal response with positive benefit in heart failure

dilatation can cause regurgitation of the mitral valve and elevated left atrial pressures. These effects accelerate the remodeling process.

Another component of ventricular remodeling includes necrosis and apoptosis of cardiac myocytes. Necrosis, accidental cell death, occurs in response to deprivation of oxygen. Apoptosis, programmed cell death, is stimulated by several factors, including angiotensin II and cytokines (Laurent, 2005). Myocyte loss in either form can facilitate slippage of myocytes. In response to slippage, a reparative fibrosis occurs that makes the ventricle stiffer.

This process of ventricular remodeling is complicated by other physiological responses beyond the scope of this chapter. Remodeling is also enhanced by the prolonged activation of the SNS, RAAS, and other neurohormonal responses, including endothelin production (Opie, 2004). In addition to norepinephrine, other substances produced in the activation of neurohormonal responses may have direct cardiotoxic effects.

ONGOING ASSESSMENT IN HEART FAILURE MANAGEMENT

Functional Capacity

The New York Heart Association (NYHA) classification is the most commonly used system to assess functional capacity (see Table 7-4).

Patients classified as NYHA class IV have 20% overall annual mortality (Hunt et al., 2005). The NYHA classification system has limitations due the subjectivity involved in the assessment process. In addition, NYHA functional capacity class assessment does not always progress in a systematic way. Patients can move between classes throughout the progression of their disease. NYHA classifications do not correspond with the ACC/AHA stages of heart failure progression. Other tools that are used to assess functional capacity include the 6-minute walk test,

maximal exercise testing, and peak oxygen consumption (Hobbs & Boyle, 2004; Hunt et al., 2005).

Clinical Application

Because patients commonly decrease their activity levels to adjust to declining functional capacity, it is important to ask specific questions regarding the level of activity the patient is able to tolerate. For example, ask, "Is there any leisure activity you are no longer able to do that you wish you still could do?"

Fluid Volume Status

Several ongoing physical parameters are assessed to determine ECF volume status, including

* weight

* amount of jugular venous distention

* edema of legs, abdomen, sacral area, or scrotum

* presence of organ congestion: hepatomegaly or rales.

The most reliable sign of ECF overload is jugular venous distention (Hunt et al., 2005). Most patients with peripheral edema also have ECF overload; however, peripheral edema also has noncardiac causes. Most patients with compensated chronic heart failure do not have audible rales or crackles in their lung fields on physical examination. Rales or crackles are generally a sign of rapid onset of heart failure.

TABLE 7-4: NEW YORK HEART ASSOCIATION FUNCTIONAL CLASSIFICATIONS

Class I	Class II	Class III	Class IV
Cardiac disease with no resulting limitation on physical activity	Cardiac disease with slight limitation on physical activity	Cardiac disease with marked limitation on physical activity	Cardiac disease resulting in inability to carry out any physical activity without discomfort
Ordinary activity free from fatigue, palpitations, dyspnea, and anginal pain	Comfortable at rest but ordinary activity results in fatigue, palpitations, dyspnea, or anginal pain	Comfortable at rest but less-than-ordinary activity results in fatigue, palpitations, dyspnea, or anginal pain	Possible symptoms of cardiac insufficiency at rest

(Hunt et al., 2001)

Therefore, the absence of pulmonary rales should not be considered an adequate measure of optimal fluid volume status. Short-term assessment of ECF volume status is best measured by a change in daily weight.

Clinical Application

Patients should be instructed to weigh themselves daily first thing in the morning, after urinating, and prior to eating. They should be instructed to use the same scale and wear the same amount of clothing. A weight gain of more than 2 lb in 24 hours or more than 3 lb in a week should be reported to the physician. Keep in mind that 1 lb of weight = 1 pt of fluid.

Many physicians have patients adjust their diuretic doses at home based on daily weights. With the assessment of daily weights and appropriate intervention, ECF volume can be managed on an outpatient basis and many hospital admissions can be avoided.

Laboratory Values

Monitoring potassium levels is particularly important in heart failure patients. Diuretics can cause hypokalemia. Many heart failure patients are also on digoxin, and hypokalemia increases the risk of digoxin toxicity. In contrast, other medications used in the treatment of heart failure, such as ACE inhibitors, angiotensin II receptor blockers (ARBs), and aldosterone antagonists, can predispose patients to hyperkalemia. Patients taking loop diuretics who experience the expected side effect of hypokalemia and who also take one or more medications that can predispose patients to hyperkalemia are unlikely to be ordered potassium supplements.

TREATMENT GOALS IN PATIENTS AT RISK FOR AND WITH HEART FAILURE

The majority of major clinical trials performed have evaluated treatment strategies for systolic dysfunction. Few large-scale clinical trials have evaluated the treatment of isolated diastolic dysfunction. Clinical practice guidelines exist for the treatment of systolic dysfunction; these guidelines are addressed in this section. However, many patients with diastolic dysfunction are on many of the same medications. Treatment goals in diastolic dysfunction aim to control hypertension, heart rate, and blood volume.

Risk Control in Patients with Structural Heart Disease

Once a patient has evidence of structural heart disease, aggressive measures should be put in place to reduce risk. Strict control of blood pressure, both systolic and diastolic, should be maintained in patients with hypertension. Blood pressure targets of less than 130/80 mm Hg should be established for patients with diabetes and renal disease. When combination drug therapy is required to manage hypertension, those medications effective in treating both heart failure and hypertension become the preferred medications. These include diuretics, ACE inhibitors or ARBs, and beta-blockers. Diabetes not only increases the risk of heart failure but also worsens outcomes for those with heart failure. ACE inhibitors have been shown to limit end-organ damage in diabetic patients even if hypertension is not present (U.S. Department of Health and Human Services, 2003). ARBs have also been shown to prevent heart failure in high risk patients, including those with vascular disease, hypertension, and diabetes (Hunt et al., 2005).

Any patient with CHD should have aggressive control of risk factors to decrease the risk of future coronary events and to reduce the risk of heart failure development. Treatment of hyperlipidemia in patients with previous MI has been shown to reduce the risk of heart failure (Braunwald et al., 2002). After an MI, all patients should be started on beta-blockers, and most patients are also started on ACE inhibitors or ARBs. These medications help reduce left ventricular remodeling after MI. Aggressive efforts to reperfuse patients during acute MI are important in preserving myocardial function in the short-term and preventing heart failure in the long-term.

Patients with contributing lifestyle habits, such as smoking, illicit drug use, or excessive alcohol consumption, should be counseled regarding the impact of these habits on the development of heart failure. Coexisting noncardiac disorders, such as thyroid disease, should be treated because untreated tachycardia associated with hyperthyroidism can cause cardiomyopathy.

Treatment in Patients with Asymptomatic Chronic Left Ventricular Systolic Dysfunction

Patients with asymptomatic chronic left ventricular systolic dysfunction should be managed with ACE inhibitors or ARBs, and beta-blockers because these two classifications of medications have been proven to slow the progression of left ventricular dysfunction. There are no data to support the use of digoxin in these patients because digoxin has minimal impact on disease progression (Hunt et al., 2005). Diuretics are not indicated because these patients show no signs or symptoms of fluid overload.

Treatment in Patients with Symptomatic Left Ventricular Dysfunction

Patients with symptomatic left ventricular dysfunction are generally considered as having active heart failure. These patients are managed with ACE inhibitors or ARBs, and beta-blockers to slow disease progression. In addition, they are placed on diuretics and moderate sodium restrictions to control ECF volume status. Daily weight can be used to guide diuret-

ic therapy. Diuretic therapy can also improve symptoms, increase cardiac function, and improve exercise tolerance (Hunt et al., 2005). However, diuretics do not improve survival and may cause renal and metabolic side effects (Hobbs & Boyle, 2004). Patients may also be on digoxin to improve symptoms and exercise tolerance. Physical activity should be encouraged in all heart failure patients, except those in an acute decompensated state. Physical activity is encouraged to prevent deconditioning, which contributes to exercise intolerance.

PHARMACOLOGICAL TREATMENT OF HEART FAILURE

Angiotensin-Converting Enzyme Inhibitors and Angiotensin II Receptor Blockers

ACE inhibitors interfere with the conversion of angiotensin I to angiotensin II in the RAAS system. In addition, they enhance the action of kinins. Both actions are responsible for their positive impact in heart failure. These medications interfere with the ventricular remodeling process, slow disease progression, and reduce the risk of death (Calclasure, Kozlowski, & Highfill, 2001; Hobbs & Boyle, 2004; Hunt et al., 2005; Laurent, 2005). ACE inhibitors also improve symptoms and contribute to a sense of well-being. Benefits are seen in all stages of heart failure, although it may take several weeks to months for the effects to be seen.

ACE inhibitors remain the first choice for interuption of the RAAS in chronic heart failure. However, ARBs are now an acceptable first-line alternative to ACE inhibitors in patients with mild to moderate heart failure. ARBs directly block angiotensin II. In addition to being an acceptable first-line agent in some patients, ARBs are indicated in patients who cannot tolerate ACE inhibitors due to cough or angioedema. Candesartan was the first ARB to be approved by the FDA for the treatment of heart failure (Hunt et al., 2005).

Beta-Blockers

Beta-blockers are indicated in heart failure to block the neurohormonal responses of chronic SNS stimulation. Multiple studies have proven a mortality benefit in patients treated with beta-blockers. Beta-blockers have several beneficial effects, including favorably affecting ventricular remodeling and apoptosis. Beta-blockers can decrease arrhythmias and ischemia by decreasing heart rate and contractility, thereby decreasing myocardial oxygen consumption.

Beta-blockers are initiated in low doses and slowly titrated upward. Beta-blockers are not initiated when the patient is in fluid overload or a decompensated state. Patients who show signs of decompensation after a maintenance dose of beta-blocker therapy has been administered generally do not have beta-blocker therapy discontinued.

Diuretics

Loop diuretics work at the loop of Henle to increase sodium and water excretion. These diuretics are usually initiated in the management of heart failure, beginning with the presentation of fluid overload. After fluid overload has been resolved, diuretics are usually continued to maintain fluid volume status. Few heart failure patients are able to maintain optimal ECF balance without the use of a diuretic.

Diuretics improve symptoms more rapidly than any other drug and can also increase cardiac function and improve exercise tolerance. Optimal use of diuretics is also key to the effectiveness of ACE inhibitor and beta-blocker therapy. ACE inhibitor therapy is less effective and patients are less likely to tolerate beta-blocker therapy if the diuretic dose is too low and ECF overload is present. The risk of hypotension and renal insufficiency are increased with ACE inhibitor use if the diuretic dose is too high.

Digoxin

Digoxin is a weak inotropic agent, but its benefits in heart failure come from its other effects, including reducing sympathetic outflow and suppressing renin secretion. Digoxin can improve symptoms and decrease the rate of hospitalization but has not been proven to reduce mortality (Hobbs & Boyle, 2004). A dose of 0.125 mg per day, lower than once thought necessary to be effective, is recommended in most patients (Hunt et al., 2005). Digoxin is recommended for heart failure patients who remain symptomatic despite treatment with ACE inhibitors, beta-blockers, and diuretics.

Other Medications

Aldosterone Antagonists

An aldosterone antagonist, such as spironolactone or eplerenone, can be beneficial in heart failure patients who experience symptoms at rest. In a large-scale, long-term trial, low-dose spironolactone reduced the risk of death in patients already taking ACE inhibitors. The greatest benefit was seen in those patients who were also taking beta-blockers and digoxin (Hunt et al., 2005). Hyperkalemia is a potential side effect, especially when patients are already on ACE inhibitors.

Medications used in the treatment of heart failure are summarized in Table 7-5. Specific medications by class are listed in Table 7-6.

Contraindicated Medications

Although ACE inhibitors, ARBs, beta-blockers, diuretics, and digoxin are used in the treatment of heart failure, certain medications should be avoided in patients with heart failure. Most antiarrhythmics are poorly tolerated in heart failure patients due to their proarrhythmic and cardiodepressant effects. Amiodarone is the only antiarrhythmic that does not adversely affect survival in heart failure patients (Hunt et al., 2005).

Calcium channel blockers, with the exception of amlodipine, adversely affect survival in patients

TABLE 7-5: SUMMARY OF HEART FAILURE MEDICATIONS BY CLASS

ACE inhibitors and ARBs	• Interrupt the neurohormonal responses of the RAAS and favorably impact disease progression • Reduce mortality and morbidity
Beta-blockers	• Interrupt the neurohormonal responses of the SNS and favorably impact disease progression • Reduce hospitalizations * Not initiated in acute decompensated state
Diuretics	• Decrease ECF load and improve symptoms in an overload state • Maintain ECF volume status and sodium balance • Have no impact on mortality *Loop diuretics with the addition of a thiazide diuretic if needed*
Digoxin	• Improves symptoms, exercise tolerance, and quality of life • Used in patients who are symptomatic on the above three medications • No mortality impact *Dosage is usually 0.125 mg; toxicity can occur with normal serum levels*
Aldosterone antagonists	• Reserved for patients with moderate to severe heart failure *Cannot be used if creatinine level is greater than 2.5 mg/dl due to risk of hyperkalemia*

TABLE 7-6: EXAMPLES OF MEDICATIONS BY CLASS

ACE inhibitors	ARBs	Beta-blockers	Loop diuretics	Aldosterone antagonists
Captopril Enalapril Lisinopril Ramipril	Candesartan	Carvedilol Metoprolol Bisoprolol	Furosemide Torsemide Bumetanide	Spironolactone (nonselective) Eplerenone (selective)

with systolic dysfunction. Amlodipine has a neutral effect in heart failure and can be used if needed to treat coexisting angina or hypertension. Patients with heart failure should be instructed to avoid the use of nonsteroidal anti-inflammatory drugs (NSAIDs) which can cause sodium retention and peripheral vasoconstriction. These medications diminish the efficacy of diuretics and ACE inhibitors while enhancing the likelihood of toxic renal effects.

NONPHARMACOLOGICAL TREATMENT STRATEGIES FOR HEART FAILURE

Exercise Training

Controlled trials have shown that exercise training improves symptoms, quality of life, and exercise capacity in patients with heart failure. This beneficial effect is additive to the effects of optimal medical therapy (Hunt et al., 2005). Exercise training in heart failure patients is best accomplished in a formally structured program, such as cardiac rehabilitation. Studies show that many of the hemodynamic abnormalities associated with chronic heart failure improve with exercise training. The physiological benefits of exercise training for patients with chronic heart failure occur in skeletal muscle as opposed to in the heart itself (Myers, 2005).

Resynchronization Therapy

Resynchronization therapy is indicated in patients with moderate to severe heart failure and those with wide QRS complexes who are symptomatic despite optimal medical therapy. In resynchronization therapy, a biventricular pacemaker is placed, with leads in both the right and left ventricles. A lead is also implanted in the right atrium to allow for atrial pacing. Resynchronization is common in heart failure because many patients have bundle branch block that causes the right and left ventricles to depolarize at different times. When this occurs, the walls of the right and left ventricles do not contract simultaneously. Resynchronization therapy with a biventricular pacemaker allows the right and left ventricles to contract simultaneously, thereby improving cardiac performance. Studies show clinical improvement in exercise tolerance and quality of life after resynchronization therapy in patients with moderate to severe heart failure (Hunt et al., 2005; Jacobson & Gerity, 2005).

SPECIAL ISSUES IN HEART FAILURE

Sudden Death

Patients with heart failure are at high risk for sudden cardiac death. They can also die of progressive pump failure and congestion or end-organ failure from systemic hypoperfusion. Although more than 50% of heart failure patients have episodes of nonsustained ventricular tachycardia, it is not necessarily the simple progression to sustained ventricular tachycardia that increases the risk of sudden death (Hunt et al., 2005). Sudden death in heart failure patients is commonly associated with an acute

ischemic event or even bradyarrhythmias. For this reason, interventions in heart failure are aimed at preventing sudden death rather than treating asymptomatic ventricular arrhythmias.

Treatments used to decrease the risk of sudden cardiac death in heart failure include:

- beta-blockers
- amiodarone
- implantable cardioverter-defibrillators (ICDs).

Most antiarrhythmic drugs are poorly tolerated in heart failure patients. However, amiodarone, although a class III antiarrhythmic, also has vasodilatory properties and is generally well tolerated in heart failure patients. Because of the toxicity associated with amiodarone, it is not routinely used in the treatment of heart failure. However, it is used in patients with a history of sudden cardiac death, ventricular fibrillation, or sustained unstable ventricular tachycardia (Hunt et al., 2005). ICDs are indicated in the following heart failure patients: survivors of cardiac arrest and those with sustained ventricular tachycardia, inducible ventricular tachycardia during an electrophysiology study, or ejection fraction less than 30% after an MI (Jacobson & Gerity, 2005).

Acute Decompensated Heart Failure

Patients with acute decompensated heart failure commonly present with the following clinical signs: tachycardia, tachypnea, pallor, diaphoresis, inspiratory crackles or rales, jugular venous distention, peripheral edema, hepatomegaly, ascites, extra heart sounds (S_3 and often S_4), and a possible mitral regurgitation murmur.

Brain Natriuretic peptide (BNP) Levels

BNP levels are used as a diagnostic indicator in patients presenting with signs of decompensation. Plasma concentrations of BNP are elevated in patients with decompensated heart failure with fluid overload. This diagnostic tool is also helpful when a patient's primary complaint is shortness of breath, yet the etiology is unclear. A BNP level of less than 100 pg/ml has a high negative predictive value; therefore, it can be used to eliminate heart failure as the cause of dyspnea. BNP levels greater than 500 pg/ml at the time discharge are highly associated with readmission within 30 days. BNP levels can remain chronically elevated in end-stage heart failure (Hunt et al., 2005).

Inotropic Therapy

Patients in acute decompensated heart failure may require intravenous (IV) administration of a positive inotrope. Dobutamine, a sympathomimetic, and milrinone, a phosphodiesterase inhibitor, are the commonly used IV inotropes. Milrinone has vasodilator properties in addition to inotropic properties.

Vasodilator Therapy

Patients in acute decompensated heart failure may also need vasodilator therapy to help reduce preload or afterload. Nesiritide, a synthetic BNP, is one vasodilator used in the treatment of acute decompensated heart failure. Nesiritide is a venous and arterial vasodilator so it reduces both preload and afterload. Other vasodilators used in acute decompensated heart failure include nitroglycerin and nitroprusside. IV nitroglycerin is usually given in low doses as a venous vasodilator, and nitroprusside is predominantly an arterial vasodilator.

End-Stage Heart Failure

Patients with end-stage refractory heart failure have special management issues. These patients need very careful control of their ECF volume status because many of their symptoms are related to sodium imbalances causes by ECF overload. ACE inhibitors and beta-blockers are effective in patients with end-stage refractory heart failure; however, these patients may not tolerate these medications well and, therefore, lower doses may need to be used. Patients should not receive these medications if systolic blood pressure is less than 80 mm Hg or if they show signs of hypoperfusion. Patients should not be initiated on beta-blockers if they have symptomatic ECF retention or require IV inotropic support.

End-stage heart failure patients may decompensate frequently and may need to be admitted for IV inotropic or vasodilator therapy. After the patient is stabilized and oral medications are resumed, the patient must be observed for a period to assure the oral regime is sufficient to avoid further decompensation. Patients unable to be weaned from IV inotropic support may be candidates for at-home, continuous, inotropic support. This measure is a final option, used only for palliative relief in end-stage disease. Intermittent inotropic therapy is not indicated in the management of end-stage heart failure because it has been shown to increase mortality.

Transplantation

Cardiac transplantation is the only established surgical treatment for refractory heart failure. Unfortunately, this treatment option is available only to a small group of patients each year. Transplantation is indicated only for patients with severe functional impairment who require continuous IV inotropic support. Candidates need to be otherwise healthy. The survival rate at 1 year is 85%, with a decline of approximately 4% each year thereafter (LeDoux & Luikart, 2005). After transplantation, patients remain on lifelong immunosuppression therapy, placing them at risk for further complications.

Left Ventricular Assist Devices

Left ventricular assist devices can be used to provide hemodynamic support to failing hearts for patients waiting for cardiac transplantation and those who are not candidates for transplantation. Some left ventricular assist devices can be surgically implanted. Complications with left ventricular assist devices are common and can be life threatening. For this reason, the use of these devices is limited.

Prognosis and Hospice Referral

Physicians should discuss end-of-life care issues with patients with end-stage heart failure while they are still able to participate in the decision-making process. Hospice care is one option for end-stage disease management that is often underutilized. A prediction of death within 6 months is traditionally a criterion for admission to hospice services. Because sudden cardiac death is one of the major causes of death in heart failure patients, the time of death is difficult to predict. Many patients with end-stage heart failure have periods of good quality of life during the final 6 months. Hospice admission policies need to be flexible enough to allow end-stage heart failure patients to participate in these palliative programs when appropriate. Heart failure health care providers also need to be more attentive to end-of-life care in this population and initiate more patient dialogue and appropriate hospice referrals.

PATIENT EDUCATION

Heart failure is the final pathway for many cardiac disorders. Heart failure care is complex and involves continuity across the continuum. Research shows that careful monitoring and follow-up make a difference. Nurses play an important role in the monitoring and follow-up of heart failure patients. Nurses also contribute substantially to patient and family education. Teaching the patient and family self-management strategies is key in the effective management of heart failure. Through discharge education, postdischarge telephone follow-up, and nurse-led heart failure clinics, nurses are making a difference in the management of heart failure.

Recognition of Signs and Symptoms

Patients need to understand how to recognize the signs and symptoms of worsening heart failure. Recognizing changes in activity tolerance is key. Some patients and families find it helpful to keep an activity diary as an objective record of their activities and tolerance. Daily weights are important in accurately assessing ECF status. A scale with large numbers for visibility is important for elderly patients. Some patients require family assistance

with weighing themselves because they cannot independently step onto and off of a scale. Scales with grab bars are beneficial but, due to their cost, may not be an option for all patients.

Clinical Application
Asking about the presence of a working scale at home is a key nursing intervention.

Nurses should instruct patients to keep a chart of daily weight and to take the chart with them to their physician office visits. Patients should also be instructed to report any gain of greater than 2 lb in 24 hours, or greater than 3 lb in 1 week. Some hospitals have programs that allow patients to call in and report their weights each day to a nurse or a computer system. Patients with weight gain and patients who do not call in are identified to receive further follow-up.

Clinical Application
It is important for patients to report their weight gain even if they do not yet have any other symptoms.

Medication Compliance

Medication compliance is critical to the effective management of heart failure. Patients are more compliant when they fully understand the benefits of therapy. Heart failure patients are on multiple medications, and this can cause a variety of compliance issues. A careful assessment of any financial concerns regarding prescribed medications is also important. Nurses should discuss any financial concerns with physicians so that every effort can be made to prescribe the most cost-effective, yet appropriate, medication regime. Social services should be consulted to assure that patients receive all available health care support services.

Physical limitations affecting compliance include poor vision and poor dexterity. Nurses should assess ability to read the small print on labels, open vials, and divide pills, if necessary. Nurses should also instruct patients to report any perceived side effects to their physician prior to stopping any medications. Because of the effects of NSAIDs on diuretic and ACE inhibitor therapy, nurses should instruct patients to avoid the use of these medications.

Patients should always carry with them a complete list of medications and their doses, especially to every physician office visit. Nurses can facilitate this practice by providing a comprehensive, legible list of medications with a current date printed on a wallet card. Nurses should review all admission and discharge medications to ensure that the necessary medications are ordered and that different physicians did not inadvertently order two medications in the same drug classification.

Sodium Restriction

Heart failure patients also need information regarding adherence to a moderate sodium restriction. In many cases, patients do not realize the hidden sodium content in processed foods. Because many food contain high amounts of sodium, patients and their caregivers must learn how to read food labels. Patients with heart failure should limit their sodium intake to less than 3 g per day, unless ordered otherwise. Fresh foods are the best choice for low sodium content. Frozen foods typically contain less sodium than do canned foods.

Physical Activity and Socialization

Physical activity should be promoted in all heart failure patients to prevent deconditioning. Most heart failure patients benefit from exercise training in a formal cardiac rehabilitation program. Participation in this type of program also provides interaction with other people and the opportunity for a health care provider to assess the patient at regular intervals.

Heart failure patients are at risk for isolation and depression if they have limited activity tolerance. Many hospitals and communities have support groups for patients and families living with heart failure. Nurses should carefully assess support systems

and opportunities for socialization in heart failure patients who are homebound.

Follow-Up

Close physician or nurse practitioner follow-up is critical to the successful management of heart failure. Patients need to understand the importance of keeping all scheduled appointments, even when they are feeling well. Many medications are titrated to optimal doses on an outpatient basis. Nurses need to assess for any barriers to keeping office appointments, such as lack of transportation or conflicting work schedules of family members. Key components of patient education for heart failure patients are summarized in Box 7-1.

BOX 7-1: PATIENT EDUCATION CHECKLIST

- Recognition of signs and symptoms
  - Activity intolerance: activity diary
  - ECF retention: daily weight
    » Assess for home scale
- Medication compliance
  - Review benefits of therapy
  - Provide wallet card with current medication list
    » Assess for and eliminate barriers to accurate and consistent administration
- Sodium limitation
  - Label reading
  - Avoiding processed and canned foods
- Physical activity plan
  - Cardiac rehabilitation
- Support system and socialization opportunities
- Follow-up with primary cardiac care providers

Additional resources for patient education can be found at the Heart Failure Society of America web site (www.hfsa.org).

CONCLUSION

Heart failure is a chronic condition in which nurses play an important role in patient management. Nurses have a tremendous opportunity to collaborate with physicians and other members of the health care team to maximize patient outcomes. Research regarding the management of heart failure is ongoing, and practice guidelines are works in progress. New pharmacological agents involved in blocking various inflammatory and neurohormonal responses are being studied. In addition, gene therapy offers exciting hope regarding the possibility of preventing the loss of, or restoring the function of, left ventricular myocytes (Laurent, 2005).

The role of nurses in the management of heart failure will continue to expand. All cardiac nurses should understand the importance of heart failure prevention strategies in patients who are at risk for CHD and those who have CHD but do not yet have heart failure.

EXAM QUESTIONS

CHAPTER 7
Questions 54-63

54. The hallmark manifestations of heart failure are

    a. rapid heart rate with syncope.

    b. chest pain with positive myocardial enzymes.

    c. dangerously low heart rate requiring a pacemaker.

    d. dyspnea and fatigue or fluid retention.

55. Heart failure is most commonly a result of

    a. digoxin toxicity.

    b. ischemic CHD.

    c. an untreated viral infection.

    d. renal failure.

56. Systolic left ventricular dysfunction is best defined as

    a. impaired ability of the left ventricle to contract and effectively eject blood.

    b. impaired ability of the left ventricle to relax and fill.

    c. heart failure with an elevated systolic blood pressure.

    d. heart failure in which the heart stops beating during systole.

57. Neurohormonal responses in heart failure which over time lead to clinical deterioration include

    a. activation of the liver to release glycogen stores.

    b. increased production of cholesterol to make more needed hormones.

    c. activation of the SNS and RAAS.

    d. increased production of hemoglobin to increase oxygen capacity.

58. The one positive neurohormonal response in chronic heart failure, which results in vasodilatation, is increased release of

    a. endothelin.

    b. cytokines.

    c. natriuretic peptides.

    d. vasopressin.

59. Medications commonly used in the treatment of heart failure to interrupt neurohormonal responses, reduce ventricular remodeling, and decrease mortality include

    a. ACE inhibitors and beta-blockers.

    b. ACE inhibitors and calcium channel blockers.

    c. calcium channel blockers and nitrates.

    d. beta-blockers and nitrates.

60. Which of the following statements is true concerning the use of diuretics in heart failure?

    a. Diuretics have common life-threatening side effects and are only used in severe decompensation.

    b. Diuretics are used in patients with past and present signs of fluid overload.

    c. Diuretics are used because they reduce mortality.

    d. Diuretics should only be used in patients who cannot tolerate ACE inhibitors.

61. Cardiac resynchronization therapy is used in heart failure to

    a. restore sinus rhythm in patients with atrial fibrillation.

    b. defibrillate patients out of life-threatening arrhythmias.

    c. restore synchrony between right and left ventricle depolarization by pacing both ventricles at the same time.

    d. restore synchrony between the heart and lungs by dilating the pulmonary artery.

62. A true statement regarding end-stage heart failure is

    a. all patients die within 6 months from the time of diagnosis of end-stage disease.

    b. most end-stage heart failure patients are candidates for and receive cardiac transplantation.

    c. most patients come to the hospital once a week for intermittent infusion of an IV inotrope.

    d. many patients can have periods of good quality of life even after they are diagnosed as having end-stage disease.

63. Key patient education nursing interventions in heart failure include instruction on

    a. recognizing signs and symptoms of hypoglycemia.

    b. the importance of daily weights and reporting weight gain.

    c. eating foods high in sodium.

    d. maintaining bed rest to avoid episodes of exacerbation.

CHAPTER 8

CARDIOMYOPATHY

CHAPTER OBJECTIVE

After completing this chapter, the reader will be able to recognize the three main types of cardiomyopathy and their physiological differences.

OBJECTIVES

After studying this chapter, the reader will be able to

1. define cardiomyopathy.

2. identify the three primary types of cardiomyopathy.

3. differentiate the pathophysiology associated with each type of cardiomyopathy.

4. identify tools utilized for the diagnosis of cardiomyopathy.

5. recognize the primary treatment goals for cardiomyopathy.

6. describe the difference between hypertrophic obstructive cardiomyopathy (HOCM) and hypertrophic nonobstructive cardiomyopathy.

7. recall one medication to avoid with HOCM that is useful in the treatment of other types of cardiomyopathy.

INTRODUCTION

The term "cardiomyopathy" refers to a group of disorders caused by dysfunction of the myocardium. These disorders are classified as primary or secondary cardiomyopathies. Primary (or idiopathic) cardiomyopathies are diseases of the myocardium that have no known cause. Secondary cardiomyopathies are diseases of the heart muscle that result from another disease process, such as a myocardial infarction (MI), valvular disease, or hypertension (Kavinsky & Parrillo, 2000). There are three main categories or types of cardiomyopathy: 1) dilated cardiomyopathy (DCM); 2) restrictive cardiomyopathy (RCM); and 3) hypertrophic cardiomyopathy (HCM) (Porth, 2004). In 1996, the World Health Organization (WHO) added two additional categories: arrhythmogenic right ventricular cardiomyopathy and peripartum cardiomyopathy (Porth, 2004). The classification of each type is based on clinical, structural, functional, and hemodynamic criteria (Kavinsky & Parrillo, 2000). The end result of all types of cardiomyopathy is dysfunction of the myocardium. As knowledge about cardiomyopathy grows, causes are identified for what was once considered idiopathic cardiomyopathy. For the purpose of this text, the discussion in this chapter is limited to the three main types of cardiomyopathy.

DILATED CARDIOMYOPATHY

Definition

An enlarged, dilated cardiac chamber is the hallmark characteristic of DCM. This dilatation can affect one or all four cardiac chambers. As the chamber enlarges, its ability to contract becomes impaired, resulting in systolic dysfunction (see Figure 8-1).

FIGURE 8-1: COMPARISON OF NORMAL LEFT VENTRICULAR MORPHOLOGY AND LEFT VENTRICULAR MORPHOLOGY IN DILATED CARDIOMYOPATHY, HYPERTROPHIC CARDIOMYOPATHY, AND RESTRICTIVE CARDIOMYOPATHY

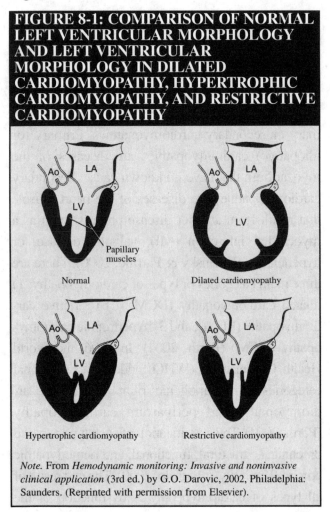

Note. From *Hemodynamic monitoring: Invasive and noninvasive clinical application* (3rd ed.) by G.O. Darovic, 2002, Philadelphia: Saunders. (Reprinted with permission from Elsevier).

Prevalence

DCM is the most common form of cardiomyopathy and represents the largest group of heart failure cases (O'Neill & Bott-Silverman, 2003). Although the exact number of people with DCM is difficult to determine, the population is large. The American Heart Association and the American College of Cardiology (ACC) stage heart failure into four categories (see Table 8-1). Most people who fall into stages B, C, or D have one type of cardiomyopathy. It has been estimated that idiopathic DCM occurs in 0.4 per 1,000 of the general population (O'Neill & Bott-Silverman, 2003). African-Americans have an increased risk of developing DCM due to increased presence of risk factors, such as hypertension. African-Americans with DCM also have a higher mortality rate than white Americans (Bozkurt & Mann, 2000).

Causes

The most common identifiable cause of DCM is ischemic cardiomyopathy that results from damage to the myocardium from MI (O'Neill & Bott-Silverman, 2003). DCM also has a variety of nonischemic causes (see Box 8-1). These causes include a variety of disease processes that result in damage to the myocardial fibers, with the end result being dilatation of the cardiac chambers (secondary causes).

Pathophysiology

The primary dysfunction in DCM involves ventricular dilatation and a decreased ability of the ventricle to contract. As the ventricular chamber enlarges, the myocardial fibers stretch to the point that they become overstretched and can no longer forcefully contract. This loss of contractile function is referred to as *systolic dysfunction*. As contractile function is lost, the ventricle is unable to eject its contents and ejection fraction decreases, as does stroke volume and cardiac output. As a result of this decreased ejection of ventricular contents, volume in the ventricle at the end of systole increases. When the left atrium empties into the left ventricle during diastole, the increased residual volume in the ventricle prevents the atrium from emptying completely. The increased volume in the left atrium subsequently increases the pressure in the left atrium. The left atrium dilates to compensate for the increased volume and subsequent pressure. This atrial dilatation

TABLE 8-1: AMERICAN HEART ASSOCIATION/AMERICAN COLLEGE OF CARDIOLOGY STAGING OF HEART DISEASE

STAGE	DESCRIPTION
A	Patients at risk for heart failure with no structural heart disease
B	Patients with structural heart disease without symptoms of heart failure
C	Patients with past or present heart failure symptoms
D	Patients with advanced disease

(Hunt et al., 2005)

BOX 8-1: CAUSES OF DILATED CARDIOMYOPATHY

- Idiopathic
- Ischemic heart disease
- Genetic disorders
- Hypertension
- Viral or bacterial infection
- Valvular heart disease
- Chemotherapy
- Peripartum syndrome related to toxemia
- Cardiotoxic effects of drugs or alcohol

can provide adequate compensation for some time. Ultimately, however, this compensation fails and the increased volume and pressure in the atrium are reflected back into the pulmonary system. Pulmonary failure occurs and symptoms of left-sided heart failure develop. As left ventricular function deteriorates, the right ventricle ultimately fails as well, resulting in right-sided heart failure.

Many compensatory mechanisms occur as dilatation of the ventricular chamber occurs. Normally, as the ventricular wall dilates, it becomes thinner. In some instances, the ventricular wall may actually increase in thickness to help maintain cardiac contraction, as seen with aortic regurgitation. This compensatory mechanism, although helpful initially, eventually results in diastolic dysfunction.

Although they maintain a normal structure, the mitral and tricuspid valves develop a "functional" regurgitation as dilatation of the ventricle increases. As the ventricle becomes larger, the valve opening dilates, resulting in an inability of the leaflets to come together completely and impairing the ability of the valve to function normally. Papillary muscle dysfunction may also occur as a result dilatation of the ventricular walls.

The neurohormonal system becomes activated in response to the decrease in forward ejection of blood. As ejection fraction decreases, the body responds to the decrease in cardiac output. The renin-angiotensin-aldosterone system (RAAS) activates, causing vasoconstriction of the arteries and retention of fluids and sodium. This vasoconstriction increases afterload and causes an already poorly contracting ventricle to pump harder as it attempts to overcome vasoconstriction and eject its contents. Fluid retention places an increased burden on the already overloaded system, and heart failure develops. A full discussion of the response of the neurohormonal system is covered in chapter 7.

Heart rate normally increases when cardiac output decreases. In the early stages of DCM, this response is adequate to maintain perfusion. However, as the disease process progresses, this response is no longer enough to compensate for the contractile defect. (See Figure 8-2 for a diagram of the basic physiologic changes in DCM.)

FIGURE 8-2: BASIC PHYSIOLOGIC PROGRESSION OF DILATED CARDIOMYOPATHY

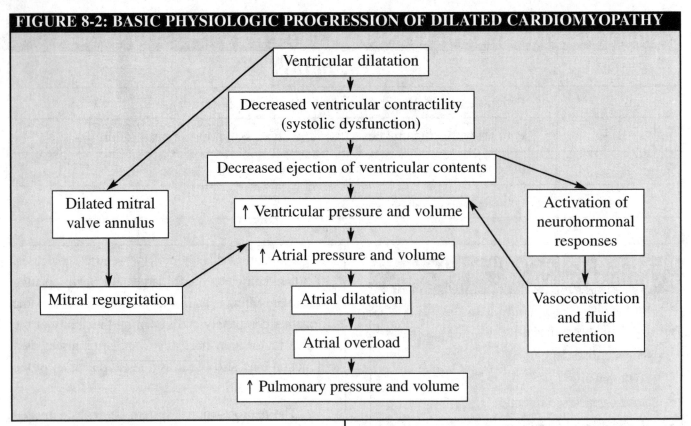

Clinical Presentation

Symptoms of DCM are directly related to the severity of the disease process and generally develop over time. Most commonly, patients present with symptoms related to low cardiac output, including weakness, fatigue, and decreased activity tolerance (Kavinsky & Parrillo, 2000). Because symptoms develop slowly, patients make adjustments in activity levels to compensate for the changes, commonly without being aware that they are doing so. Shortness of breath, dyspnea on exertion, and orthopnea occur as pulmonary edema develops. Because failure of the left ventricle generally occurs before failure of the right ventricle, left-sided heart failure symptoms appear before right-sided symp-

toms (see Table 8-2). Symptoms of right-sided failure are usually a late development. Some conditions, such as right ventricular infarctions and pulmonary hypertension, can cause direct damage to the right ventricle. In these cases, right ventricular failure may occur without any damage to the left ventricle.

Clinical Application
It is important to question patients about their normal level of activity to determine exercise intolerance. Those having symptoms with minimal activity are more seriously ill than those who can participate in activities on a regular basis.

TABLE 8-2: HEART FAILURE SYMPTOMS: RIGHT-SIDED VERSUS LEFT-SIDED

Right-Sided Heart Failure	Left-Sided Heart Failure
Dependent edema	Dyspnea
Distended jugular veins	Paroxysmal nocturnal dyspnea
Enlarged, tender liver	Orthopnea
Ascites	Crackles in lungs

Physical Examination

Findings during the physical examination vary depending on the severity of the disease (see Table 8-3). The severity of DCM depends on the degree of systolic dysfunction. Patients are usually alert until the end stages of the disease process. As perfusion decreases over time, eventually cerebral perfusion will be effected and changes in mental status will occur. The skin may be cool and pale, and cyanosis may be present late in the disease process. When palpating a pulse, the examiner may note an irregularity in the strength. Pulsus alternans, an alternation between weak and strong beats, can occur. Heart rate rises in an attempt to compensate for decreased stroke volume. Heart rates of 120 to 130 beats per minute may be tolerated; however, sustained heart rates greater than 140 beats per minute usually result in rapid decompensation. Heart rate may also be irregularly irregular if the patient is in atrial fibrillation, which is not uncommon. Blood pressure is generally low, with a narrowed pulse pressure. As pulse pressure narrows, systolic and diastolic blood pressure readings move closer to each other. Patients may also experience orthostatic hypotension.

Examination of the heart reveals a displaced apical impulse. At the apex of the heart, a pulse can normally be palpated with each beat. The apical impulse is normally palpable at the fourth or fifth intercostal space, at the left midclavicular line. As the ventricle dilates and changes shape and size, the location of the apex of the heart shifts to the left and down. The apical impulse also decreases in force as the force of contraction decreases with disease progression. During auscultation, normal first (S_1, or "lub") and second heart sounds (S_2, or "dub") are present. Additionally, an extra, third (S_3) heart sound may be audible immediately after the second heart sound. The third heart sound is best discovered with the bell of the stethoscope when the patient is lying on his or her left side. This sound is loudest at the fourth intercostal space to

TABLE 8-3: PHYSICAL EXAMINATION FINDINGS IN DILATED CARDIOMYOPATHY	
Neurological	• Alert and oriented
Skin	• Cool and dry • Cyanotic (late)
Pulse	• Pulsus alternans
Heart rate	• Elevated
Blood pressure	• Normal to low • Narrowed pulse pressure
Heart examination	• Apical impulse displaced • Additional heart sounds (S_3 or S_4) • Mitral or tricuspid regurgitation murmur
Lung sounds	• Crackles
Jugular vein	• Distended
Liver	• Enlarged • Hepatojugular reflux
Edema	• Peripheral • Ascites

the left of the sternum if the patient has right-sided heart failure and at the fifth intercostal space at the midclavicular line if the patient has left-sided heart failure (Cray, Kothare, & Weinstock, 1999). The third heart sound is an indication of an increase in extracellular fluid (ECF) volume and should resolve if the overload is corrected. In addition to the extra heart sound, mitral and tricuspid regurgitation murmurs may be audible. As stated earlier, dilatation of the ventricle increases the size of the valve annulus, resulting in mitral and tricuspid regurgitation. These are systolic murmurs, best heard with the diaphragm of the stethoscope, and occur between the first and second heart sounds. Mitral regurgitation murmur is a blowing murmur that is best heard at the apex of the heart. Tricuspid murmur is a blowing or scratchy murmur best heard at the fourth intercostal space, left of the sternal boarder (Cray, Kothare, & Weinstock, 1999).

Lung sounds are clear early in the disease process. However, as the disease progresses and heart failure occurs, crackles develop, indicating pulmonary edema. Dullness to percussion or diminished breath sounds could indicate pleural effusion, which can also occur with heart failure.

Other examination findings consistent with right-sided heart failure include jugular venous distension, hepatojugular reflux, liver engorgement, edema, and ascites. All of these findings are directly related to the amount of failure present. Jugular veins are distended when the patient lies with the head elevated at a 45-degree angle. The liver is enlarged and often times tender. Hepatojugular reflux is present when pressure is applied to the liver and the jugular veins become distended. Peripheral edema is generally present, and ascites may also occur.

Clinical Application

Confusion and disorientation should be carefully evaluated because patients with DCM commonly develop atrial fibrillation and are at high risk for the development of emboli.

Clinical Application

Asking patients to tightly squeeze your hand while listening to their hearts enhances murmurs and the additional heart sound in DCM.

Diagnosis

Chest X-ray Film

An enlarged cardiac silhouette is visible on chest X-ray film. Pulmonary congestion and pleural effusion, may also be visible, if present.

Echocardiogram

The echocardiogram is very useful in the diagnosis of DCM. Echocardiography can provide information about the size of the hearts chambers as well as wall thickness. In DCM, all four chambers may be enlarged; however, the left ventricle is the largest of all the chambers and may also be the only chamber enlarged. Myocardial wall thickening is usually not present because the chamber walls are normal and often thin.

The echocardiogram is also useful in assessing ventricular function. Assessment of ventricular wall motion and ejection fraction provides valuable information about the ability of the dilated heart to contract. Normal ejection fraction is 55% to 65% (Bond, 2005). In DCM, ejection fraction is less than 40% when cardiac compromise has occurred (Kumar, Abbas, & Fausto, 2005). Echocardiography can also indicate the presence of thrombi in the ventricular cavity.

Cardiac Catheterization (arteriogram)

Cardiac catheterization is beneficial only if it is necessary to determine whether the patient has coronary heart disease (CHD). Although catheterization provides information about wall motion and ejection, noninvasive cardiac echocardiography is a better choice.

Electrocardiogram

An electrocardiogram (ECG) will most commonly show sinus tachycardia and arrhythmias, such as atrial fibrillation and ventricular ectopy. Left bundle branch block may be noted as the dilated ventricle causes changes in the conduction pattern through the bundle branches. Large QRS complexes characteristic of ventricular hypertrophy may be present as well.

Clinical Application

Hypertrophic changes on the ECG may cause ST-segment and T wave changes that mimic myocardial ischemia. Careful patient assessment and ECG analysis is needed to differentiate between ischemia and these changes.

Medical Therapy

Medical therapy for DCM is essentially the same as therapy for heart failure. The chapter on heart failure (chapter 7) covers the treatment options in full detail.

Medical therapy has three primary goals in addition to trying to provide symptom relief:

1. reduction of preload
2. reduction of afterload
3. increased contractility.

Preload Reduction

Reduction of preload is accomplished with diuretics. Decreased ECF volume allows the ventricle to become less dilated. The smaller ventricle decreases some of the regurgitation that occurs due to overstretched valve rings. As increased ECF volume is decreased, the stretch on the heart decreases, as does myocardial oxygen demand.

Venous vasodilators, such as nitrates, also decrease preload by dilating the veins, allowing more blood to remain in the vascular system and sending less to the heart. Angiotensin-converting enzyme (ACE) inhibitors help reduce volume by blocking the RAAS effects that have been activated.

Aldosterone antagonists, such as spironolactone and eplerenone, may be added to help with the diuretic effect if the patient continues to have symptoms at rest. More importantly, newer studies show that the addition of this class of medication can reduce mortality, especially in patients with ejection fractions less than 35% (Loghin, 2001).

Afterload Reduction

Reduction of afterload is accomplished with arterial vasodilators. Arterial dilatation reduces the work of the ventricle as it attempts to eject its contents. Arterial vasoconstriction is a normal response to decreased cardiac output. This response makes the process of ejecting blood from the ventricle more difficult and puts a greater strain on an already struggling heart. Hydralazine (Apresoline) and ACE inhibitors are the medications of choice for decreasing afterload. In fact, any patient with an ejection fraction less than 40%, with or without symptoms, should be started on an ACE inhibitor because these drugs have been shown to decrease long-term mortality (Loghin, 2001).

Clinical Application

Arterial vasodilators decrease blood pressure. Patients on arterial vasodilators should be instructed to report any symptoms of low blood pressure, such as dizziness when standing up.

Contractility

Increased contractility is achieved first by decreasing afterload. Usually, as afterload decreases, contractility increases. Digoxin is the oral medication of choice to assist with contractility. Digoxin does not improve mortality rates but it does improve exercise capacity, improve quality of life, and decrease hospitalizations. This medication is most effective in patients who have low ejection fractions.

Other Considerations in Medical Therapy

Beta-blockers

Standard treatment for patients with left ventricular dysfunction includes the administration of beta-blockers. Although beta-blockers should not be initiated during an episode of acute heart failure, they should be started once the failure is under control. Carvedilol (Coreg), metoprolol (Lopressor), and bisoprolol (Zebeta) have been found in multiple studies to decrease mortality and morbidity in heart failure (Kavinsky & Parrillo, 2000; Loghin, 2001).

Antiarrhythmic therapy

Patients with DCM may experience ventricular arrhythmias that require treatment. Medication choices should be made carefully because some medications can cause further depression of the myocardium. Currently, amiodarone is the medication of choice. Attempts should be made to convert patients from atrial fibrillation by either mechanical or pharmacological options. If conversion cannot be achieved, then rate control is essential. Digoxin and beta-blockers can be helpful in rate control.

Anticoagulation therapy

The utilization of anticoagulation therapy is controversial. Patients with DCM are at increased risk for embolization due to insufficient contraction of the large ventricular chambers. Additionally, these patients are also at high risk for the development of atrial fibrillation. Anticoagulation is recommended for patients with evidence of a left ventricular thrombus, a previous embolic event, or atrial fibrillation. Some literature supports anticoagulation for any patient with an ejection fraction less than 30% (Loghin, 2001).

Dietary restrictions

A salt restriction of 2 to 4 g per day, depending on the severity of the disease process, may be necessary. Excessive salt leads to retention of ECF. Simply eliminating table salt can decrease salt intake by 1 to 2 g per day. Fluid restrictions are only necessary in late stages of the disease process, when medical therapy is no longer effective in controlling volume.

> ### *Clinical Application*
> *Patients with DCM are commonly prescribed multiple medications. It is essential to ensure that the patient understands the importance of each medication and the value of compliance with the medication regime.*

Exercise

A sedentary lifestyle in this population leads to cardiac deconditioning. Exercise should be encouraged. Cardiac rehabilitation programs can be very beneficial in helping develop appropriate exercise programs.

Surgical Therapy

Cardiac Resynchronization Therapy

One of the newest therapies available for patients with DCM is cardiac resynchronization therapy (CRT). This therapy is reserved for patients with New York Heart Association (NYHA) heart failure class III or IV. These patients must also be on maximum medical therapy without benefit and have ejection fractions less than 35% (Jessup, 2004). The final key criterion is evidence that the right and left ventricles are not contracting at the same time. This dysynchrony is evident by a bundle branch block pattern (wide QRS complexes) on an ECG. As ventricular dilatation becomes greater, the ventricles no longer contract at the same time. Pacemaker wires are placed in the normal location of the right atrium for atrial pacing and in the right ventricle for right ventricular pacing. A third wire is placed on the left ventricle so that the right and left ventricles can contract simultaneously. This resynchronization of the right and left ventricle has shown improvement in exercise tolerance and quality of life.

Implantable Cardioverter-defibrillators

Patients at high risk for sudden death from ventricular arrhythmias may need implantable cardioverter-defibrillators (ICDs). As the ventricle become larger and ejection fraction decreases, the risk of sudden death increases. Patients with ejection fractions less than 35% and a history of MI are candidates for ICD placement (Ganz, 2004). ICDs are commonly implanted as part of the procedure for CRT.

Other Surgical Procedures

One surgical procedure that has demonstrated some benefit is left ventricular reduction surgery (Batista procedure). This procedure involves cutting out part of the left ventricle and sewing the remaining walls together to decrease the size of the ventricle. Another surgical option, called *cardiac myoplasty,* involves wrapping a muscle from the patient's back around the heart. A pacemaker wire is placed in the muscle and the muscle is stimulated to contract in conjunction with the heart, assisting contraction. Left ventricular assist devices may be implanted to support the patient until cardiac transplant is available. Ultimately, cardiac transplant is the final option because DCM has no cure.

Outcomes

DCM is the final disease process for many other disorders and diseases that effect the myocardium. Once diagnosed, 50% of patients diagnosed with heart failure die within 5 years (Loghin, 2001). Death is usually due to progressive heart failure but can also be caused by sudden cardiac death, pulmonary emboli, or embolic stroke. The lower the ejection fraction, the poorer the prognosis. Patient follow-up and compliance with treatment regimes seems to impact outcomes. Chapter 7 outlines the nurse's role in educating patients with heart failure. Patient understanding impacts compliance and, therefore, outcomes in this disease process.

RESTRICTIVE CARDIOMYOPATHY

Definition

RCM is characterized by rigidity of the myocardial wall. This rigidity results in a decreased ability of the chamber walls to expand during cardiac filling (see Figure 8-1).

Prevalence

RCM is the least common form of cardiomyopathy and accounts for approximately 5% of all primary heart muscle diseases (Goswami & Reddy, 2003). Men and women are equally affected. This process can be seen in children as well as adults; however, it appears to be better tolerated by adults.

Causes

As with other cardiomyopathies, RCM has both primary and secondary causes (see Box 8-2). Each cause results in different processes that restrict the myocardium. Some patients present with hemodynamics representative of RCM, but no cause can be determined. Amyloidosis is responsible for 90% of RCM cases in North America (Darovic, 2002). In this disease process, protein fibrils (amyloid) deposits in the tissues of the body and impair organ function. These protein fibrils are deposited throughout the myocardium, resulting in a firm, rubbery heart with thick, but not dilated, ventricular walls. Not all patients with amyloidosis develop cardiac involvement; however, amyloid heart disease has a very poor prognosis.

BOX 8-2: CAUSES OF RESTRICTIVE CARDIOMYOPATHY

Primary Causes
- Endomyocardial fibrosis
- Löffler's endocarditis
- Idiopathic RCM

Secondary Causes
- Infiltrative disorders
  - Amyloidosis
  - Sarcoidosis
  - Radiation carditis
- Storage diseases
  - Hemochromatosis
  - Glycogen storage disorders
  - Fabry's disease

(O'Neill & Bott-Silverman, 2003)

Although not prevalent in North America, endomyocardial fibrosis is relatively common in children and young adults in Africa and the Tropics. Fibrosis of the ventricular endocardium and subendocardium that extends to the mitral and tricuspid valves greatly decreases ventricular chamber function. Patients who have undergone radiation treatments may develop radiation-induced myocardial fibrosis. This fibrosis is not evident until several years after treatment.

Pathophysiology

Normally, as ventricular diastole begins, the atrioventricular valves open and the contents of the atria passively empty into the ventricles. At the end of ventricular diastole, the atria contract and add an additional volume of blood to the ventricles. During ventricular filling, the ventricular walls expand, stretching the cardiac muscle fibers and allowing for adequate filling.

In patients with RCM, the ability of the ventricular walls to expand is limited due to the disease process occurring in the myocardium. This limitation in chamber expansion decreases the heart's ability to adequately fill the ventricle during diastole. This decrease in diastolic filling results in a decrease in the volume of blood the ventricle is then able to eject during systole, and stroke volume is decreased. Generally, the ability of the myocardium to contract is not affected. If the disease process is infiltrative, contractile function can become impaired as the disease progresses. In addition to decreased stroke volume, a concurrent decrease in the forward flow of blood occurs because the ventricle is unable to accept all the contents from the atrium. Therefore, an increase in intravascular volume occurs and blood backs up into the lungs (left-sided failure) and the body (right-sided failure), resulting in heart failure.

Clinical Presentation

Patients with RCM experience an inability to complete normal daily activities due to fatigue and weakness. These symptoms are due to decreased stroke volume and an inability to compensate for increased metabolic demands. Normally, any increase in activity causes heart rate to increase. This increase in heart rate provides an increase in circulating blood volume to support the increase in demand. For patients with RCM, an increase in heart rate decreases cardiac output because it decreases the amount of time the ventricle has to fill during diastole. RCM patients already have a decreased ability to fill during diastole due to the restriction of the myocardial wall. Decreased cardiac output results in symptoms of fatigue and weakness.

Clinical Application

Anything that would normally cause the heart rate to increase, including activity, decreased blood pressure, fever, shivering, and low blood volume, results in a further decrease in stroke volume in patients with RCM.

Hypotension and syncope may be present in patients with amyloidosis. Other symptoms are caused by the heart failure that occurs. The patient experiences biventricular failure, because the disease process is not limited to one ventricle. Right-sided failure may be more prominent early because the impaired function of the right ventricle helps decrease the load on the left side of the heart, therefore decreasing the left-sided failure.

The patient may experience palpitations caused by atrial fibrillation, which is common with RCM. Disturbances in cardiac conduction are not uncommon in infiltrative disorders.

Physical Examination

On physical examination, signs of heart failure are present with associated signs of low cardiac output, including cool extremities, hypotension, and possibly lethargy, depending on the progression of the disease. Hypotension is not uncommon in amyloidosis. Peripheral pulses are decreased and become weaker as the disease progresses and stroke volume continues to decrease.

Auscultation of the heart reveals normal first and second heart sounds and the presence of a third heart sound that is caused by decreased compliance of the ventricle. Systolic murmurs of mitral or tricuspid insufficiency may be audible, because the valve opening dilates in conjuction with atrial dilatation from volume overload. Amyloidosis may also infiltrate the papillary muscles, resulting in regurgitation of the mitral or tricuspid valve.

Diagnosis

Aortic stenosis, cardiac tamponade, HCM, and hypertensive heart disease should all be ruled out when considering a diagnosis of RCM (Goswami & Reddy, 2003). The most important process that must be differentiated is constrictive pericarditis because this disease process can mimic RCM; the clinician must differentiate these two processes so appropriate intervention can be started (see Table 8-4).

Chest X-ray Film

The size of the ventricles on chest X-ray film appears normal, although the atria may be dilated. If the patient is presenting with congestive heart failure, pulmonary congestion may be present. In constrictive pericarditis a calcified pericardium may be seen on lateral chest X-ray film.

Echocardiogram

In RCM, cardiac echocardiography shows enlarged atria. The ventricles are normal in size without thickened walls unless an infiltrative disease process is present that causes increased wall mass. Normal contractility is also noted. The ventricular cavity size appears normal or reduced. In patients with amyloidosis, abnormal myocardial textures, such as a speckled appearance of the myocardium, may be noted (Carroll & Crawford, 2003). The echocardiogram also shows any mitral and tricuspid regurgitation caused by atrial enlargement.

Clinical Application
The echocardiogram is most helpful in differentiating constrictive pericarditis from RCM.

Cardiac Catheterization (angiogram)

A complete cardiac catheterization may not be necessary unless CHD is suspected. Invasive hemodynamic measurements provide valuable information about the hemodynamics associated with the disease process. As restriction occurs, filling pressure of each ventricle increases and stroke volume

TABLE 8-4: CLINICAL FEATURES OF CONSTRICTIVE PERICARDITIS AND RESTRICTIVE CARDIOMYOPATHY

Clinical Features	Constrictive Pericarditis	Restrictive Cardiomyopathy
History	Prior history of pericarditis or condition that causes pericardial disease	History of systemic disease (such as amyloidosis or hemochromatosis)
General exam		Peripheral stigmata of systemic disease
Heart sounds (non-murmurs)	Pericardial knock, high frequency sound	Presence of loud diastolic filling sound, third heart sound, low frequency sound
Murmurs	No murmurs	Murmurs of mitral and tricuspid insufficiency
Chest X-ray	Pericardial calcification	No change from prior normal X-ray film

(Goswami & Reddy, 2003)

decreases. Again, differentiating between constrictive pericarditis and RCM is important, and the measurements of pressures on the right and left sides of the heart assist in the differential diagnosis. In RCM, the right- and left-sided ventricular filling pressures are increased; however, left-sided filling pressures are generally higher than those of the right side by 5 mm Hg or greater. In constrictive pericarditis, filling pressures are generally equal.

Endomyocardial Biopsy

An endomyocardial biopsy obtained from the septal wall of the right ventricular is essential for the diagnosis of RCM for a variety of disease processes, including amyloidosis, hemochromatosis, and sarcoidosis. Multiple specimens must be obtained from multiple sites because many of these disease processes spread in a patchy, scattered pattern. A biopsy can positively identify infiltrative disorders and provide a definitive diagnosis of RCM (see Figure 8-3).

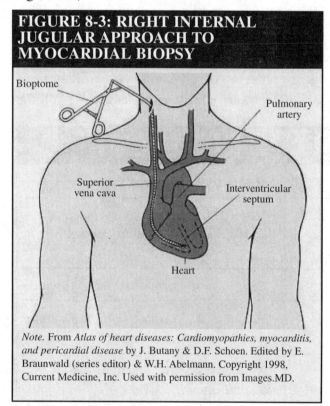

FIGURE 8-3: RIGHT INTERNAL JUGULAR APPROACH TO MYOCARDIAL BIOPSY

Bioptome

Pulmonary artery

Superior vena cava

Interventricular septum

Heart

Note. From *Atlas of heart diseases: Cardiomyopathies, myocarditis, and pericardial disease* by J. Butany & D.F. Schoen. Edited by E. Braunwald (series editor) & W.H. Abelmann. Copyright 1998, Current Medicine, Inc. Used with permission from Images.MD.

Electrocardiogram

Generally, QRS voltage is low and the ECG shows some nonspecific ST-segment and T wave changes. Large P waves are indicative of atrial enlargement. This change, however, is a late sign of atrial enlargement. Cardiac conduction abnormalities occur as the infiltrative disease infiltrates the conduction system. Atrial fibrillation is common in patients with RCM. Ventricular arrhythmias are common in patients with cardiac amyloidosis.

Medical Treatment

Medical treatment is supportive and aimed at the reduction of symptoms, with a focus on:

* reduction of diastolic dysfunction
* treatment of arrhythmias
* treatment of thromboembolic complications
* treatment of the underlying disease process.

Reduction of Diastolic Dysfunction

Although no medications directly affect restriction, treatment is aimed at reducing the effects of the restriction. Those effects include increased ECF volume and decreased stroke volume. Diuretics are the medication of choice to reduce increased ECF volume. Careful assessment of volume status is essential in the treatment of RCM. Reduction of ECF volume is necessary to prevent symptoms of heart failure; however, overreduction of volume further decreases the already decreased filling of the ventricle. Patients with severe RCM have a very narrow range of acceptable volume.

Clinical Application
Patients with RCM should be closely monitored for signs of decreased cardiac output that may result from overdiuresis. Signs include hypotension, especially orthostatic hypotension; lethargy; increased heart rate; and increased blood urea nitrogen levels.

Arterial vasodilators, such as ACE inhibitors, may be useful in decreasing afterload and allow for a more effective contraction by the ventricle. However, ACE inhibitors also contribute to diuresis, so volume status must be considered when utilizing ACE inhibitors with diuretics. Any vasodilator that affects the veins decreases the volume entering the heart (preload). This decrease in volume decreases the amount of volume available for ventricular filling. In many cases, treatment should be initiated with very low doses, with the patient being carefully monitored.

Treatment of Arrhythmias

Atrial fibrillation is the most common arrhythmic complication in RCM (Carroll & Crawford, 2003). Loss of atrial contraction can contribute to a decrease in ventricular filling; therefore, a normal sinus rhythm is preferable to atrial fibrillation. A variety of antiarrhythmic medications proven to treat atrial fibrillation may be used. Digoxin may be used cautiously for ventricular rate control. Patients with amyloidosis are particularly susceptible to digoxin-induced arrhythmias and heart blocks (Carroll & Crawford, 2003). As RCM worsens, conduction system abnormalities develop. Heart blocks, including complete heart blocks, may develop, resulting in the need for a permanent atrioventricular pacemaker. Ventricular arrhythmias may also develop. Treatment of these arrhythmias is based on the patient's hemodynamic response and whether the arrhythmias are sustained or life threatening. These arrhythmias should be treated in a usual manner, with no specific treatment differences for RCM.

Treatment of Thromboembolic Complications

Patients with endocardial fibrosis are at highest risk for thromoembolism. However, many patients with RCM are at risk for thrombus formation (Carroll & Crawford, 2003). In patients with atrial fibrillation, thrombi can form in the enlarged atrium at the location of the atrial appendage. Thrombi are also a concern in patients with low cardiac output states and mitral or tricuspid valve regurgitation. In these patients, anticoagulation with warfarin should be considered.

Treatment of Underlying Disease Process

Treatment of the underlying disease process varies. Although amyloidosis has no cure, steroids and chemotherapy may be helpful in slowing the progression of the disease. Cardiac transplantation has limited benefits in amyloidosis because the amyloid infiltrates the transplanted organ. Chelation therapy or phlebotomy can be used to treat hemochromatosis, depending on the cause of the iron overload (Kavinsky& Parrillo, 2000).

Clinical Application
Inotropic assistance (medications that increase contractility) is not usually beneficial in RCM because ventricular contraction is not impaired.

Surgical Treatment

Cardiac transplant is beneficial in idiopathic and familial RCM (Goswami & Reddy, 2003). Transplant of both the heart and liver is indicated in hemochromatosis. Its usefulness in infiltrative disorders, such as amyloidosis and sarcoidosis, is questionable because these disorders affect the new organ once transplant is completed. In fibrotic endocarditis, excision of the fibrotic endocardium may provide symptomatic relief. Replacement of regurgitant valves may also provide symptomatic relief; however, both of these procedures have a fairly high mortality rate.

Outcomes

Prognosis is poor in patients with RCM, with a 90% mortality rate at 10 years (Kavinsky & Parrillo, 2000). Amyloidosis carries the highest mortality, with a 2-year mortality rate being greater than 80% (Darovic, 2002).

HYPERTROPHIC CARDIOMYOPATHY

Definition

HCM is characterized by hypertrophy of the myocardium (see Figure 8-1). Associated with this increase in muscle mass is a decrease in ventricular filling and a decrease in cardiac output. Other causes of ventricular hypertrophy, including long-standing hypertension and aortic stenosis, must be ruled out before a diagnosis of HCM can be made. This disease process has had many names in the past, including *idiopathic hypertrophic subaortic stenosis*. The WHO's recommendation of "hypertrophic cardiomyopathy" as the correct terminology for this disease process has been widely accepted. HCM is a general term that covers all cases; however, a subgroup of patients with HCM develop HCM with obstruction. Once obstruction develops, the process is referred to as hypertrophic obstructive cardiomyopathy (HOCM).

Prevalence

HCM is found in one in every 500 people and effects women and men equally (Maron et al., 2003). It is the most common reason for sudden cardiac death in young adults.

Causes

The cause of HCM is unknown; however, more than 50% of HCM cases are transmitted genetically (Kavinsky & Parrillo, 2000). An abnormal sympathetic nervous system response or abnormal catecholamine levels may cause the other half of the cases (Shah, 2003).

Pathophysiology

In HCM, a generalized disarray of the cardiac myofibrils occurs, along with hypertrophy of the myocytes (see Figure 8-4). Cardiac cells take on a variety of shapes, and myocardial scarring and fibrosis occur. These changes result in myocardial walls that become very thin and stiff. The left ventricle is usually affected, with little affect on the right ventricle. The changes may be symmetrical; however, in many cases, asymmetrical septal hypertrophy is the most common finding (see Figure 8-5). In asymmetrical septal hypertrophy, the ventricular septum experiences the greatest increase in wall thickness, often times up to twice its normal size. Involvement of the septum may be limited to the upper one third, the lower two thirds, or the entire length of the septum (see Figure 8-6).

Ventricular chamber size decreases as the enlarging ventricular walls close in on the ventricular chamber. The thick, stiff walls resist filling. The

FIGURE 8-4: NORMAL MUSCLE STRUCTURE VERSUS MUSCLE STRUCTURE IN HCM

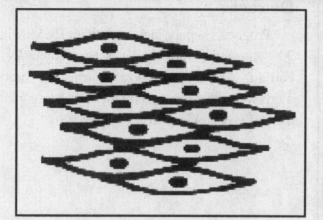

Normal Muscle Structure

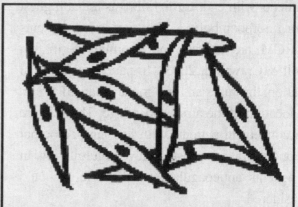

Myocardial Disarray

Note. From Hypertrophic Cardiomyopathy Association. Reprinted with permission. Retrieved December 31, 2004, from http://www.4hcm.org/wcms/index.php?overview

FIGURE 8-5: HCM WITH ASYMMETRICAL SEPTAL HYPERTROPHY

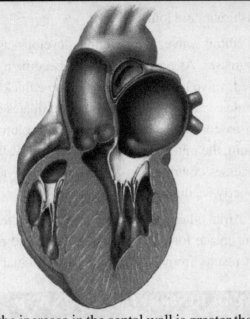

Note the increase in the septal wall is greater than the lateral wall of the left ventricle.

FIGURE 8-6: HCM WITH ASYMMETRICAL SEPTAL HYPERTROPHY INVOLVING THE UPPER PORTION OF THE SEPTAL WALL

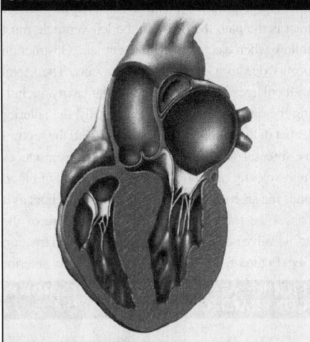

most prominent hemodynamic effect is decreased ventricular filling. This decreased ability to fill during diastole is referred to as *diastolic dysfunction*. As ventricular diastole begins, the mitral valve opens and the contents of the left atrium passively empty into the left ventricle. Normally, 70% to 75% of left ventricular filling occurs during this passive stage. In the presence of HCM, early passive filling is slowed due to the stiff, small left ventricle. The second part of diastole is atrial contraction, when the atrium contracts (atrial kick) and delivers an additional volume (25% to 30% of total volume) to the ventricle. A normal ventricle can hold approximately 150 ml of volume and normally ejects 55% to 65% of that volume with each beat. A stiff, noncompliant ventricle can neither hold 150 ml of volume nor accept the amount of volume (70% to 75% of total) normally provided during passive filling due to the high pressure in the left ventricle.

Therefore, atrial kick becomes essential in delivering the volume needed to fill the ventricle.

Clinical Application

ECF volume balance in patients with HCM is critical. Because the ventricular chamber is no longer able to expand during filling, the ventricle must fill fully in order to produce adequate stroke volume.

Clinical Application

The development of atrial fibrillation results in a loss of atrial kick. Without atrial kick, ventricular filling (preload) decreases, with an associated decrease in stroke volume.

To compensate for the decreased volume in the ventricle, systolic function becomes hyperdynamic. The ejection fraction that is normally 55% to 65% rises and a greater portion of the ventricular contents are ejected. Ejecting 70% to 80% of a smaller volume helps maintain normal stroke volume.

HOCM occurs when the upper one third of the intraventricular septum becomes hypertrophied and narrowed and obstructs the left ventricular outflow tract (see Figure 8-7). The left ventricular outflow tract is the path the blood in the left ventricle must follow when ejected from the ventricle. Obstruction occurs due to a combination of events. The septal wall enlarges into the left ventricular cavity, including the outflow tract area. Additionally, the anterior leaflet of the mitral valve is drawn toward the septum as forceful left ventricular contraction produces high-velocity blood flow. The rapid current of blood pulls the anterior leaflet toward the outflow tract as it passes the leaflet, resulting in early closure of the aortic valve and a greatly decreased ejection fraction (see Figure 8-7). Referred to as systolic anterior

motion (SAM), this obstruction by the anterior leaflet can be life threatening. It is estimated that 30% to 50% of patients with HCM have obstruction (Nishimura & Holmes, 2004).

Mitral valve regurgitation develops as HCM progresses. As papillary muscles become hypertrophied, valve leaflets may also become thick and the annulus calcified. As the left atrium dilates to compensate for the increased pressure and volume in the atrium, the mitral valve ring enlarges as well. These processes contribute to a valve that does not close properly, leading to regurgitation.

Atrial dilatation occurs as the atrium attempts to compensate for the increased volume and pressure that results from decreased left ventricular filling.

FIGURE 8-7: HYPERTROPHIC CARDIOMYOPATHY DURING RELAXATION AND CONTRACTION

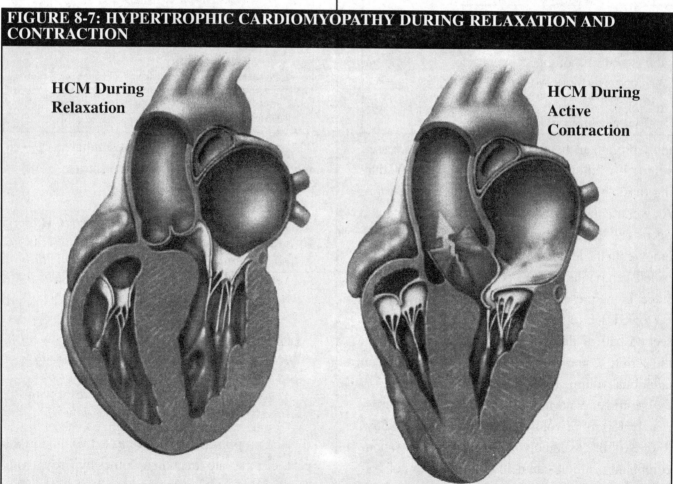

HCM During Relaxation

HCM During Active Contraction

Note the protrusion of the septum into the outflow tract at rest. As the ventricle contracts (shown in the picture on the right), the anterior leaflet of the mitral valve pulls into the outflow tract and nearly touches the septal wall, causing a nearly complete occlusion of outflow.

Note. From Mayo Foundation for Medical Education and Research. All rights reserved. Reprinted with permission. Retrieved December 31, 2004, from http://www.mayoclinic.org/hypertrophic-cardiomyopathy/obstruction.html

As hypertrophy of the left ventricle increases, forward flow decreases, resulting in decreased cardiac output. Additionally, ECF overload occurs with a backup of the additional volume in the lungs.

Clinical Presentation

Many patients with HCM remain asymptomatic for years. In many cases, HCM is first identified during routine screening of relatives of a known HCM patient. An episode of sudden death is frequently the first clinical presentation of HCM in children and young adults. Symptoms usually develop as the disease progresses. However, not always does the severity of the disease process relate to the severity of symptoms. Symptoms may be closer related to the severity of the diastolic dysfunction or mitral regurgitation. The most common symptoms are dyspnea, chest pain, syncope or pre-syncope, and sudden death.

Dyspnea

Ninety percent of patients presenting with symptoms cite dyspnea as the most prevalent problem (Loghin, 2001). As the size of the left ventricular chamber becomes smaller, the pressure in the left ventricle increases because the left ventricle is unable to accept the full volume from the left atrium. Left atrial pressure consequently increases, and the left atrial chamber dilates in an attempt to compensate for the increased volume in the atrium. The increase in pressure is ultimately referred back to the pulmonary system. As pulmonary pressures increase, the patient is predisposed to bouts of pulmonary congestion, resulting in dyspnea. Dyspnea is commonly related to activity. Any increase in activity normally increases heart rate to provide an increase in circulating blood volume to support the increase in demand. As with RCM, the normal cardiac response of an increase in heart rate is detrimental to patients with HCM. Increased heart rate decreases the amount of time the ventricle has to fill during diastole, and HCM patients already have a decreased ability to fill due to restriction of the myocardial wall. An increase in heart rate further decreases diastolic filling time. The hyperdynamic walls of the heart continue to eject a larger-than-normal percentage of the volume in the ventricle, which is helpful to a point. As filling decreases, so does the total volume available for ejection. More important in HCM patients is the increase in the backup of volume. Increased heart rate allows less and less volume to move forward through the left ventricle. The volume coming from the right side of the heart ends up in the pulmonary system because the left atrium is already full, and pulmonary edema develops.

Chest Pain

Chest pain caused by an imbalance in myocardial oxygen supply and demand is a common symptom of HCM. The increased left ventricular wall mass and hypercontractile state of the ventricle causes an increase in left ventricular myocardial oxygen demand. Several factors contribute to a decrease in myocardial oxygen supply. First, the decrease in cardiac output caused by decreased left ventricular filling does not deliver the oxygenated blood needed. Second, the increased myocardial mass requires more oxygenated blood due to its size. Finally, the coronary arteries are small and have difficulty dilating due to the increased myocardial mass; therefore, they are less able to deliver the needed oxygenated blood. While the patient is at rest, blood supply may be adequate to meet the body's needs. However, with increased stress or exercise, the increased myocardial oxygen demand of the thickened ventricular wall can no longer be met, resulting in angina. Angina can be caused by coronary heart disease (CHD) in addition to increased wall mass, but CHD does not usually occur in HCM.

Syncope

Normally, during exercise, arterial blood vessels dilate to increase blood flow to the system and blood pressure decreases. The normal compensatory mechanism of the heart is to increase cardiac output to compensate for the decreased pressure.

The body increases heart rate to increase cardiac output. This system keeps blood pressure in a normal range and allows a patient to tolerate the exercise. As noted earlier, in patients with HCM, increased heart rate does not increase cardiac output because diastolic filling time is decreased, actually decreasing cardiac output. Patients with HCM experience decreased blood pressure during exercise, resulting in dizziness, light-headedness, and blackout spells. Exercise can also cause ventricular or atrial arrhythmias, resulting in syncopal episodes.

Sudden Death

Sometimes, the first indication of HCM is a sudden cardiac death event. The degree of hypertrophy generally relates with the incidence of arrhythmias. A ventricular wall thickness of 30 mm or greater is associated with an increased risk of sudden death arrhythmias (Maron et al., 2003), whereas a wall thickness less than 15 mm is associated with no risk of sudden death arrhythmias. Life-threatening arrhythmias tend to occur in patients under 40 years of age. Undiagnosed HCM is one of the most common causes of sudden death in young adults. These life-threatening arrhythmias generally occur when the young adult engages in strenuous activity.

Other Symptoms

Patients may also present with complaints of fatigue and activity intolerance, which are caused by decreased cardiac output. Palpitations are also a common concern. Often times, palpitations are due to hyperdynamic contraction of the heart. Due to the forcible heartbeat, the patient can actually feel each contraction of the ventricle. An irregular heart rate may also be noted because atrial fibrillation can occur as a result of atrial dilatation. Atrial fibrillation results in a loss of atrial kick. Atrial kick provides active filling during ventricular diastole. This loss results in a large decrease in cardiac output because the hypertrophic ventricle counts on atrial kick for ventricular filling. Therefore, atrial fibrillation is poorly tolerated and the patient exhibits signs of low cardiac output and decreased perfusion.

Physical Examination

A bisferious carotid pulse is characteristic of patients with HOCM. The initial upstroke of the carotid pulse is brisk because there is initially no difficulty ejecting blood through the outflow tract. As systole progresses, left ventricular outflow tract obstruction may occur. This obstruction results in a collapse of the pulse and then a secondary rise.

Clinical Application

Because HCM may be confused with aortic stenosis, it is important to note that, in aortic stenosis, the carotid pulse has a delayed upstroke and amplitude.

During cardiac examination, the point of maximal impulse, located at the apex, is forceful and brisk due to the force of contraction. Upon auscultation of the heart, an additional sound is heard (S_4) just before the first heart sound. This fourth heart sound is not audible in patients with atrial fibrillation. Patients with HOCM have a classic crescendo-decrescendo systolic murmur. This murmur is best heard at the apex of the heart, at the fifth intercostal space to the left of the sternum or at the fifth intercostal space to the left of the midclavicular line. This murmur can be heard equally well with the bell or diaphragm of the stethoscope and is described as harsh or rough (Cray et al., 1999). Proper identification of the murmur assists in differentiating aortic stenosis from HOCM. The HOCM murmur becomes louder during Valsalva's maneuver, whereas the aortic stenosis murmur becomes quieter. Decreased venous return during Valsalva's maneuver decreases ventricular size and increases the obstruction, therefore increasing the sound of the murmur. Any factor that decreases venous return to the heart increases the murmur in HOCM (see Box 8-3).

Mitral regurgitation is not uncommon in HCM. This blowing murmur is heard throughout systole (holosystolic) and is best heard at the fifth intercostal space to the left of the midclavicular line.

BOX 8-3: FACTORS THAT DECREASE VENOUS RETURN TO THE HEART

- Valsalva's maneuver
- Position change from squatting to standing
- Tachycardia
- Venodilating drugs (such as nitroglycerin)
- Decreased ECF volume from blood loss or diuretics

This murmur does not change in the way a left ventricular outflow obstruction murmur does. This murmur may also radiate to the axillae, whereas left ventricular outflow obstruction murmurs do not.

Crackles may be present in the lung bases if the patient is experiencing heart failure. Right-sided heart failure is a late sign because left-sided failure generally occurs first. Other possible findings on examination include tachypnea and tachycardia. Apical irregularities may be noted if the patient is in atrial fibrillation or experiencing ventricular ectopy.

Diagnosis

Chest X-ray Film

In most cases, chest X-rays are not helpful because HCM does not usually increase ventricular size. The heart generally appears normal in size.

The left atrium may be slightly larger than normal and increases in size as the disease progresses. Signs of pulmonary congestion may be present.

Echocardiogram

Echocardiography is the tool of choice for diagnosing HCM. The diagnosis of HCM is easily established utilizing echocardiography. A wide variety of information can be obtained during echocardiography that leads to a diagnosis of HCM (see Table 8-5).

Cardiac Catheterization

For diagnosis of HCM, echocardiography has become the diagnostic tool of choice. Cardiac catheterization provides no additional information for the diagnosis. Most patients with HCM do not have CHD. They may have small vessels due to the increased muscle mass. A mismatch occurs as the small vessels are unable to supply the enlarged myocardium with the needed oxygen. This mismatch, although a supply and demand issue, is not CHD. Cardiac catheterization is useful in patients at high risk for CHD. If cardiac catheterization is necessary, the ventricular cavity and left ventricular outflow tract gradients can be assessed.

TABLE 8-5: ECHOCARDIOGRAM FINDINGS IN HYPERTROPHIC CARDIOMYOPATHY	
Echocardiogram Parameters Evaluated	**Echocardiogram Findings in HCM/HOCM**
Wall thickness	Increased
Symmetry of septal wall thickness	Septal wall greater than other walls of left ventricle
Left ventricular size	Usually normal
Hyperdynamic left ventricular function	Ejection fraction > 70%
Left atrial size	Usually dilated
Mitral valve leaflets	Systolic anterior motion of anterior mitral leaflet (in obstructive cases) Thickened, elongated anterior leaflet Mitral regurgitation
Left ventricular outflow tract	Obstruction to flow may be present

Electrocardiogram

On a 12-lead ECG, changes consistent with left ventricular hypertrophy are usually present. These changes include large QRS complexes with abnormal T waves. The absence of ECG changes does not rule out HCM. Deep symmetrical inversion of T waves in leads V_1 to V_6 usually accompanies the large QRS complexes in patients with HCM. In patients experiencing chest pain, these T-wave inversions need to be carefully evaluated by a physician experienced in 12-lead ECG interpretation because these changes may indicate myocardial ischemia. The ECG may also show bundle branch blocks, including left anterior hemiblock, right bundle branch block, and left bundle branch block. Cardiac arrhythmias, such as atrial fibrillation, may also be discovered using an ECG.

Medical Treatment

Treatment for HCM is aimed at relieving symptoms, preventing complications, and reducing the risk of sudden death. No clinical evidence supports treating nonsymptomatic patients. The data for this population are small because many patients are unaware of the disease process until symptoms appear.

Beta-blockers

The medication type of choice in the initial treatment of HCM with or without obstruction is beta-blockers. They provide symptomatic improvement and can increase exercise tolerance. The greatest benefit is seen with patients who are only experiencing symptoms with exertion or exercise. The normal beta response to sympathetic stimulation is an increase in contractility, heart rate, and conduction of impulses from the atrium to the ventricle. Beta-blockers block these normal responses. As previously stated, the primary problem associated with HCM is filling of the ventricle during diastole. The ventricles in patients with HCM are actually hyperdynamic so there is no issue with contractility. Beta-blockers slow heart rate. By decreasing heart rate, the diastolic filling time of the ventricle lengthens, providing more time for the atrium to fill the ventricle. Beta-blockers not only decrease the resting heart rate but also limit the ability of the heart rate to increase in response to stimulation such as exercise. In addition to preventing an increase in contractility, beta-blockers actually allow for ventricular relaxation. This relaxation again allows for better diastolic filling, especially passive filling. This decrease in contractility and heart rate with increased filling also benefits the patient by decreasing myocardial oxygen demand. A decrease in myocardial oxygen demand should also decrease any myocardial ischemia that is occurring from the increase in muscle mass and decrease in coronary artery size.

Clinical Application
Beta-blockers can cause fatigue, impotence, and sleep disturbances, especially with initial dosing. These symptoms, especially the fatigue, generally ease over time as the patient's body adjusts to the medication. Patients should be made aware of these effects and should be encouraged to continue taking the medication as the body adjusts to the changes.

Calcium Channel Blockers

Another type of medication used in both obstructive and nonobstructive HCM is calcium channel blockers. This class of medications has been shown to decrease symptoms, particularly chest pain. Calcium channel blockers also assist in decreasing contractility. Verapamil is the calcium channel blocker of choice because it decreases ventricular contractility and improves myocardial relaxation, resulting in increased ventricular filling.

Clinical Application
Nifedipine is a calcium channel blocker that should be avoided in patients with HCM because it is a potent vasodilator that may have detrimental effects.

Generally, beta-blockers are the first medication of choice. If beta-blockers do not provide symptom relief, calcium channel blockers are substituted. There is currently no evidence that supports utilizing beta-blockers with calcium channel blockers.

Antiarrhythmic Therapy

Treatment of arrhythmias in HCM has traditionally included disopyramide (Norpace) because it is a negative inotrope (decreases contractility) as well as a class I antiarrhythmic. In addition to the negative inotropic effect of decreasing outflow obstruction and mitral regurgitation, disopyramide helps control atrial and ventricular arrhythmias to some degree. Disopyramide should be used in conjunction with a beta-blocker because it may cause an increase in ventricular rate in atrial fibrillation. Disopyramide also has the ability to prolong the QT interval and cause an increase in ventricular arrhythmias. The utilization of disopyramide should be limited to patients with severe obstructive disease.

Atrial fibrillation is the most common arrhythmia associated with HCM. Every attempt should be made to convert atrial fibrillation back to normal sinus rhythm. The loss of atrial contraction and potentially high ventricular heart rates contribute to decreased ventricular filling and, quite often, rapid hemodynamic deterioration. Either pharmacologic conversion or mechanical cardioversion is acceptable. Beta-blockers help control ventricular rate. Amiodarone is also useful in both obstructive and nonobstructive disease with ventricular or atrial arrhythmias. Digoxin should be avoided in patients with HOCM because it increases contractility, thereby increasing the obstruction. Anticoagulation protocol should be followed as with anyone who may have atrial fibrillation.

Other Medications

Diuretics should be used cautiously in patients with HCM because volume status is very important. With the hypertrophy that has developed, preload is already decreased due to the ventricle's inability to expand during filling. Any further loss of filling can result in a decrease in cardiac output.

ACE inhibitors and nitroglycerin preparations should be avoided in patients with HOCM due to their ability to vasodilate and their ability to decrease preload. Both of these effects can increase the outflow obstruction and greatly decrease cardiac output.

Clinical Application

Any medication that increases contractility should be strictly avoided in patients with HOCM. An increase in contractility increases any outflow obstruction and greatly decreases cardiac output. This effect can be life threatening. Examples of drugs that increase contractility include digoxin, dobutamine, dopamine, epinephrine, and norepinephrine.

Nonobstructive Disease Progression

Some patients never develop obstructive disease. These patients can be more difficult to treat, and therapy may be less effective in providing symptom relief. Beta-blockers and calcium channel blockers are beneficial in decreasing heart rate and improving diastolic function. However, over time, the hypertrophic heart evolves into a dilated myocardium and the clinical picture becomes similar to DCM with the development of systolic dysfunction. As patients develop symptoms of heart failure, diuretics, ACE inhibitors, and digoxin may be helpful. Ultimately, cardiac transplant may be considered as the heart deteriorates.

Endocarditis Prophylaxis

Infective endocarditis prophylaxis is recommended by the ACC in patients with evidence of outflow obstruction, both resting and with exercise, before dental work or surgical procedures (Maron et al., 2003). There is no evidence that supports the use of prophylaxis in nonobstructive disease.

Pregnancy

Because many patients with HCM are young, the issue of pregnancy must be addressed. According to the ACC and the European Society of Cardiology (ESC) Clinical Expert Consensus Document on

Hypertrophic Cardiomyopathy (Maron et al., 2003), there is currently no evidence that pregnancy should be avoided in patients with HCM. The mortality risk may be slightly higher; however, that risk is generally associated with women who are already at high risk for other reasons. Normal vaginal deliveries may occur without difficulties.

Surgical Treatment

Cardiac Pacemakers

Dual-chamber cardiac pacing (pacing both the atrium and ventricle) has been utilized to assist in symptom relief. Although dual-chamber pacing is not a primary treatment, some patients report improvement in symptoms with cardiac pacing. There has been a particular benefit noted for elderly patients older than age 65 (Maron et al., 2003). Dual-chamber pacing allows for more aggressive treatment with medications that can decrease heart rate.

Ventricular Septal Myectomy

Patients with marked outflow obstruction may be considered for surgical removal of a portion of the hypertrophied septum that is contributing to the outflow obstruction. This surgical procedure is reserved only for those patients on maximum medical therapy who continue to experience severely limiting symptoms and are classified as NYHA functional class III or IV (Maron et al., 2003).

During the procedure, a small amount of the septum is removed from just below the base of the aortic valve, resulting in an enlarged outflow tract (see Figure 8-8). This procedure immediately decreases outflow tract obstruction and SAM of the anterior leaflet of the mitral valve. Mitral valve replacement or repair may also occur during the procedure, depending on the situation. Myectomy without valve replacement is becoming a low-risk procedure with a relatively low operative mortality rate among all age-groups (Maron et al., 2003). Symptoms immediately improve and some literature suggests that improvements are sustained for as much as 30 years. Most patients improve from NYHA class III or IV to class

II or III. Survival rates are greater than 83% at 10 years (Salberg, 2004). Patients may develop left bundle branch block as a result of the procedure but pacemakers are rarely necessary.

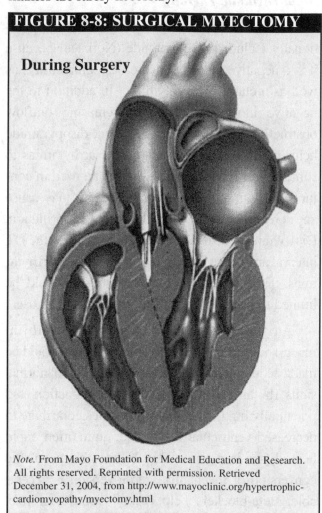

FIGURE 8-8: SURGICAL MYECTOMY

During Surgery

Percutaneous Alcohol Septal Ablation

A second nonsurgical alternative to septal myectomy is percutaneous alcohol septal ablation (PASA). This procedure is relatively new but has become an acceptable treatment option. Candidates for PASA are symptomatic patients with obstruction who are NYHA class III or IV on maximum medical therapy (Maron et al., 2003). However, if mitral valve involvement is advanced and requires repair or replacement, then surgery is the preferable option. PASA is a noninvasive procedure without the risks associated with a major surgery. This procedure may be appropriate for elderly patients who are not good operative candidates.

PASA is performed in the cardiac catheterization laboratory. A catheter is placed in the left anterior descending coronary artery. The catheter is then advanced into one of the septal perforator branches, which provide blood flow to the septum. Once the appropriate septal perforator is located, ethyl alcohol is injected (see Figure 8-9). The alcohol infiltrates the surrounding myocardial tissue as a toxic agent and a controlled MI occurs. The enlarged septal tissue eventually shrinks and the outflow obstruction is relieved. This reduction in tissue size does not occur immediately and may actually continue to occur for up to 1 year after the procedure. In young patients, the benefits of the surgical procedure outweigh the postprocedure arrhythmia risk of PASA. A larger percentage of patients require permanent pacing after PASA than after myectomy.

FIGURE 8-9: ALCOHOL SEPTAL ABLATION

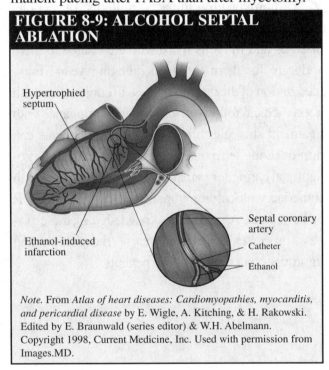

Hypertrophied septum

Ethanol-induced infarction

Septal coronary artery

Catheter

Ethanol

Note. From *Atlas of heart diseases: Cardiomyopathies, myocarditis, and pericardial disease* by E. Wigle, A. Kitching, & H. Rakowski. Edited by E. Braunwald (series editor) & W.H. Abelmann. Copyright 1998, Current Medicine, Inc. Used with permission from Images.MD.

Sudden Cardiac Death

On the whole, life expectancy in patients with HCM is normal; however, sudden cardiac death is the most serious complication of HCM. In most cases, sudden cardiac death is the event that leads to a diagnosis of HCM. Sudden cardiac death occurs most frequently in young people (less than age 35) who are asymptomatic or mildly symptomatic.

However, the risk is not limited to this age-group. Researchers continue to attempt to predict the HCM population that is at high risk for sudden cardiac death so that ICDs can be implanted (see Box 8-4). As risk criteria continue to be evaluated, most literature agrees that ICDs should be placed in any patient with an episode of sudden cardiac death, sustained ventricular tachycardia, or a family history of sudden cardiac death. Patients with other risk factors should not be eliminated from ICD consideration because multiple risk factors may warrant placement of a device. Medication to treat the ventricular arrhythmias should be utilized in conjunction with the ICD; amiodarone is the drug of choice.

BOX 8-4: RISK FACTORS FOR SUDDEN CARDIAC DEATH IN HCM OR HOCM

- One or more first-degree relatives with an episode of sudden cardiac death
- Left ventricular wall thickness greater than 35 mm
- Prolonged or repetitive nonsustained ventricular tachycardia on Holter monitor
- Hypotensive blood pressure response to exercise
- Syncope or near syncope

(Maron et al., 2003)

Clinical Application
Implantation of an ICD is a very emotional process and patients should be provided with emotional support. Many facilities that place ICDs are aware of an ICD support group that can be helpful to patients dealing with the emotions associated with the risk of sudden death and implantation of this device.

Activity Recommendations

Patients with HCM should be restricted from intense competitive sports. HCM is the most common cause of sudden cardiac death in young athletes, especially in football and basketball. Not all sudden cardiac death occurs with intense activity; in fact, sudden cardiac death can occur at rest. However, the incidence of sudden cardiac death increases with the intensity of the activity in the presence of HCM. Patients do not need to restrict activity all together but should avoid "burst" exertion, such as sprinting, and isometric exercises, such as heavy lifting. No evidence supports the exclusion from competitive sports of athletes with a family history of HCM but no personal evidence of the disease.

Clinical Application
Patient response to activity provides a guide for determining the level of activity that is acceptable. Development of chest pain, overt shortness of breath, and syncope may indicate that the activity is too strenuous.

Family Evaluation

HCM is largely a genetic disease process. If HCM is diagnosed or an HCM-related death occurs, all first-degree relatives should be screened for the disease and other blood relatives should be encouraged to undergo screening. The ACC/ESC Clinical Expert Consensus Document on Hypertrophic Cardiomyopathy recommends genetic testing if available. If genetic testing is not feasible, a variety of other tests are appropriate for screening (see Box 8-5). These screenings should occur annually from age 12 through 18. Delayed adult onset is also possible; therefore, relatives with normal studies through age 18 should have an evaluation every 5 years. Children younger than age 12 need not undergo evaluation unless there is a high-risk family profile or the child is involved in intense competitive sports.

BOX 8-5: SCREENING METHODS FOR FAMILIAL HCM

- History and physical examination
- 12-lead ECG
- Echocardiography

Outcomes

The majority of patients with HCM can expect a normal life span if they survive past the age of 35 (Shah, 2003). Once diagnosed with the disease, routine follow-up every 12 to 18 months is recommended. Sudden cardiac death continues to be the primary cause of shortened life spans. Prevention and identification of risk for sudden cardiac death is a major area of focus. Many studies continue to increase the understanding of the genetic code and its impact on the disease process. Hopefully, these studies will provide the key to successful treatment in the future.

CONCLUSION

Cardiomyopathy impacts millions of people, including those who are diagnosed with these diseases and millions more who are related to them and care for them during debilitating years. Early recognition of the disease process in conjunction with good medical follow-up and patient compliance with treatment strategies and risk factor adjustments can improve long-term outcomes. Every health care professional caring for patients will come in contact with someone with cardiomyopathy at some point in his or her career. A good base knowledge of these disease processes helps with early recognition and improves outcomes for these patients.

EXAM QUESTIONS

CHAPTER 8
Questions 64-70

64. Cardiomyopathy is a group of disorders caused by dysfunction of the

    a. pericardium.

    b. endocardium.

    c. myocardium.

    d. epicardium.

65. The primary types of cardiomyopathy are dilated, restrictive, and

    a. alcoholic.

    b. hypertrophic.

    c. peripartum.

    d. arrhythmogenic.

66. The primary pathophysiological change associated with DCM is

    a. decreased ventricular filling.

    b. decreased ventricular chamber size with decreased ventricular filling.

    c. obstruction of the left ventricular outflow tract.

    d. ventricular dilatation with decreased ventricular contraction.

67. The most useful diagnostic tool in all cardiomyopathies is

    a. chest X-ray.

    b. echocardiography.

    c. cardiac catheterization.

    d. ECG.

68. The primary treatment goals for DCM include treatment of arrhythmias, thromboembolic complications, and the underlying disease process and

    a. reduction of diastolic dysfunction.

    b. reduction of preload.

    c. reduction of contractility.

    d. increased afterload.

69. HOCM occurs when there is obstruction of the

    a. left atrial outflow tract.

    b. right atrial outflow tract.

    c. left ventricular outflow tract.

    d. right ventricular outflow tract.

70. Medications that should be avoided once obstructive cardiomyopathy has developed include medications that

    a. increase contractility.

    b. decrease contractility.

    c. decrease heart rate.

    d. decrease impulses from the atrium to the ventricle.

CHAPTER 9

AORTIC VALVE DISEASE

CHAPTER OBJECTIVE

After completing this chapter, the reader will be able to recognize aortic valve disease and identify its impact on the body.

LEARNING OBJECTIVES

After studying this chapter, the reader will be able to

1. identify the pathophysiology that occurs with aortic stenosis.

2. describe key signs and symptoms of aortic stenosis.

3. explain the medical and surgical treatment options available for patients with aortic stenosis.

4. identify the pathophysiology that occurs with aortic regurgitation.

5. describe key signs and symptoms of aortic regurgitation.

6. define the key differences between acute and chronic aortic regurgitation.

7. explain the medical and surgical treatment options available for patients with aortic regurgitation.

INTRODUCTION

The aortic valve is the gateway to the circulatory system of the body. Proper functioning of the valve allows blood to flow from the left ventricle to the aorta when open and prevents backflow of blood from the aorta to the ventricle when closed. Valve dysfunction occurs when the valve does not open properly or close completely. Blood flow from the left ventricle to the aorta is key in delivering the required oxygenated blood to the body.

AORTIC VALVE FUNCTION

The normal aortic valve consists of an annulus and three cusps (see Figure 9-1). The aortic valve functions by pressure changes in the left ventricle and the aorta. During diastole, the aortic valve is closed while the left ventricle fills with blood from the left atrium. As the pressure in the left ventricle rises, the mitral valve closes between the left atrium and left ventricle. Systole begins when the left ventricle begins to contract. Once the pressure in the left ventricle is greater than the pressure on the other side of the aortic valve, the valve is forced open and blood is ejected out of the ventricles into the aorta. After ejection is complete, the pressure in the left ventricle becomes less than the pressure in the aorta and the aortic valve snaps shut. The aortic valve closes tightly to prevent the backflow of blood from the aorta to the left ventricle, and the cycle

FIGURE 9-1: AORTIC VALVE SHOWING THE THREE CUSPS

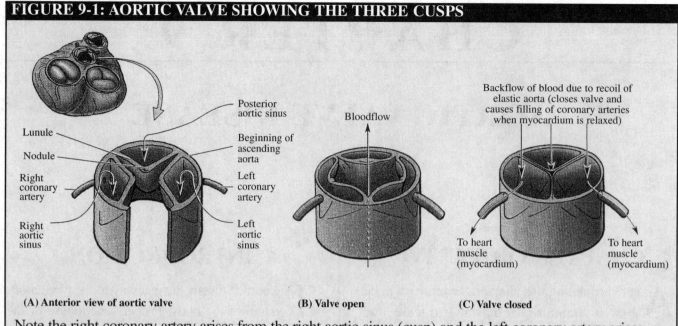

(A) Anterior view of aortic valve   **(B) Valve open**   **(C) Valve closed**

Note the right coronary artery arises from the right aortic sinus (cusp) and the left coronary artery arises from the left aortic sinus (cusp).

Note. From *Clinically Oriented Anatomy* (4th ed.), by K.L. Moore and A.F. Dalley, 1999, Philadelphia: Lippincott Williams & Wilkins. Reprinted with permission from Lippincott Williams & Wilkins.

begins again. Normal aortic valve function is essential for normal cardiac output. Impedance of forward flow, or backflow of volume that should be moving forward, can greatly affect cardiac output. A more detailed description of the cardiac valves is discussed in chapter 1.

Abnormal Valve Function

Basically, two functional valve alterations are responsible for valvular heart disease: stenosis and regurgitation. Valve stenosis occurs when a constriction or narrowing of the valve opening impedes the free flow of blood across the valve. Regurgitation occurs when the valve leaflets do not close completely to form a tight seal, resulting in backward flow of blood. Other terms used to refer to backward blood flow include *prolapse, insufficiency,* and *incompetence.* Although these terms refer to differences in the anatomical process, they all represent a valve that does not close properly.

AORTIC STENOSIS

Definition

Aortic stenosis is said to exist when there is obstruction of flow at the level of the aortic valve. Opening of the aortic valve leaflets is usually restricted.

Causes

Aortic valve stenosis is classified as *congenital* or *acquired.* Congenital valve disease occurs when an abnormal number of valve cusps (unicuspid, bicuspid, tricuspid, or even quadricuspid) are present. It is the most common cause of aortic stenosis in patients younger than age 70. Congenital valve disease is more prevalent in men. Symptoms can appear between ages 40 and 60 in male patients who have had a murmur for years (Novaro & Mills, 2004).

Acquired aortic stenosis caused by rheumatic heart disease or senile degenerative calcification accounts for most symptom-producing aortic stenosis in patients older than age 70 (Havranek & Adair, 2001). Aortic disease that is secondary to rheumatic heart disease is almost always accompanied by mitral valve disease (Darovic, 2002). Aortic stenosis without the presence of mitral valve disease is generally considered nonrheumatic in origin. The incidence of rheumatic aortic valve disease has decreased appreciably with the decrease in the incidence of rheumatic heart disease in this country.

The most common cause of aortic stenosis is senile degenerative calcification (Carabello & Crawford, 2003). Senile degenerative calcification is the result of progressive calcification of the valve leaflets. As calcification progresses, the valves become very stiff and noncompliant (see Figure 9-1). This calcification progression results in severe aortic stenosis and is the most common reason for aortic valve surgery (Carabello & Crawford, 2003). Aortic stenosis resulting from senile degenerative calcification has been associated with individuals over age 70 (men more than women), patients with elevated lipoprotein and low-density lipoprotein cholesterol levels, hypertension, diabetes, elevated serum calcium levels, and elevated serum creatinine levels (LeDoux, 2005).

Pathophysiology

The primary process occurring with rheumatic heart disease is progressive fibrosis of the valve leaflets with fusion of the commissures (points where the valve leaflets connect) and occasionally calcification. In senile degenerative calcification, the valve leaflets thicken and develop calcified nodules that restrict their movement, resulting in valve leaflets that do not open easily or fully (see Figure 9-2).

As the aortic valve opening narrows, due to damaged valve leaflets, blood flow through the valve becomes turbulent and less efficient. The left ventricle must work harder in order to eject blood across the stiff, noncompliant valve. As valve compliance decreases, afterload increases. Afterload is the pressure the left ventricle must overcome to eject blood. In an effort to compensate for the increase in afterload, the left ventricular wall mass (myocardial wall

FIGURE 9-2: DEGENERATIVE AORTIC VALVE DISEASE

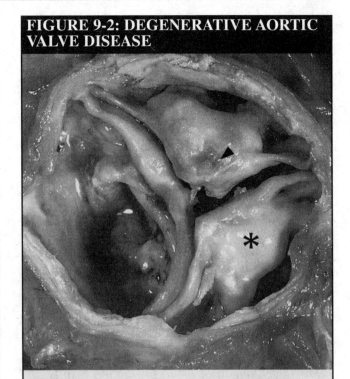

This photo shows severe stenosis of the aortic valve with marked calcific deposits on the left (*) and the posterior noncoronary (▲) cusps without commissural fusion.

Note. From Atlas of heart diseases: Valvular heart disease by R. Virmani, A. Burke, & A. Farb. Edited by E. Braunwald (series editor) & S.H. Rahimtoola. Copyright 1997, Current Medicine. Used with permission from Images.MD.

thickness) increases in size, resulting in progressive concentric left ventricular hypertrophy. Concentric hypertrophy is characterized by increasing left ventricular wall mass with no increase in ventricular chamber size. In fact, the increasing muscle mass actually begins to encroach on the chamber and actually decreases the size of the intraventricular chamber. As the left ventricular wall becomes thicker, an associated decrease in ability of the ventricular wall to expand normally during ventricular filling occurs. Referred to as *diastolic dysfunction,* this inability to expand results in decreased ventricle filling during diastole. With less volume entering the ventricle, there is less volume available for ejection during systole. The ventricle normally ejects 55% to 65% of its contents with each beat. Now, however, the thickened myocardium compensates with a stronger contraction and ejects a larger percentage of the decreased volume, thereby maintaining good cardiac output. As the disease progresses, the left ventricle's attempt to compensate ultimately fails and left ventricular contractile function begins to decrease. This decrease in contractile function results in decreased stroke volume, leaving the ventricle with an excess volume at the end of each contraction. This overload is transferred to the left atrium and ultimately the lungs as signs of heart failure begin.

Clinical Application

Intravascular fluid balance in patients with severe aortic stenosis is critical because the ventricular chamber is no longer able to expand during filling. In order to produce an adequate stroke volume, complete filling of the ventricular chamber is essential.

Clinical Application

The development of atrial fibrillation results in the loss of atrial kick. A loss of atrial kick results in a decrease in ventricular preload (ventricular filling) and an associated decrease in stoke volume.

Clinical Presentation

As the obstruction to flow from the left ventricle continues to increase, so does left ventricular mass. This ability to compensate can last many years before symptoms appear. Symptoms generally begin to appear when the valve opening is one third its normal size. Once symptoms appear, mortality rates rise greatly. Patients with moderate to severe aortic stenosis treated medically observe a 50% mortality rate 2 to 3 years from the onset of symptoms (Darovic, 2002). Generally, after the sixth decade of life, a trio of classic symptoms occurs:

1. angina pectoris

2. syncope

3. heart failure.

(Lewis, Heitkemper, & Dirksen, 2004)

Angina

Increased left ventricular wall mass (hypertrophy) increases left ventricular myocardial oxygen demand. While the patient is at rest, blood supply may be adequate to meet the body's needs. However, with stress or exercise, the increased myocardial oxygen demand of the thickened ventricular wall can no longer be met, resulting in angina. Commonly, angina during exercise is the first presenting symptom in aortic stenosis. Angina can, of course, be caused by coronary heart disease (CHD) in addition to increased wall mass. Approximately one half of aortic stenosis patients presenting with angina also have CHD (Massie & Amiodon, 2004).

Clinical Application

Patients with little or no considerable CHD still have angina as a result of a thickened myocardial wall. These patients benefit from the same measures that increase supply to the myocardium, such as oxygen and adequate hemoglobin levels.

Syncope

During exercise, total systemic vascular resistance (ventricular afterload) normally decreases to allow for better flow of blood out of the ventricle. This decrease in systemic vascular resistance results in decreased blood pressure. The normal compensatory mechanism of the heart is to increase cardiac output to compensate for decreased pressure. This system keeps blood pressure in a normal range and allows patients to tolerate exercise while providing the body with an increased flow of oxygenated blood. However, with a narrowed valve opening, it is essentially impossible to increase cardiac output because the restriction of the valve does not allow for increased blood flow. Patients with severe aortic stenosis experience decreased blood pressure during exercise, resulting in light-headedness, dizziness, and blackout spells. In patients with aortic stenosis, exercise can also cause ventricular or atrial arrhythmias, resulting in syncopal episodes.

Patients should be reminded not to make any sudden position moves. They should be taught to move from a lying to standing position slowly as well as be aware that exercise may result in syncope.

Patients with mild aortic stenosis are not restricted in activity levels or exercise. Patients with moderate aortic stenosis should avoid strenuous activities and competitive sports. Patients with severe aortic stenosis should be advised to limit their activity to low levels.

Heart Failure

Patients with severe aortic stenosis ultimately develop diastolic and systolic failure. Left ventricular hypertrophy results in diastolic dysfunction as the thick-walled ventricle becomes noncompliant and loses its ability to expand during filling. This inability to expand decreases the amount of blood that can enter the left ventricle from the left atrium and results in a back up of blood into the left atrium. The subsequent overload in the left atrium is transferred back to the pulmonary veins, and pulmonary edema results.

Additionally, over time, the hypertrophy that has been compensating for the increased afterload causes the myofibrils to stretch beyond the point of returning to a normal state. The ability of the ventricle to contract decreases and ejection fraction begins to decline. This decrease in ejection fraction again results in a state of extracellular fluid (ECF) overload because the ventricle is unable to empty properly. The patient experiences dyspnea on exertion, orthopnea, and paroxysmal nocturnal dyspnea as well as other signs of volume overload.

Physical Examination

A stenotic aortic valve may produce a murmur before causing any noteworthy hemodynamic changes. The systolic ejection murmur of aortic stenosis is best heard over the second intercostal space, left of the sternal border. The murmur is described as a medium-pitched murmur heard equally with the bell or diaphragm of the stethoscope (Cray et al., 1999). The murmur is described as rough and may become harsh as stenosis worsens. The murmur radiates to the right shoulder and both carotid arteries. In elderly patients with calcific aortic stenosis, the murmur may also radiate to the apex (fifth intercostal space, left midclavicular line) resulting in a misinterpretation of mitral regurgitation. The intensity of the murmur does not correspond with the severity of the stenosis. As aortic stenosis increases in severity, the murmur actually decreases in intensity.

In addition to the murmur and normal first and second heart sounds (S_1 and S_2, or "lub" and "dub" respectively), a fourth heart sound (S_4) may be audible just prior to the first heart sound. As left ventricular mass increases, the compliance of the ventricle decreases along with the ventricles ability to expand during diastolic filling. With this decrease in compliance, the fourth heart sound can be heard late in ventricular diastole, when atrial kick ejects blood into the already full ventricle. When aortic stenosis is advanced and systolic failure occurs, a third heart sound S_3 can also be heard.

The normal pulse is sharp and quick. As aortic stenosis worsens, it becomes more difficult for the left ventricle to quickly push the valve open. As the valve slowly opens, the rush of blood through the valve is delayed, resulting in a decrease in the sharpness of the upstroke of the pulse.

Diagnosis

Echocardiography

The cardiac echocardiogram is the primary tool utilized to confirm the diagnosis of aortic stenosis and quantify its severity. During echocardiography, pressure gradient difference from one side of the valve to the other can be assessed. As valve stenosis worsens, the pressure gradient increases. Additionally, aortic valve area is calculated. Normal valve area ranges from 3 to 4 cm². It is not until the valve area is approximately one fourth the normal size that any changes in flow occur. A valve area of 0.8 to 1.0 cm² indicates severe stenosis (Bonow et al., 1998). Left ventricular mass, valve leaflet mobility, and systolic and diastolic function can also be assessed using echocardiography.

Cardiac Catheterization

Patients with symptomatic aortic stenosis require cardiac catheterization to determine the extent, if any, of CHD. If valve replacement is questionable, the presence of treatable CHD answers the question and moves the patient toward surgery. A valve area of less than 0.8 cm² on cardiac catheterization indicates critical aortic valve stenosis and supports a decision for valve replacement (Havranek & Adair, 2001).

Electrocardiogram

An electrocardiogram (ECG) demonstrates an increased QRS voltage with associated ST-segment and T wave abnormalities. The increased QRS voltage is due to the increase in myocardial mass. Atrial abnormalities, demonstrated by abnormal P waves, indicate atrial enlargement. Theses ECG changes are neither sensitive nor specific to aortic stenosis and always require other testing for confirmation.

Chest X-ray Film

On chest X-ray film, the heart usually appears normal in size. The shape, however, demonstrates a rounded left ventricular border, representing concentric hypertrophy. The aortic shadow may become enlarged, and occasionally, calcification of the valve is visible on the lateral view.

Medical Therapy

Medical treatment beyond the occasional need for rate control with atrial fibrillation is rarely needed early in the disease process. Medication temporarily resolves heart failure; however, if the valve is not replaced, failure worsens and death is the end result.

ACE Inhibitors

Although indicated for heart failure, angiotensin-converting enzyme (ACE) inhibitors are generally contraindicated in patients with *severe* aortic stenosis. ACE inhibitors decrease systemic vascular resistance, which decreases blood pressure (LeDoux, 2005). The normal response to this change is an increase in heart rate to compensate for the decrease in blood pressure. A stenotic valve prevents large volumes of blood from being forced through, resulting in an inability to increase cardiac output. The patient develops hypotension and, ultimately syncope could result.

Nitroglycerin

Nitrates should be used cautiously in patients with severe disease. It is important to remember that low-dose nitroglycerin decreases preload. With the hypertrophy that has developed, preload is already decreased due to the ventricles inability to expand during filling. Any further loss of filling would result in a decrease in stroke volume. Nitroglycerin at high doses could further complicate the issue by causing a decrease in systemic vascular resistance similar to the effects of ACE inhibitors (Balentine & Eisenhart, 2005).

Beta-blockers

Beta-blockers are contraindicated because they block the normal adrenergic response that has been occurring to compensate for decreased cardiac output (increased heart rate and contractility) and lessen the ability of the ventricle to overcome the pressure gradient that has developed (LeDoux, 2005).

Endocarditis Prophylaxis

Antibiotic prophylaxis for endocarditis is essential in all patients with aortic stenosis, regardless of age or symptoms. The damaged valve causes hemodynamic turbulence, which is an environment for infection in which endocarditis can result. Therefore, all patients with aortic valve disease with a murmur should be treated prophylactically with antibiotics for endocarditis (Darovic, 2002).

Surgical Intervention

With the onset of symptoms, mortality rates dramatically increase. Survival rates of patients with symptomatic aortic stenosis without surgical intervention are 50% at 2 to 3 years (Darovic, 2002). Once symptoms appear, the need for surgical repair becomes imminent. Surgical outcomes improve with early detection. Therefore, close follow-up of patients with aortic stenosis, with an early decision to treat once symptoms begin, is imperative. Patients with mild aortic stenosis should have follow-up echocardiography every 2 years. After severe stenosis develops, but while the patient remains asymptomatic, evaluations should occur every 6 to 12 months (LeDoux, 2005). Several options are available once the patient becomes symptomatic.

Percutaneous Balloon Valvuloplasty

A balloon inflated in the valve orifice can be used to fracture calcium deposits in the leaflets and stretch the aortic annulus. This procedure is considered palliative and should be reserved for patients who are not surgical candidates but are seeking relief from symptoms. The American College of Cardiology (ACC) and American Heart Association (AHA) recommendations for aortic balloon valvuloplasty in adults with aortic stenosis are reviewed in Box 9-1. This procedure has no effect on long-term mortality rates. Six months after the procedure, about half of the patients have lost all benefit of the procedure (LeDoux, 2005). Prior to the procedure, patients should be evaluated for aortic regurgitation. Aortic regurgitation is an expected postoperative result after valvuloplasty. The procedure should not be performed if the patient has 2+ or greater aortic valve regurgitation.

Aortic Valve Replacement

Surgery is the treatment of choice in most adults with calcific aortic stenosis once symptoms develop (see Box 9-2). There has been no demonstrated benefit from surgery for nonsymptomatic patients (Carabello & Crawford, 2003). Therefore, surgery is

---

> **BOX 9-1: ACC/AHA RECOMMENDATIONS FOR AORTIC BALLOON VALVULOPLASTY**
>
> - A bridge to surgery in hemodynamically unstable patients with severe aortic stenosis who are too unstable to undergo surgery
> - Palliative care in patients with serious comorbid conditions
> - Asymptomatic patients with severe aortic stenosis who require urgent noncardiac surgery
>
> (Bonow et al., 1998)

not indicated until symptoms appear. Prior to surgery, the mitral valve is also evaluated because quite frequently, mitral regurgitation also exists and mitral valve replacement may also be necessary. Cardiac catheterization should also be performed to determine the need for coronary artery bypass surgery. A preoperative assessment of left ventricular function determines systolic and diastolic dysfunction. Surgical mortality risk is lowest in those with normal left ventricular function and increases as systolic function decreases (Darovic, 2002).

> **BOX 9-2: ACC/AHA RECOMMENDATIONS FOR AORTIC VALVE REPLACEMENT**
>
> - Symptomatic patients with severe aortic stenosis
> - Patients with severe aortic stenosis (with or without symptoms) undergoing coronary artery bypass surgery
> - Patients with severe aortic stenosis (with or without symptoms) undergoing surgery on the aorta or other heart valves
> - Asymptomatic patients with severe aortic stenosis and one of the following:
>   - left ventricular systolic dysfunction
>   - abnormal response to exercise
>   - marked or excessive left ventricular hypertrophy
>   - prevention of sudden death in asymptomatic patients with none of the findings listed under asymptomatic patients with severe aortic stenosis
>
> (Bonow et al., 1998)

Clinical Application

Patients with aortic valve disease should be aware of signs of decompensation. With early recognition, the appropriate treatment can take place before any permanent damage to the ventricle has occurred.

The type of valve prosthesis used is determined by the anticipated longevity of the patient and the patient's ability to tolerate anticoagulants. Mechanical valves have better durability than tissue valves that come from human or pig donors (bioprosthetics). Mechanical valves require lifelong anticoagulation, which is not necessary for tissue valves. They are generally best suited for young patients with no contraindications to anticoagulation. However, young female patients who wish to become pregnant require tissue valves because the utilization of anticoagulation during pregnancy increases fetal mortality (Carabello & Crawford, 2003). Elderly patients with a life expectancy less than that of the tissue valve (7 to 10 years) are better suited for tissue valves and can then avoid the need for anticoagulation and its associated complications.

Some centers also perform the Ross procedure, which involves placing a patient's pulmonic valve in the aortic valve position and placing a tissue valve in the pulmonic valve location. It has been noted that tissue valves last longer in the lower pressure right heart and the need for anticoagulation is avoided (Carabello & Crawford, 2003).

Outcomes

After successful aortic valve replacement, decreased left ventricular systolic pressure and decreased afterload result in improved ejection fraction and increased cardiac output. Left ventricular hypertrophy actually regresses, with most of that regression occurring in the first year but continuing to improve for up to 10 years (Carabello & Crawford, 2003) . However, diastolic function most likely never returns to normal due to the increase in collagen content in the myocardial tissue.

AORTIC REGURGITATION

Definition

Aortic regurgitation occurs when the valve cusps do not close tightly and blood is allowed to travel retrograde, or backward, through the valve during ventricular systole. A variety of processes can affect the valve cusps, the aortic root, or both, resulting in aortic regurgitation (see Figure 9-1).

Causes

Aortic regurgitation can be classified as acute or chronic. Symptoms depend on the severity and rapidity of onset. With the decreased incidence of rheumatic valve disease, chronic nonrheumatic causes now account for the majority of isolated cases of aortic regurgitation. Causes of nonrheumatic valve disease include congenital bicuspid valve, infective endocarditis, and connective tissue diseases as well as calcifications that affect the valves cusps. Many patients with chronic aortic regurgitation have processes that affect the aortic root, including Marfan's syndrome, aortic dissection, inflammatory diseases, and syphilis (LeDoux, 2005). Acute aortic regurgitation is seen with trauma, acute bacterial endocarditis, and acute aortic dissection (Bonow et al., 1998). Additionally, severe systemic hypertension has been noted to cause aortic regurgitation (Bonow et al., 1998).

Because the presentation of acute aortic regurgitation is entirely different than that of chronic aortic regurgitation, the two are discussed separately.

CHRONIC AORTIC REGURGITATION

Pathophysiology

Normally, as the ventricle ejects blood through the aortic valve, the aorta expands to accept the volume. When the pressure in the ventricle becomes less than the pressure in the aorta, the aortic valve closes. The aorta relaxes and blood is dispersed to the area of least resistance. This expansion and relaxation of the aorta are known as the *elastic and recoil properties* of the aorta. With a competent aortic valve, blood moves forward. The closed valve stops blood from moving backward toward the aortic valve (see Figure 9-3).

FIGURE 9-3: NORMAL FUNCTIONING OF THE AORTA DURING SYSTOLE AND DIASTOLE

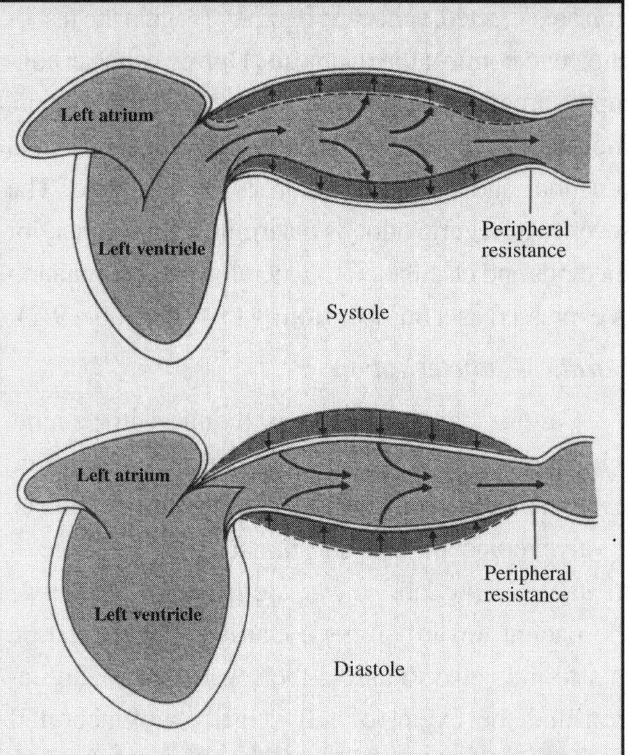

Note. From *Critical care nursing: Diagnosis and management* (2nd ed.), by L.A. Thelan, J.K. Davie, L.D. Urden, & M.E. Lough, 1994, St. Louis: Mosby. Reprinted permission from Elsevier.

In aortic regurgitation blood enters the left ventricle normally from the left atrium. Blood also enters the left ventricle from the aorta because the valve does not close properly and backflow occurs from the aorta through the aortic valve into the left ventricle. This results in a larger-than-normal volume in the left ventricle. To compensate, left ventricular chamber size increases to allow for the additional volume. Left ventricular wall thickness also increases to help maintain normal wall stress. The enlarged left ventricular chamber size maintains a normal or near-normal preload and the increase in wall thickness helps increase stroke volume. This increased stroke volume is necessary because a portion of the blood ejected to the aorta with each beat returns to the left ventricle during ventricular diastole through the regurgitant valve. If the ventricle can eject a larger-than-normal volume with each beat, the cardiac output needs should be met. While maintaining preload, normal wall stress, and contractility, ejection fraction remains the same. This phase of the disease process is considered the *chronic compensatory phase* and lasts for many years or even decades. As with aortic stenosis, patients remain asymptomatic for years with very low morbidity.

Eventually, however, the compensatory mechanisms begin to fail and the enlarged heart begins to show signs of decompensation. As dilatation of the left ventricle continues, contractility eventually decreases because the myocardium has been overstretched. Left ventricular ejection fraction also decreases, resulting in decreased cardiac output (systolic dysfunction). As ejection fraction decreases, left ventricular volume (preload) increases due to the inability of the ventricles to empty appropriately. Additionally, afterload increases to compensate for decreased cardiac output. Heart rate also increases to compensate for the decrease in cardiac output; however, this increased rate is often ineffective. After decades without any difficulties, patients begin to develop symptoms of ECF overload.

Clinical Presentation

Although patients commonly remain asymptomatic for years, the initial symptoms noted most frequently are exertional dyspnea and fatigue due to the failing left ventricle. As the disease progresses, patients can also develop paroxysmal nocturnal dyspnea and orthopnea with pulmonary edema. Angina can result from an inability of the coronary arteries to supply the volume of oxygenated blood needed for the increased myocardial mass. Patients with aortic regurgitation commonly experience ischemia without associated CHD. The incidence of concurrent CHD with aortic regurgitation is less common than with aortic stenosis.

Physical Examination

A variety of signs can lead a health care professional toward a diagnosis of aortic regurgitation. A diastolic murmur, displaced left ventricular impulse, wide pulse pressure, and specific peripheral findings are characteristic signs of chronic aortic regurgitation. The characteristic murmur of aortic regurgitation is a soft, diastolic murmur best heard at the third intercostal space to the left of the sternum. The murmur is loudest at end-expiration and is better recognized with the patient sitting and leaning forward (Cray et al., 1999). If the patient has aortic root disease (Marfan's syndrome), then the murmur is best heard to the right of the sternum (Cray et al., 1999). Occasionally, the murmur is described as a diastolic rumble heard best at the apex; in this case, it is referred to as an Austin Flint murmur (Zoghbi & Afridi, 2003). The apical impulse (normally at the apex of the heart) is displaced leftward and downward due to the hypertrophy and is forceful due to increased stroke volume.

As regurgitation progresses, diastolic blood pressure decreases, resulting in a widened pulse pressure. Diastolic blood pressure decreases as more blood is returned to the left ventricle; it is generally less than 60 mm Hg (Hilkert & Yoo, 2002). Additionally, systolic pressure increases as a result of increased stroke volume. Pulse pressure is commonly greater than 100 mm Hg. The same physiological changes that are responsible for widened pulse pressure also result in a variety of peripheral signs that have been associated with chronic aortic regurgitation (see Table 9-1).

Diagnosis

Echocardiography

Once the characteristic signs of aortic regurgitation are detected, echocardiography is again the test of choice to confirm the diagnosis. During echocardiography, an assessment of the severity of regurgitation, morphology of the valve, left ventricular size and function, and the aortic root can all be made. The severity of regurgitation is determined by a variety of methods and calculations. Generally, the regurgitation is expressed as a number from 1 to 4 (see Table 9-2).

Cardiac Catheterization

Cardiac catheterization is required in patients with symptomatic aortic regurgitation to determine the extent, if any, of CHD. As with aortic stenosis, if valve replacement is questionable, the presence of treatable CHD can answer the question and move the patient toward surgery. Cardiac catheterization is also indicated to assess the severity of regurgitation and the extent of left ventricular function if noninvasive tests are inconclusive.

TABLE 9-1: PERIPHERAL SIGNS OF CHRONIC AORTIC REGURGITATION

Sign	Description
Water-hammer pulse (Corrigan's pulse)	A rapid rise and collapse of the pulse upon palpation of the peripheral pulse
Musset's sign	Bobbing of the head with each heart beat
Traube's sign (pistol-shot sounds)	Booming systolic and diastolic sounds heard over the femoral artery
Duroziez's sign	Systolic murmur heard over the femoral artery when compressed proximally and diastolic murmur heard over the femoral artery when compressed distally

(Zoghbi & Afridi, 2003)

TABLE 9-2: AORTIC REGURGITATION SEVERITY

Rating	Definition
1+	Mild aortic regurgitation
2+	Moderate aortic regurgitation
3+	Moderately severe aortic regurgitation
4+	Severe aortic regurgitation

(Hilkert & Yoo, 2002)

Chest X-ray Film

A chest X-ray film shows left ventricular hypertrophy (enlarged heart) and pulmonary congestion, as would be expected in a patient with heart failure.

Electrocardiogram

A 12-lead ECG demonstrates the increased QRS voltage that is seen with left ventricular hypertrophy. These ECG changes are neither sensitive nor specific to aortic regurgitation and always require other testing for confirmation.

Stress Test

Stress testing can be useful in patients with mild symptoms. The test provides an assessment of exercise tolerance with both symptomatic response and hemodynamic effects. This test assists in determining the need for intervention.

Medical Therapy

Patients may remain asymptomatic for many years. If patients with mild aortic regurgitation remain asymptomatic and have normal left ventricular function, no treatment is necessary. Vasodilators are useful in asymptomatic patients with moderately severe to severe aortic regurgitation who continue to have normal left ventricular function and good exercise tolerance. Vasodilators (hydralazine, nifedipine, and ACE inhibitors) can be helpful by decreasing left ventricular afterload (Bonow et al., 1998). A decrease in afterload decreases regurgitant volume by making it easier for blood to move forward through the aorta and less apt to move backward

through the malfunctioning valve. These medications can actually help slow the progression of the disease (Bonow et al., 1998). Patients with aortic regurgitation should also receive prophylactic antibiotic treatment for endocarditis (Darovic, 2002).

Patients with chronic aortic regurgitation should have regular follow-up serial testing that includes echocardiograms to assess left ventricular function. The frequency of follow-up increases as valve disease progresses. Since mortality with valve replacement worsens as ejection fraction worsens, careful assessment of left ventricular function is essential. Once patients develop left ventricular dysfunction, with or without symptoms, with an ejection fraction less than 50%, valve replacement surgery should be considered (Bonow et al., 1998).

Clinical Application

Although utilized in acutely ill patients, intra-aortic balloon pumping is contraindicated in patients with aortic regurgitation because it grossly increases aortic regurgitation. As the balloon inflates in the aorta during ventricular diastole, blood in the aorta is forced to return to the ventricle through the regurgitant valve.

Surgical Intervention

Once symptoms begin, patients should be evaluated for surgical replacement of the aortic valve (see Box 9-3). Surgical intervention is indicated if ejection fraction is abnormal, with or without the presence of symptoms. As the severity of left ventricular dysfunction increases, so does mortality rate with surgery; therefore, early intervention is indicated (Darovic, 2002).

Surgical options for replacement of the aortic valve in patients with aortic regurgitation are the same as those for aortic stenosis. The elderly commonly have aortic stenosis and aortic regurgitation as well as CHD. According to the ACC/AHA guidelines, the determination for surgery should be based on quality of life and not longevity. Symptom

BOX 9-3: ACC/AHA RECOMMENDATIONS FOR AORTIC VALVE REPLACEMENT IN PATIENTS WITH AORTIC REGURGITATION

- Symptomatic patients with normal left ventricular function and New York Heart Association functional class III or IV symptoms
- Symptomatic patients with left ventricular dysfunction (ejection fraction 25% to 49%)
- Asymptomatic patients with left ventricular dysfunction (ejection fraction less than 50%)

(Bonow et al., 1998)

relief should be the most important guide in making the decision for aortic valve replacement.

Outcomes

Left ventricular function generally improves for up to 2 years after surgery, with a gradual decline in ventricular hypertrophy (Zoghbi & Afridi, 2003). These results vary depending on the preoperative condition of the left ventricle. An echocardiogram should be performed shortly after surgery. If the initial echocardiogram shows improvement, then serial echocardiograms are not necessary. Patients who continue to demonstrate left ventricular dysfunction should be treated as are others with left ventricular dysfunction, including the use of ACE inhibitors. Follow-up echocardiography is necessary at 6 or 12 months to assess left ventricular function.

ACUTE AORTIC REGURGITATION

Pathophysiology

Acute aortic regurgitation is most noted with trauma, aortic dissection, and acute cases of infective endocarditis (Bonow et al., 1998). When acute aortic regurgitation occurs, a volume of blood suddenly returns to the left ventricle from the aorta. This acute regurgitation occurs with no ability of the left ventricle to make adjustments to the sudden increase. The volume overload is transferred backward to the left atrium and, ultimately, the pulmonary veins. This results in the development of acute pulmonary edema. The left ventricle is unable to increase stroke volume because it has no time to adapt. Stroke volume dramatically decreases because much of the blood is returned to the ventricle with each cardiac cycle. The body attempts to compensate for this decrease in cardiac output by increasing heart rate; however, this compensation is generally ineffective. Additionally, peripheral vasoconstriction occurs to compensate for the decrease in cardiac output. As the volume travels to the area of least resistance, vasoconstriction only increases afterload and results in a worsening of the acute aortic regurgitation.

Clinical Presentation

Patients with acute aortic regurgitation generally present with acute pulmonary edema and possibly cardiogenic shock. They complain of severe dyspnea, orthopnea, and weakness. The onset of symptoms is generally abrupt.

Physical Examination

Examination of the lungs reveals bilateral rales indicative of pulmonary edema. The patient is tachycardic and hypotensive. Because the long-term compensatory mechanisms have not had time to occur, not all of the peripheral signs associated with chronic aortic regurgitation are present.

Clinical Application
Patients with acute aortic regurgitation are acutely ill and generally in a life-threatening situation, especially in the presence of aortic root dissection.

Diagnosis

Cardiac echocardiography is utilized to quickly confirm the diagnosis of aortic regurgitation as well as determine the extent of the problem. A transesophageal echocardiogram may be done if aortic dissection is suspected. Cardiac catheterization may be done, if there is time, to further evaluate the aortic regurgitation and aortic dissection.

Medical Therapy

Early surgical treatment is necessary because patients with acute aortic regurgitation often die from pulmonary edema, ventricular arrhythmias, or cardiogenic shock (Bonow et al., 1998). While patients are being prepared for surgery, sodium nitroprusside (Nipride) is helpful because it decreases preload and afterload (Zoghbi & Afridi, 2003). Dobutamine assists with ventricular contractility and helps increase cardiac output. If the patient has developed acute aortic regurgitation as a result of infective endocarditis, 48 hours of antibiotics are preferred if the patient can tolerate the delay in surgery (LeDoux, 2005). However, surgery should not be delayed if the patient is hemodynamically unstable.

Surgical Replacement

For an unstable patient, surgical intervention resolves the instability. Valve replacement with a mechanical or bioprosthetic valve should be done as quickly as possible. If the patient has aortic dissection, repair of the aorta is also necessary.

Outcomes

Once a patient with acute aortic regurgitation has the valve successfully replaced, outcomes are very good. If left ventricular function was normal prior to the acute event, there should be no long-term effects on the ventricle. Follow-up is the same as with all valve surgeries.

CONCLUSION

The aortic valve is the gateway to the body from the left ventricle. If this gate does not function correctly, it can have long-term effects on the body as the structures surrounding the valve attempt to compensate. Health care professionals should assist the patient in understanding the disease progression associated with aortic valve disease. With a full understanding, the patient can recognize symptoms of decompensation early and intervention can take place in a timely manner.

EXAM QUESTIONS

CHAPTER 9
Questions 71-78

71. Fibrosis of the valve leaflets with fusion of the commissures is the primary pathophysiologic change that occurs in which type of aortic stenosis?

    a. congenital valve disease

    b. rheumatic heart disease

    c. senile degenerative fibrosis

    d. senile degenerative calcification

72. The classic trio of symptoms noted in symptomatic patients with aortic stenosis is

    a. angina, syncope, and heart failure.

    b. hypotension, palpitations, and angina.

    c. murmurs, hypotension, and palpitations.

    d. palpitations, syncope, and angina.

73. The primary tool used for diagnosing valvular heart disease is

    a. echocardiography.

    b. ECG.

    c. cardiac catheterization.

    d. cardiac stress testing.

74. The class of medications that is contraindicated in patients with severe aortic stenosis due to its effect of decreasing systemic vascular resistance is

    a. beta-blockers.

    b. ACE inhibitors.

    c. low-dose nitrates.

    d. aspirin.

75. In patients with chronic aortic regurgitation, a physiological change that is the direct result of the heart compensating for the regurgitation is

    a. left atrial enlargement.

    b. left ventricular enlargement.

    c. aortic enlargement.

    d. decreased contractility.

76. The most frequently noted first symptoms of chronic aortic regurgitation include

    a. hypotension, syncope, and angina.

    b. systolic murmur and head bobbing with each heart beat.

    c. exertional dyspnea and fatigue.

    d. edema and systolic murmur.

77. Signs and symptoms specific to patients with acute aortic regurgitation include

    a. decreased activity tolerance.

    b. bradycardia.

    c. water-hammer pulse.

    d. abrupt onset of shortness of breath.

78. Surgical replacement of the aortic valve for aortic regurgitation should occur when the patient develops left ventricular dysfunction with an ejection fraction less than

    a. 65%.

    b. 60%.

    c. 55%.

    d. 50%.

CHAPTER 10

MITRAL VALVE DISEASE

CHAPTER OBJECTIVE

After completing this chapter, the reader will be able to recognize mitral valve disease and identify its impact on the body.

LEARNING OBJECTIVES

After studying this chapter, the reader will be able to

1. identify the pathophysiology that occurs with mitral stenosis.

2. describe key signs and symptoms of mitral stenosis.

3. explain the medical and surgical treatment options available for patients with mitral stenosis.

4. identify the pathophysiology that occurs with mitral regurgitation.

5. describe key signs and symptoms of mitral regurgitation.

6. explain the medical and surgical treatment options available for patients with mitral regurgitation.

INTRODUCTION

The mitral valve is the gateway between the left atrium and ventricle. Proper function of the valve allows blood to move from the atrium to the ventricle. Its normal function plays a key role in the volume in the left ventricle before ejection. This volume is essential for systemic perfusion. A dysfunctional valve can alter ventricular preload and, consequently, perfusion.

MITRAL VALVE FUNCTION

The mitral valve opens passively during the beginning of diastole, allowing blood to flow passively from the atrium to the ventricle. At the end of diastole, the atrium contracts (atrial kick) and sends an additional volume to the ventricle. As the pressure in the ventricle increases, the mitral valve begins to close. Isovolumic contraction begins, and further pressure in the ventricle builds, forcing the mitral valve to snap shut. The papillary muscles contract, preventing the mitral valve leaflets from prolapsing into the left atrium during systole. The closed mitral valve forms a tight seal to assure that the blood being ejected from the ventricle flows forward through the aortic valve and not backward into the left atrium. Once ventricular ejection is complete and the pressure in the left ventricle becomes less than the pressure in the left atrium, the mitral valve opens and the cycle begins again (see Figure 10-1). A more detailed description of the cardiac valves is covered in chapter 1. Definitions of stenosis and regurgitation are provided in chapter 9.

FIGURE 10-1: NORMAL MITRAL VALVE

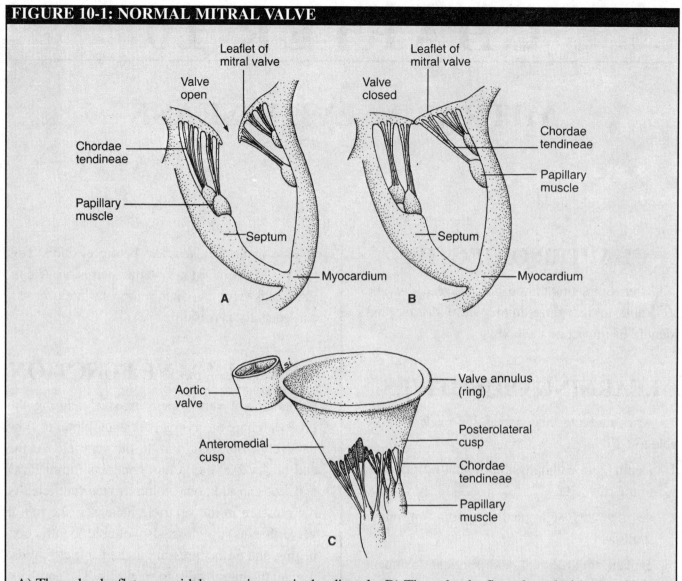

A) The valve leaflets are widely open in ventricular diastole. B) The valve leaflets close during ventricular systole. C) The mitral valve annulus and cusps form a funnel-like structure when the mitral valve is open.

Note. From *Hemodynamic monitoring: Invasive and noninvasive clinical application* (3rd ed.), by G.O. Darovic, 2002, Philadelphia: Saunders. Reprinted with permission from Elsevier.

MITRAL STENOSIS

Definition

Mitral stenosis occurs when the mitral valve no longer opens normally, causing an obstruction of blood flow from the left atrium to the left ventricle (see Figure 10-2).

Causes

Mitral stenosis is most commonly caused by rheumatic fever (Darovic, 2002). As the incidence of rheumatic fever decreases in the United States, so does the incidence of mitral stenosis. Congenital mitral stenosis, atrial myxoma, systemic lupus erythematosus, and bacterial endocarditis can also cause mitral stenosis, but these causes are rare (Swain, 2001). Mitral stenosis is more common in women than in men. Forty percent of all patients with rheumatic heart disease develop mitral stenosis, and this accounts for 60% of all cases of mitral stenosis. (Bonow et al., 1998). Many patients with rheumatic mitral stenosis have no recollection of having rheumatic fever.

FIGURE 10-2: MITRAL VALVE STENOSIS

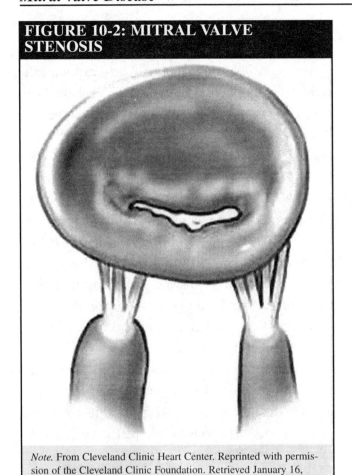

Note. From Cleveland Clinic Heart Center. Reprinted with permission of the Cleveland Clinic Foundation. Retrieved January 16, 2005, from http://www.clevelandclinic.org/heartcenter/pub/guide/disease/valve/balloon_valve.htm

Pathophysiology

The rheumatic mitral valve develops fibrosis and calcification of the valve leaflets. The valve commissures fuse together, and the chordae tendineae thicken and shorten. The combination of some or all of these changes results in a valve orifice that is much smaller than normal. The normal mitral valve area is 4 to 5 cm² (Bonow et al., 1998). As the valve opening becomes smaller, it becomes more difficult for blood to flow passively from the atrium to the ventricle. Because the ventricle depends on diastolic filling to maintain stroke volume, left atrial pressure must rise in an attempt to maintain normal flow across the valve. This increase in left atrial pressure is transferred back to the pulmonary vascular bed as pulmonary pressure subsequently increases. As the obstruction worsens, the chronic increase in left atrial pressure results in pulmonary hypertension and, ultimately, right ven-

tricular failure. The left atrium dilates in response to the increased pressure and volume, and it becomes increasingly more difficult to empty the atrium. The enlarged left atrium puts the patient at risk for the development of thrombi in the atrium.

Clinical Presentation

The development of symptoms could begin as long as 40 years after the development of rheumatic fever (Bonow et al., 1998). After the onset of initial symptoms, another 10 years may pass before symptoms that change the patient's lifestyle occur. Symptoms at rest are usually absent until the valve orifice is less than 1.5 cm² (Griffin & Hayek, 2004). Generally, the valve area is less than half the normal size before any symptoms occur (Bonow et al., 1998). Once symptoms begin, they develop slowly and patients make adjustments in activity levels to compensate for the changes, often without being aware that they are doing so. Dyspnea with exertion with no symptoms at rest is the most common initial finding. Conditions that increase heart rate, such as pregnancy, new-onset atrial fibrillation, hyperthyroidism, or fever, commonly result in symptoms that alert the physician to the possibility of mitral stenosis. An increased heart rate shortens diastole and, therefore, decreases ventricular filling time. Decreased filling time results in decreased stroke volume, which contributes to decreased cardiac output. When cardiac output is insufficient, symptoms of dyspnea and fatigue occur.

As valve dysfunction increases and the valve orifice decreases (1 cm² to 1.4 cm²), symptoms increase. Pulmonary symptoms such as orthopnea and paroxysmal nocturnal dyspnea develop. With the development of severe mitral stenosis (valve orifice less than 1 cm²), the patient develops dyspnea at rest and is essentially confined to a bed or chair, as the complications of pulmonary hypertension worsen. Cough and hemoptysis develop as the disease progresses. Ultimately, the failure of the system affects the right side of the heart, and signs of right ventricular failure appear.

Clinical Application

Patients with severe mitral stenosis may develop acute pulmonary edema with exercise because the narrowed mitral opening cannot handle the increased blood flow produced by the normal increase in heart rate and venous return that occurs with exercise.

Clinical Application

Although patients with mild to moderate mitral stenosis should be counseled to avoid unusually stressful exercise, they should be encouraged to maintain a low-level aerobic exercise program to maintain cardiovascular fitness. The limits of this exercise should be determined by individual patient tolerance.

With the atrium enlarging and cardiac output decreasing, the risk of thrombi development in the atrium increases, as does the risk for embolization. In many cases, stroke caused by an embolus is the first indication of mitral stenosis. The probability of a stroke exists if the patient is in sinus rhythm but increases with the development of atrial fibrillation. Atrial fibrillation is noted in more than one half of patients with mitral stenosis due to atrial enlargement (Massie & Amiodon, 2004).

Clinical Application

Patients with mitral stenosis are dependent on atrial contraction for a large portion of ventricular filling because stenosis slows the passive filling phase. Therefore, the development of atrial fibrillation in patients with mitral stenosis can quickly result in symptoms of decreased perfusion, because atrial contraction is lost with the onset of atrial fibrillation.

Physical Examination

On cardiac auscultation, the first heart sound (S_1, or "lub") is louder than normal unless the valve is heavily calcified; then the sound is diminished (Griffin & Hayek, 2004). The second heart sound (S_2, or "dub") is associated with closure of the aortic and pulmonic valves. At the same time, the mitral and tricuspid valves open. Opening of a stenotic mitral valve results in a sound that may be heard immediately after the second heart sound. This sound is called an *opening snap* and is best heard at the cardiac apex (fifth intercostal space, at the midclavicular line) with the diaphragm of the stethoscope. At the same location, a low-pitched rumbling diastolic murmur can be heard with the bell of the stethoscope. The murmur occurs during ventricular diastole and can be heard after the second heart sound and before the first heart sound. The more severe the disease process, the longer the murmur lasts throughout diastole. The murmur is best heard with the patient lying on the left side and increases with exercise (Cray et al., 1999). Patients may also present with signs of right ventricular failure, including crackles, jugular venous distension, hepatomegaly, and peripheral edema. Mitral facies is a pinkish purple discoloration of the cheeks that is common in patients with severe mitral stenosis (Darovic, 2002).

Diagnosis

Echocardiography

Cardiac echocardiography is the method of choice for diagnosing mitral stenosis. With echocardiography, the mitral valve orifice can be measured to assist in the determination of stenosis severity (see Table 10-1). Valve motion, leaflet thickness, and calcification can also be evaluated with echocardiography. In addition to an evaluation of the valve itself, left atrial size and pulmonary artery pressures are measured. Patients with mitral stenosis may also benefit from transesophageal echocardiography to detect valve vegetation or thrombi in the left atrium.

Cardiac Catheterization

Cardiac catheterization allows for assessment of the need for coronary artery revascularization if valve replacement is needed. During cardiac catheterization, left atrial pressure can be measured to assist in the evaluation of the progression of the

TABLE 10-1: MITRAL STENOSIS STAGES

Mitral Valve Area	Stage of Progression
> 2.5 cm^2	Minimal
1.4 to 2.5 cm^2	Mild
1.0 to 1.4 cm^2	Moderate
< 1.0 cm^2	Severe
(Stoltz & Bryg, 2003)	

disease. However, cardiac catheterization is not as useful in determining the severity of the stenosis as is echocardiography.

Chest X-ray Film

The presence of signs of mitral stenosis on chest X-ray film depends on the extent of the disease. As the disease progresses and pulmonary hypertension develops, the pulmonary arteries are more visible on the X-ray film. An elevation of the left mainstem bronchus, with left atrial enlargement, may also be noted. Signs of pulmonary edema are noted if the patient is in a volume overload state.

Electrocardiogram

The electrocardiogram (ECG) demonstrates signs of left atrial enlargement with abnormal P waves (wide, notched P waves in lead II.) If right ventricular hypertrophy is present, a QRS axis shift to the right may be visible. These ECG changes are neither sensitive nor specific to mitral stenosis and always require other testing for confirmation.

The ECG may also show atrial fibrillation. New-onset atrial fibrillation is a treatable rhythm that can be identified by comparing the patient's current ECG to previous ECGs.

Clinical Application

Clinicians should be particularly alert for the development of atrial fibrillation because the incidence of stroke is high with this rhythm. Many patients are unaware of the development of an irregularly irregular heart rhythm, but astute practitioners can recognize the changes of atrial fibrillation and begin appropriate treatment.

Medical Therapy

Endocarditis Prophylaxis

Antibiotic prophylaxis for endocarditis is appropriate in patients with anatomical changes in the valve. Antibiotics should also be given prior to surgical or dental procedures. Patients with mitral stenosis are at moderate risk for the development of bacterial endocarditis.

Rhythm Control

Medical management is of limited use in asymptomatic patients with normal sinus rhythm. Once symptoms begin, treatment is directed to alleviation of symptoms. Calcium channel blockers, beta-blockers, or digoxin can be useful in the treatment of atrial fibrillation to maintain a ventricular rate of less than 100 beats per minute (Griffin & Hayek, 2004). Because atrial fibrillation is poorly tolerated, it is reasonable to attempt to return the patient to normal sinus rhythm with cardioversion, either electrical or chemical (with medications). Continued use of antiarrhythmics after successful cardioversion to sinus rhythm has proven to be helpful in maintaining a normal rhythm.

Anticoagulation

Anticoagulation is necessary for patients with mitral stenosis and either sustained or intermittent atrial fibrillation. There is controversy in the literature over the benefits of anticoagulation in patients with mitral stenosis and normal sinus rhythm. Patients with mitral stenosis and normal sinus rhythm who have a history of embolic events have experienced some benefits on anticoagulation.

Currently, no clinical trials support the use of anti-coagulants in patients without a history of embolic events (Griffin & Hayek, 2004).

Beta-blockers

By decreasing contractility, beta-blockers can help decrease ventricular pressure and improve filling from the atria. Decreased heart rate can benefit patients experiencing symptoms from high heart rates during activity. The decrease in heart rate provides a longer diastolic time, resulting in better diastolic filling of the ventricle and emptying of the atrium. Beta-blockers may also help to control atrial fibrillation.

Diuretics

Diuretics and sodium restrictions provide symptomatic support for patients who develop symptoms of extracellular fluid (ECF) overload. These measures reduce volume and, ultimately, venous return to the heart (preload).

Surgical Intervention

When the valve area becomes less than 1.5 cm^2, most patients with mitral stenosis begin to experience symptoms at rest and lifestyle is affected. Once these symptoms occur, surgical options should be considered.

Mitral Valvuloplasty

Valvuloplasty of the mitral valve has better long-term results than that of the aortic valve. In this procedure, a balloon is passed through the valve and inflated, causing the fused leaflets to split. Valvuloplasty is greatly beneficial to patients with only fusion of the valve commissures. If calcification of the valve is present, the results will be suboptimal. The American College of Cardiology and American Heart Association (ACC/AHA) guidelines recommend valvuloplasty as described in Box 10-1. Mitral valvuloplasty should not be performed on patients who also have mitral regurgitation of 2+ or more because the procedure increases the amount of regurgitation (Griffin & Hayek, 2004).

BOX 10-1: ACC/AHA RECOMMENDATIONS FOR MITRAL BALLOON VALVULOPLASTY

- Symptomatic patient with moderate or severe mitral stenosis, pliable leaflets, and no atrial clot or significant mitral regurgitation

- Asymptomatic patient with moderate or severe mitral stenosis, pliable leaflets, no atrial clot or significant mitral regurgitation, presence of pulmonary hypertension (pulmonary artery pressure > 50 mm Hg at rest or > 60 mm Hg with activity)

- Symptomatic patient with moderate or severe mitral stenosis, no atrial clot or significant mitral regurgitation, and nonpliable calcified valve and who is a high-risk surgical candidate

(Bonow et al., 1998)

Mitral Commissurotomy

As stenosis develops, the commissures (points where valve leaflets come together) begin to fuse together. During mitral commissurotomy, commissures are cut apart to allow for increased movement of the leaflets. This procedure is beneficial to patients with pliable leaflets that have no calcification. ACC/AHA recommendations for mitral valve repair are listed in Box 10-2. Mitral commissurotomy can be performed as a closed heart repair or an open heart repair. However, open heart repair is becoming the preferred method because the surgeon can visualize the valve and remove calcium deposits as well as left atrial clots (Bonow et al., 1998). *Open mitral commissurotomy* is the term for an open heart procedure requiring the use of cardiac bypass.

Mitral Valve Replacement

Patients with extensive calcification and mitral regurgitation in addition to stenosis and pulmonary hypertension are candidates for mitral valve replacement. If the valve is replaced with a mechanical valve, lifelong anticoagulation therapy is required. Anticoagulation therapy is not required if the patient in sinus rhythm receives a bioprosthetic

BOX 10-2: ACC/AHA RECOMMENDATIONS FOR MITRAL VALVE COMMISSUROTOMY

- Symptomatic patients with moderate or severe mitral stenosis and pliable valves <u>with</u> no valvotomy available

- Symptomatic patients with moderate or severe mitral stenosis, pliable valves, <u>and</u> left atrial clot despite anticoagulants

- Symptomatic patients with moderate or severe mitral stenosis and nonpliable or calcified valves (decision to repair or replace made during surgery)

(Bonow et al., 1998)

valve. (Chapter 9 includes a more in-depth discussion of valve replacement options.)

Outcomes

As cardiovascular technology and skill continue to advance, patients undergoing valvuloplasty and open heart commissurotomy continue to experience excellent short- and long-term results (Stoltz & Bryg, 2003). Patients who have the correct valve anatomy should undergo valvuloplasty to avoid the risks associated with bypass surgery. The operative risk for surgery increases with age but continues to remain fairly low (Bonow et al., 1998). Patients begin to experience an improvement in symptoms as soon as the valve is replaced or repaired. An echocardiogram should be completed no sooner than 72 hours after the procedure. Patients should follow up yearly with a physical examination, chest X-ray film, and ECG. Further echocardiograms are only indicated if patients develop recurrent symptoms (Bonow et al., 1998).

MITRAL VALVE REGURGITATION

Definition

Mitral regurgitation (insufficiency) occurs when a backward flow of blood occurs from the left ventricle to the left atrium during ventricular systole. This backward flow of blood is caused by inadequate closure of the mitral valve.

Causes

Mitral valve prolapse is the most common form of valvular heart disease that can result in regurgitation and occurs in 2% to 6% of the population (Bonow et al., 1998). Young women are most commonly affected by mitral valve prolapse. Mitral valve prolapse can be familial and passed from generation to generation. Patients with Marfan syndrome and other connective tissue diseases also have an increased prevalence of mitral valve prolapse (Massie & Amiodon, 2004).

Rheumatic heart disease, bacterial endocarditis, ischemic heart disease, left ventricular dilatation, and hypertrophic cardiomyopathy are some of the primary causes of mitral regurgitation (LeDoux, 2005). As the incidence of rheumatic heart disease in the United States decreases, so does the incidence of mitral regurgitation. However, rheumatic heart disease is still prevalent in underdeveloped countries.

The causes of mitral regurgitation can be classified as organic or functional (Crawford, 2003). Organic processes are considered to be disease processes that involve the structure of the valve itself. The mitral valve is a unique, complex structure and normal function of the mitral valve depends on normal valve leaflets, chordae tendineae, and papillary muscles that stretch and contract appropriately, as well as normal ventricular tissue where the papillary muscle attaches to the ventricular wall. Functional abnormalities include changes in other structures that result in changes in valve function. These abnormalities can include left ventricular or left atrial dilatation.

Mitral valve prolapse occurs when changes in the valve leaflets and chordae tendineae result in lengthening of the chordae tendineae. The papillary muscle, functioning normally during ventricular systole, contracts. This contraction applies pressure to the chordae tendineae. As contraction occurs, the chordae tendineae pull on the valve leaflets to prevent them from prolapsing into the atria as the force of ventricular contraction and ejection pushes against the leaflets (see Figure 10-1). In mitral valve prolapse, the lengthened chordae tendineae cannot keep the valve leaflet in its proper place and the valve leaflets are forced into the left atrial chamber (see Figure 10-3). Mitral valve prolapse that occurs in young, otherwise healthy women may cause only mild mitral regurgitation with little effect on the heart.

FIGURE 10-3: MITRAL VALVE PROLAPSE

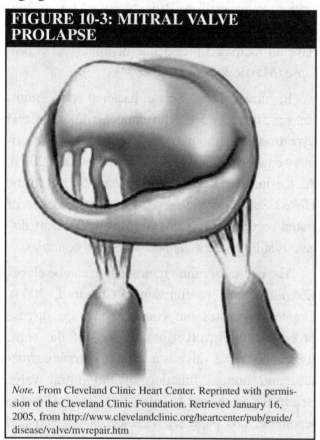

Note. From Cleveland Clinic Heart Center. Reprinted with permission of the Cleveland Clinic Foundation. Retrieved January 16, 2005, from http://www.clevelandclinic.org/heartcenter/pub/guide/disease/valve/mvrepair.htm

In rheumatic heart disease, the valve leaflets become fibrotic and shorten. Inflammation of the valve from the disease process may also lead to calcification. Once marked calcification occurs, the leaflets become very stiff and remain in a fixed open position.

Myocardial infarction (MI) can result in impairment or rupture of a papillary muscle. Once the myocardial wall becomes damaged, attachment of the papillary muscle to that ventricular wall can become impaired. As the heart continues to pump,

the papillary muscle continues to contract. With each contraction of the papillary muscle, the attachment to the ventricle can weaken. If enough damage to the myocardial wall or papillary muscle has occurred, the papillary muscle can disconnect from the ventricular wall (see Figure 10-4). This results in an acute mitral regurgitation state, and emergency measures are necessary to prevent death.

Clinical Application

Inferior wall MIs greatly increase the risk of acute papillary muscle ruptures. Papillary muscle ruptures do not generally occur at the onset of the infarct but may develop 48 to 72 hours later.

FIGURE 10-4: RUPTURED PAPILLARY MUSCLE

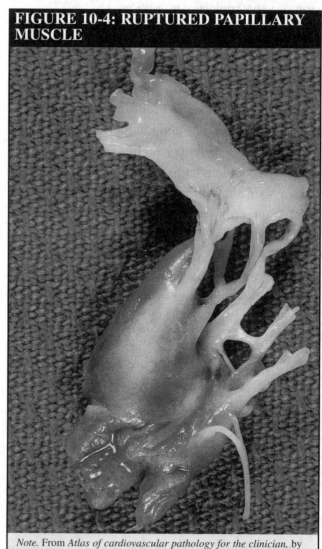

Note. From *Atlas of cardiovascular pathology for the clinician,* by J. Butany & A. Gotlieb. Edited by E. Braunwald & B.M. McManus. Copyright 2000, Current Medicine, Inc. Used with permission from Images.MD.

Bacterial invasion of the heart with the development of endocarditis can cause chordae tendineae or papillary muscle dysfunction or rupture. Vegetation can also develop on the valve leaflets themselves, disrupting their ability to close properly.

Without damage to the valve leaflets, changes in the size of the left atrium or left ventricle can affect the mitral valve annulus. Dilatation of the left ventricle or left atrium can stretch the mitral annulus, preventing the leaflets from closing properly.

Mitral valve regurgitation has a variety of causes; however, the pathophysiological results are the same no matter what the cause. Rather, the development of regurgitation, be it acute or chronic, changes the clinical picture. Therefore, chronic and acute mitral regurgitation are discussed separately.

CHRONIC MITRAL REGURGITATION

Pathophysiology

During ventricular systole, the contracting left ventricle forces blood forward through the aortic valve. In the presence of mitral regurgitation, some of that forward blood flow is diverted retrograde (backward) through the dysfunctional mitral valve. This retrograde flow decreases the normal stroke volume (forward flow) by the percentage of blood that is diverted backward. As the left atrium continues to fill normally from the pulmonary system, the volume of blood returning through the abnormal mitral valve increases the normal volume of blood in the left atrium. This increase in left atrial volume results in an increase in pressure in the left atrium. The left atrium responds to this increased volume and pressure by dilating. If this dilatation is not adequate to handle the increased volume and pressure, the effects are transferred backward to the pulmonary system and pulmonary hypertension develops.

Since the left atrium has a larger volume, the left ventricle ultimately receives this larger volume from the atrium during diastole. The ventricle adjusts to this increased volume by enlarging. Additionally, left ventricular contractions actually may become stronger for a period of time. The purpose of these changes (increase in left ventricular filling and an increase in contraction) is to compensate for the volume of blood that is returned to the atrium with each beat. As ejection occurs, normal stroke volume is ejected forward with the additional volume being returned to the left atrium through the regurgitant valve. This compensatory mechanism functions well for many years, until the myocardial fibers have been stretched beyond their physical limitations and systolic ventricular dysfunction occurs.

Clinical Presentation

Patients with chronic mitral regurgitation remain asymptomatic for many years. As symptoms develop, the patient most frequently reports fatigue and dyspnea, initially on exertion. These symptoms progress to include paroxysmal nocturnal dyspnea, orthopnea, and even palpitations from atrial fibrillation. In many cases, the initial diagnosis of mitral regurgitation is made when patients present with new-onset atrial fibrillation. Patients with mitral valve prolapse early on may report symptoms of tachycardia, orthostatic hypotension, or panic attacks.

Clinical Application
Patients with mitral valve prolapse should avoid caffeine and other stimulants because they can increase the incidence of tachycardia and anxiety attacks.

Physical Examination

The classic murmur of mitral regurgitation is a systolic, blowing, high-pitched murmur that is best heard at the apex of the heart with the diaphragm of the stethoscope. Occasionally, due to the leaflet that is prolapsed, the murmur is louder at the aortic area (second intercostal space, right sternal border). The murmur generally radiates to the axillae but may also be heard over the spine, again depending on the leaflet that is defective. In addition to the murmur, an extra heart sound (S₃) is audible due to the increased left ventricular volume.

Increased heart rate is noted in patients with atrial fibrillation or heart failure. As stroke volume decreases, pulse pressure narrows and the carotid pulse volume may decrease. The apical impulse, normally at the apex, becomes displaced due to dilatation of the left ventricle. If the patient is in heart failure, assessment findings may include increased respiratory rate with audible crackles. If left ventricular failure has progressed enough to reflect failure on the right side of the heart, then jugular venous distension, hepatomegaly, and edema will be present.

Diagnosis

Echocardiogram

Echocardiography is the recommended standard for assessment of mitral valve disease. An echocardiogram can determine left ventricular and left atrial volumes, left atrial ejection fraction, and an approximation of the severity of regurgitation. The cause of the mitral regurgitation is commonly determined during this study. Echocardiography is a good baseline study that can be utilized for many years to monitor the progression of the disease.

Cardiac Catheterization

Cardiac catheterization is necessary to determine the presence of coronary artery disease in patients facing mitral valve surgery. Ventricular function and ejection fraction can be assessed as well as pulmonary pressures. However, echocardiography remains the gold standard for this diagnosis.

Chest X-ray Film

An enlarged left atrium and left ventricle are noted on chest X-ray film. If pulmonary hypertension has developed, right ventricular and pulmonary artery enlargement are also present. Patients in a volume overload state show signs of pulmonary edema.

Electrocardiogram

The 12-lead ECG shows evidence of left atrial hypertrophy with abnormal P waves (wide, notched P waves in lead II). Left ventricular hypertrophy is also demonstrated by large QRS complexes with associated ST-segment abnormalities. Atrial fibrillation or ectopic beats may be noted. These ECG changes are neither sensitive nor specific to mitral regurgitation and always require other testing for confirmation.

Medical Therapy

For asymptomatic patients with normal ventricular function, no treatment has been found to decrease the progression of the disease process (Darovic, 2002). Once patients have been diagnosed with mitral valve regurgitation, they should be monitored on a regular basis. The ACC/AHA guidelines recommend an initial echocardiogram and yearly physical exams for asymptomatic patients with mild mitral regurgitation and no evidence of left ventricular dysfunction or enlargement (Bonow et al., 1998). Patients should be instructed to report any signs of physical deterioration to their physicians. Once symptoms develop, a yearly echocardiogram may be needed and should be completed if moderate mitral regurgitation is present. If patients have asymptomatic severe mitral regurgitation, they should follow up with an echocardiogram every 6 to 12 months (Bonow et al., 1998).

Clinical Application

Regular follow-up for patients with mitral regurgitation becomes important in determining the correct timing for valve replacement. Appropriate timing of replacement can prevent irreversible ventricular damage.

Rhythm Control

Digoxin and beta-blockers can provide ventricular rate control for atrial fibrillation. Attempting to return the patient to a regular rhythm with cardioversion, either electrical or chemical, is reasonable if the normal guidelines are followed regarding anticoagulation.

Anticoagulation

Anticoagulation therapy is the same as with mitral stenosis. There is some evidence in the literature indicating that the occurrence of embolization in patients with atrial fibrillation and mitral regurgitation is lower than in those with mitral stenosis (Bonow et al., 1998). However, this information should not change the normal treatment patterns.

Endocarditis Prophylaxis

Endocarditis prophylaxis recommendations for patients with mitral regurgitation are the same as for the mitral stenosis population.

Fluid Control

If the patient exhibits signs of heart failure, a low-sodium diet and fluid restriction may be beneficial. However, liberal salt and water intake can benefit mitral valve prolapse patients who are experiencing orthostatic hypotension.

ACE Inhibitors

If patients are not surgical candidates due to increased risk or a desire not to have surgery, vasodilators, especially angiotensin-converting enzyme (ACE) inhibitors, have been found to be helpful in decreasing regurgitation. ACE inhibitors decrease afterload and preload. The decrease in afterload decreases the resistance to ejection, thereby decreasing regurgitation and allowing blood to move forward.

Surgical Intervention

Once symptoms of heart failure develop, surgery should be considered. With careful monitoring of the patient to assess for development of left ventricular dysfunction, the decision for surgery can be made quickly. If surgical intervention occurs before marked damage, the ventricle can be preserved and pulmonary hypertension should improve. As the severity of left ventricular dysfunction increases, so does operative mortality.

The mitral valve can either be replaced or repaired. Repair is more difficult because, in many cases, structures other than the leaflets require repair. Mitral valve repair surgeries take longer than mitral valve replacement, and therefore, results in longer cardiopulmonary bypass time. Repairs also require very skilled surgeons. Repaired valves offer patients the opportunity to avoid anticoagulants if they are not in atrial fibrillation and prevent the need for future replacements.

If valve replacement is required, the chordae tendineae and papillary muscles may be left in place and attached to the new valve. Mechanical valves are preferred over bioprosthetic valves for their longevity; however, lifelong anticoagulation is required. Bioprosthetic valves may be appropriate for patients who need to avoid anticoagulation.

Outcomes

Patients who have developed mitral regurgitation due to myocardial ischemia or MI have a poorer prognosis than others (Crawford, 2003). These patients generally have left ventricular dysfunction from the MI. Rheumatic heart disease patients have better results, but those with mitral valve prolapse have the best outcomes.

ACUTE MITRAL REGURGITATION

Pathophysiology

In contrast to the progressive development of chronic mitral regurgitation, acute mitral regurgitation occurs when a sudden event causes the immediate development of mitral regurgitation. In many cases, a papillary muscle tears away from the ventricular wall. With the papillary muscle free, the attached valve leaflet does not close, leaving a gaping hole through which blood ejects.

With each ejection of blood from the ventricle, blood moves to the area of least resistance, or lowest pressure. With only 50% of the mitral valve area closing, a very large volume of blood is ejected retrograde into the atrium and stroke volume is greatly decreased. Decreased stroke volume and subsequently decreased cardiac output result in increased systemic vascular resistance (afterload). As the vessels constrict in an attempt to compensate for the decreased forward flow of blood, the resistance against which the ventricle must pump increases. With an increase in systemic vascular resistance, even more blood is ejected retrograde into the atrium and less is available for cardiac output (forward flow).

Clinical Presentation

Because of the acute changes that occur during acute mitral regurgitation, the heart has no time to compensate. With no time for the left atrium to dilate, the pulmonary system quickly becomes overloaded. Pulmonary edema ensues and patients present with acute dyspnea. Blood pressure may initially be normal but quickly deteriorates because the body cannot continue to compensate. Heart rate is rapid, with a decreased pulse amplitude. Cardiac arrhythmias can develop as perfusion decreases. Patients with acute regurgitation have the same murmur as those with chronic regurgitation. However, a new murmur in an acutely ill patient is a key finding because the patient most likely did not have chronic mitral regurgitation prior to this event.

Diagnosis

With acute mitral regurgitation, there is usually no time for extensive testing. Therefore, the most reliable diagnostic tools should be utilized. Echocardiogram is the key diagnostic tool in this acute situation. This test quickly identifies the primary valve problem. Cardiac catheterization is indicated when ischemia may be causing the problem. However, patients are rarely stable enough to undergo cardiac catheterization. The decision to use cardiac catheterization should be made based on the patient's stability.

Surgical Intervention

Valve replacement is the treatment of choice and is most often performed urgently. While preparing the patient for surgery, vasodilators may prove helpful. Venous vasodilators decrease preload and, therefore, decrease the volume overload state. More importantly, however, arterial vasodilators decrease systemic vascular resistance, allowing more blood to propel forward. Intra-aortic balloon pumping may also be beneficial in assisting to decrease afterload (Crawford, 2003). Antibiotics are necessary in patients with acute regurgitation to prevent endocarditis. It is always beneficial to provide as many days as possible of antibiotic therapy before surgery if the patient can tolerate waiting; however, surgery should never be held because of antibiotics.

Outcomes

If surgical valve replacement is successful, patients can do well depending on the cause of the acute event. In patients with acute MI, the outcomes are less promising because it is usually a large infarction that results in papillary muscle rupture. Postoperative follow-up is the same as with mitral stenosis.

CONCLUSION

The mitral valve is an essential part of the functioning heart. Abnormal valve function causes the heart to make adjustments in an attempt to compensate. Over time, these adjustments have detrimental effects. In many cases, the first inkling of valve disease comes through the ears of a cognizant health care professional. Early recognition of cardiac murmurs can result in the chance to educate patients early in the disease process so intervention can be taken before it is too late.

EXAM QUESTIONS

CHAPTER 10
Questions 79-85

79. The heart's compensatory responses to chronic mitral stenosis include

    a. increased ventricular contractility.

    b. increased left ventricular wall thickness.

    c. dilated left atrium.

    d. loss of atrial kick.

80. Symptoms of mitral stenosis generally occur after the valve orifice is

    a. greater than 2.5 cm².

    b. 2 cm² to 2.5 cm².

    c. 1.5 cm² to 1.9 cm².

    d. less than 1.5 cm².

81. The development of high heart rates with exercise in patients with mitral stenosis can be detrimental. The class of medications that can help control heart rate even with exercise is

    a. beta-blockers.

    b. angiotensin-converting enzyme (ACE) inhibitors.

    c. angiotensin receptor blockers.

    d. class III antiarrhythmics.

82. The most common form of mitral regurgitation is

    a. rheumatic heart disease.

    b. mitral valve prolapse.

    c. mitral valve insufficiency.

    d. bacterial endocarditis.

83. When assessing heart sounds in a patient with symptomatic mitral regurgitation, the examiner can expect to find

    a. diastolic murmur and a fourth heart sound.

    b. systolic murmur and a fourth heart sound.

    c. diastolic murmur and a third heart sound.

    d. systolic murmur and a third heart sound.

84. If a patient with mitral regurgitation is not a candidate for surgical valve replacement, the class of medication that can be helpful in decreasing regurgitation by reducing afterload is

    a. beta-blockers.

    b. ACE inhibitors.

    c. diuretics.

    d. digoxin.

85. Forty-eight hours after admission, a patient who is hospitalized with an inferior wall MI reports that he suddenly started to have difficulty breathing. During your assessment, you notice that his respiratory rate and heart rate are increased. You also discover a new systolic murmur that was not present during earlier assessment. As you call the physician, you anticipate that these symptoms are caused by

    a. recurrent myocardial infarction (MI).

    b. pulmonary embolism.

    c. papillary muscle rupture.

    d. pericardial effusion.

CHAPTER 11

ATRIAL FIBRILLATION

CHAPTER OBJECTIVE

After reading this chapter, the reader will be able to discuss the implications of atrial fibrillation and the current management strategies for it.

LEARNING OBJECTIVES

After studying this chapter, the reader will be able to

1. describe the difference between atrial fibrillation and the normal heart rhythm of sinus rhythm.

2. list several acute and temporary causes of atrial fibrillation.

3. define paroxysmal, persistent, and permanent atrial fibrillation.

4. contrast the pathophysiology of paroxysmal atrial fibrillation with persistent and permanent atrial fibrillation.

5. describe the major complications associated with atrial fibrillation.

6. define the difference between ventricular rate control and rhythm control in atrial fibrillation.

7. define the unique side effects and special nursing considerations associated with amiodarone therapy.

8. discuss the importance of anticoagulation prior to cardioversion.

INTRODUCTION AND DEFINITION

Atrial fibrillation is rapid, chaotic activity of the atria, resulting in the deterioration of atrial mechanical activity. This rapid, unorganized atrial activity produces irregular atrial fibrillation waves with an atrial rate greater than 350 beats per minute. Atrial fibrillation is the most common of all sustained cardiac arrhythmias. The prevalence of atrial fibrillation increases as the population ages. In the United States, atrial fibrillation affects more than two million people annually (Dresing & Schweikert, 2002).

In a normal rhythm, the sinoatrial (SA) node acts as the heart's pacemaker. The electrical impulse then travels through the right and left atria, depolarizing both atria before it reaches the atrioventricular (AV) node. After conduction passes through the AV node, it passes down both bundle branches to the Purkinje fibers, depolarizing both ventricles. On an electrocardiogram (ECG), sinus rhythm is identified by a P wave, representing atrial depolarization, followed by a QRS complex, representing ventricular depolarization. Figure 11-1 shows a normal sinus beat. Figure 11-2 shows consecutive sinus beats, or a regular sinus rhythm. In atrial fibrillation, the P wave on the ECG is replaced with atrial fibrillation waves (see Figure 11-3).

Atrial fibrillation has variable ventricular conduction, resulting in an irregularly irregular ventric-

FIGURE 11-1: NORMAL SINUS BEAT

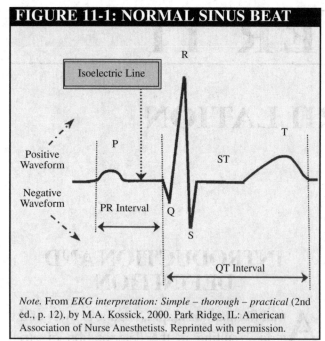

Note. From *EKG interpretation: Simple – thorough – practical* (2nd ed., p. 12), by M.A. Kossick, 2000. Park Ridge, IL: American Association of Nurse Anesthetists. Reprinted with permission.

ular rhythm (also seen in Figure 11-3). In atrial fibrillation, the AV node is bombarded with atrial depolarization waves and, when AV nodal conduction is intact, a very rapid ventricular response rate can result. A slow ventricular response in the presence of untreated atrial fibrillation is a sign of an underlying conduction abnormality.

Clinical Application

It is important to remember that atrial fibrillation is not the only cause of an irregular rhythm, so an irregular pulse alone cannot be used to diagnose atrial fibrillation. Also, a patient in atrial fibrillation with an implanted pacemaker may have a regular ventricular response and therefore a regular pulse; however, atrial fibrillation remains the underlying rhythm.

An ECG reading in at least one lead is necessary to confirm the presence of atrial fibrillation waves for proper diagnosis of atrial fibrillation.

CAUSES

There are many acute and temporary noncardiopulmonary causes of atrial fibrillation, including surgery, hyperthyroidism, electrocution, and alcohol use. Acute cardiopulmonary causes include pulmonary embolism, myocardial infarction (MI), myocarditis, pericarditis, and cardiac or thoracic surgery (Clark, 2004; Fuster, Ryden, et al., 2001).

FIGURE 11-2: REGULAR SINUS RHYTHM

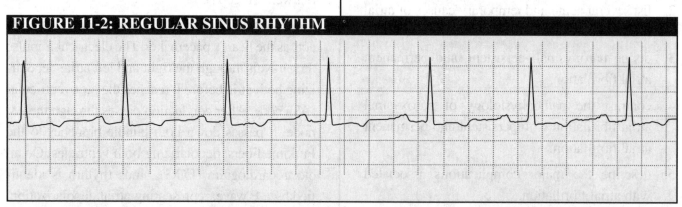

FIGURE 11-3: ATRIAL FIBRILLATION

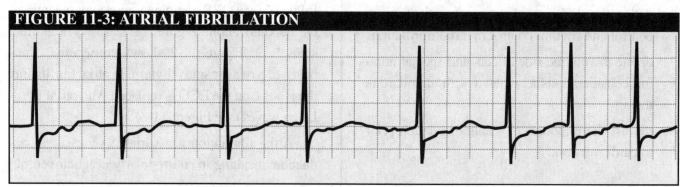

The incidence of atrial fibrillation increases with age, and atrial fibrillation is commonly associated with chronic cardiovascular conditions, including mitral valve stenosis, hypertension, heart failure, cardiomyopathy, coronary heart disease (CHD), and Wolff-Parkinson-White (WPW) syndrome (Clark, 2004; Fuster, Ryden, et al., 2001). Lung pathology in chronic lung disease is also a common cause of atrial fibrillation because any irritation of the lungs also causes irritation of the heart. This relationship between the heart and lungs is due to their connection in the cardiopulmonary circuit.

CLASSIFICATIONS

Atrial fibrillation can be classified as paroxysmal, persistent, or permanent (Fuster, Ryden, et al., 2001). Paroxysmal atrial fibrillation comes on spontaneously and terminates itself. To be classified as paroxysmal, atrial fibrillation cannot last longer than 7 days, and it usually lasts less than 24 hours. Persistent atrial fibrillation is defined by a rhythm that lasts longer than 7 days. Both paroxysmal and persistent atrial fibrillation can be seen with first time presentation. They can also both be recurrent. Permanent atrial fibrillation is diagnosed when the rhythm is accepted as permanent or when it lasts longer than one year. Further attempts to restore sinus rhythm are not indicated in permanent atrial fibrillation.

PATHOPHYSIOLOGY

Atrial fibrillation usually starts with a premature atrial contraction (PAC), an ectopic beat (beat beginning outside the SA node). This PAC is usually the source of paroxysmal atrial fibrillation. Premature atrial beats are usually caused by trigger beats coming from one or more of the superior pulmonary veins located near the junction of the left atrium (Dresing & Schweikert, 2002). These trigger beats occur due to enhanced automaticity of the tissue. Other sources for ectopic beats triggering

paroxysmal atrial fibrillation include the right atrium and, less commonly, the superior vena cava or coronary sinus.

Structural disease of the atria is usually responsible for maintaining atrial fibrillation, such as occurs in persistent and permanent atrial fibrillation. The existence of atrial fibrillation contributes to the development of this structural damage of the atria, with the end result being atrial scarring, fibrosis, and myopathy. Various pathological processes are thought to be involved in the development of these structural changes, including inflammation, fatty infiltration, atrial hypertrophy, and progressive atrial dilatation (Fuster, Ryden, et al., 2001). Atrial hypertrophy and progressive atrial dilatation can be either a cause or a consequence of atrial fibrillation. Pathological changes, such as fibrosis of the atria, occur with aging and may explain the increased incidence of atrial fibrillation in the elderly population (Folkeringa, Tieleman, & Crijns, 2004). In patients with structural disease of the atria, a reentrant mechanism, rather than a focal mechanism, is usually responsible for the maintenance of atrial fibrillation. Reentrant mechanisms in atrial fibrillation can involve one or more circuits.

Classifications of Atrial Fibrillation Based on Pathophysiology

Lone Atrial Fibrillation

Lone atrial fibrillation is defined as atrial fibrillation in patients with normal cardiac and pulmonary function and with no known predisposing factors.

Nonvalvular Atrial Fibrillation

Nonvalvular atrial fibrillation is atrial fibrillation in the absence of rheumatic heart disease that causes mitral stenosis or the absence of a prosthetic heart valve. Patients with mitral stenosis are at increased risk for atrial fibrillation because the left atrium enlarges as a result of contracting against the stenotic mitral valve. The enlarged left atrium places the patient at increased risk for the development of atrial fibrillation.

Neurogenic Atrial Fibrillation

Neurogenic atrial fibrillation accounts for atrial fibrillation in a small number of patients. In these patients, either increased vagal tone or increased adrenergic tone triggers the onset of atrial fibrillation.

SYMPTOMS

Symptoms of atrial fibrillation are commonly related to the fast ventricular rate. The duration of the episode of atrial fibrillation also impacts the symptoms. If ventricular rate is controlled and the patient is still symptomatic, symptoms are related to the loss of atrial kick. Patients who already have decreased ventricular function experience more symptoms from loss of atrial kick than those with normal left ventricular function. Common symptoms of atrial fibrillation include palpitations, dyspnea, fatigue, light-headedness, diaphoresis, and chest pain. Patients in atrial fibrillation may also experience polyuria due the increased release of atrial natriuretic peptide from overstimulation of the atria (Fuster, Ryden, et al., 2001).

Many patients with atrial fibrillation are asymptomatic. These patients are at risk for developing tachycardia-induced cardiomyopathy from poor ventricular rate control. These patients may also present for the first time with more serious complications such as stroke or heart failure.

Clinical Application
Patients who present with symptoms of stroke or transient ischemic attack (TIA) should be assessed for the presence of asymptomatic, undiagnosed atrial fibrillation.

When patients experience hemodynamic compromise due to atrial fibrillation, then more serious symptoms, such as syncope and pulmonary edema, can occur. Syncope is a rare symptom and usually indicates additional underlying pathology compromising cardiac output, such as aortic valve stenosis or hypertrophic cardiomyopathy (HCM).

COMPLICATIONS

Atrial fibrillation is rarely immediately life threatening but does cause long-term complications. The two major complications associated with atrial fibrillation are hemodynamic compromise and an increased risk of thromboembolic events, particularly stroke.

Stroke

Patients with atrial fibrillation are at increased risk for thromboembolism due to an increased risk of thrombus formation in the left atrium and left atrial appendage. Embolization of a thrombus in the left atrium or left atrial appendage can cause stroke. Patients in atrial fibrillation may also have other independent risk factors for stroke. Those at highest risk are those with:

- hypertension
- previous stroke or TIA
- diabetes mellitus
- heart failure
- moderate to severe left ventricular systolic dysfunction
- age greater than 65 years.

(Fuster, Ryden, et al., 2001)

Patients in atrial fibrillation who are younger than age 60 and who have no existing cardiac or pulmonary diseases are at lowest risk for stroke. Patients with atrial fibrillation with rheumatic heart disease have an even higher risk of stroke than those with nonvalvular heart disease (Fuster, Ryden, et al., 2001).

In patients with atrial fibrillation, thrombi most commonly form in the left atrial appendage and are the source of clots in stroke. In atrial fibrillation, the velocity of blood flow through the left atrium and left atrial appendage is decreased. This decrease in velocity increases the risk of thrombus formation. Atrial fibrillation is commonly diagnosed for the first time in patients presenting with new thrombotic stroke. Prevention of thrombotic complications is a major goal in the treatment of atrial fibrillation.

Patients in permanent atrial fibrillation require lifelong warfarin therapy to decrease the risk of stroke. Warfarin has been shown to substantially reduce the risk of stroke in patients with atrial fibrillation (Dresing & Schweikert, 2002). Antiplatelet therapy alone, such as aspirin or clopidogrel, is not generally used for stroke prevention in patients with atrial fibrillation. In certain young patients with lone atrial fibrillation and no other stroke risk factors, antiplatelet therapy may be used (Dresing & Schweikert, 2002).

Age is an important risk factor for the development of stroke with atrial fibrillation. All patients older than age 65 should be anticoagulated with warfarin unless contraindicated (Dresing & Schweikert, 2002). Unfortunately, elderly patients have a increased risk of bleeding complications from oral anticoagulation and are less likely to receive therapy with warfarin. Aspirin therapy should be considered older patients with contraindications to warfarin therapy.

In patients receiving oral anticoagulation for stroke prevention, International Normalized Ratio (INR) should be between 2 and 3. If a patient needs anticoagulation for another reason, such as a prosthetic valve, INR may need to be higher. INR is checked at least weekly during the initiation phase. After INR is therapeutic and stable, it can be reassessed monthly. Aspirin is used only in young, low-risk patients or as an alternative for patients with contraindications to oral anticoagulation. Patients in atrial flutter have the same antithrombotic prevention strategies as those in atrial fibrillation.

Hemodynamic Complications

Hemodynamic complications of atrial fibrillation are associated with rapid ventricular rate, irregular ventricular response, and loss of atrial contraction (kick). Atrial fibrillation can cause a loss in cardiac output of up to 20% because atrial con-

traction is lost (Dresing & Schweikert, 2002). People become more dependent on atrial kick with age. Loss of atrial kick can lead to increased left atrial pressure and, in turn, can lead to increased pulmonary pressure. The irregularity of the R-R interval (irregularity of the QRS complexes) on the cardiac rhythm also adversely impacts hemodynamic performance.

Some patients are at high risk for experiencing a substantial decrease in cardiac output with atrial fibrillation. These patients are those with conditions that impair diastolic filling at baseline, including mitral stenosis, HCM, restrictive cardiomyopathy, and hypertension with diastolic dysfunction.

Another long-term complication of atrial fibrillation is the development of ventricular dilated cardiomyopathy from an accelerated ventricular rate. This complication is also called *tachycardia-induced cardiomyopathy*. Control of ventricular rate can lead to complete or partial reversal of this complication.

TREATMENT CONSIDERATIONS

If a patient presents with an initial episode of paroxysmal (self-terminating) atrial fibrillation, no additional treatment may be needed. If paroxysmal atrial fibrillation is recurrent and the patient is symptomatic, then antiarrhythmic therapy may be prescribed to keep the patient in sinus rhythm or to limit the number of episodes. If the patient has continued paroxysmal episodes, then rate control medication and antithrombotic medication may also be given.

Historically, the goal of treatment in atrial fibrillation has been to restore and maintain sinus rhythm; however, this is now controversial. New research compares the benefits of rhythm control (restoration and maintenance of sinus rhythm) and rate control (allowing atrial fibrillation but controlling the rate and treating with antithrombotic therapy). For example, the AFFIRM trial compared rate control to rhythm control in patients with atrial fibrillation and found no survival benefit in the rhythm control treatment arm (Wyse et al., 2002). Ongoing research and current controversy continue regarding the optimum treatment strategies for those in atrial fibrillation.

When patients first present with persistent atrial fibrillation, a decision must be made between these two treatment arms. The maintenance of sinus rhythm generally requires the use antiarrhythmic pharmacology, so the benefits of sinus rhythm have to be weighed against the adverse or toxic effects of antiarrhythmic medications. For this reason, rate control may be considered acceptable in patients who are not symptomatic. Whether patients with no symptoms benefit from cardioversion is currently a topic of debate. If symptoms of atrial fibrillation are present with effective rate control, then cardioversion is attempted.

Rate Control

It is very important to control the ventricular rate in atrial fibrillation to avoid the development of tachycardia-induced cardiomyopathy. Without proper rate control in atrial fibrillation, ventricular rate can be rapid. Ventricular rate is considered controlled when it is between 60 and 100 beats per minute at rest and between 90 and 115 beats per minute with moderate exercise (Fuster, Ryden, et al., 2001). Rate control is accomplished by medications that slow conduction through the AV node, including beta-blockers, calcium channel blockers (such as verapamil and diltiazem), and digoxin. Calcium channel blockers and beta-blockers are the most commonly used medications for rate control in atrial fibrillation.

Patients with paroxysmal atrial fibrillation who receive rate-control medications may experience sinus bradycardia or heart block as a complication when they are in a normal sinus rhythm. Other patients may too slowly develop a ventricular response and become symptomatic even while in atrial fibrillation. These patients may require insertion of a permanent pacemaker to maintain a minimum ventricular rate (prevent sinus bradycardia and

heart block) while on sufficient doses of medications to control the ventricular rate.

If medication therapy does not adequately control ventricular rate, the AV node can be ablated. AV node ablation results in complete heart block and requires the placement of a permanent pacemaker. Although this strategy can be helpful in preventing tachycardia-induced cardiomyopathy, it has potential downsides. Because atrial fibrillation remains the underlying rhythm, the patient needs continued anticoagulation. With ablation of the AV node, permanent loss of AV synchrony occurs and the patient has continued pacemaker dependence.

Many patients who have experienced at least one unsuccessful attempt to restore and maintain their rhythm to sinus rhythm (rhythm control) are left in atrial fibrillation with appropriate rate control and receive antithrombotic therapy.

Rhythm Control

Potential benefits of restoring sinus rhythm include prevention of thrombus formation, prevention of atrial myopathy, and relief of patient symptoms. When a patient presents for the first time with persistent atrial fibrillation and the decision is made to restore and maintain sinus rhythm, cardioversion (electrical or pharmacological) is performed. For the first cardioversion, antiarrhythmic drug therapy generally is not used unless the patient has been in atrial fibrillation for longer than 3 months (Fuster, Ryden, et al., 2001).

If the first cardioversion is unsuccessful or if there is early recurrence of atrial fibrillation, repeat electrical cardioversion with antiarrhythmic drug therapy is performed. The use of antiarrhythmic drug therapy with electrical cardioversion increases the long-term success rate. However, all antiarrhythmic medications, including those used for pharmacological cardioversion and those used to maintain sinus rhythm, have the potential for toxic side effects.

Antiarrhythmic Medications

This chapter focuses on antiarrhythmic agents used in the treatment of atrial fibrillation. These agents are assessed by their classification and also by their role in both the pharmacological cardioversion of atrial fibrillation and the maintenance of sinus rhythm. According to the Vaughan Williams classification system, antiarrhythmic drugs can be grouped into four classifications.

Class II medications are beta-blockers, and class IV medications are calcium channel blockers. These medications have been discussed in chapter 3. Their role in the treatment of atrial fibrillation is primarily that of rate control by slowing conduction through the AV node. Beta-blockers may also be used to help maintain sinus rhythm in lone atrial fibrillation and prevent recurrence of atrial fibrillation due to adrenergic stimulation. Beta-blockers work by blocking the sympathetic nervous system and are the only group of medications in this classification system that do not affect the cardiac action potential.

Class I antiarrhythmic agents are sometimes called *sodium channel blockers* because they work in the fast sodium channel of the cardiac action potential. Class I agents have three distinct subgroups: Class Ia, Ib, and Ic. Class III agents are sometimes called *potassium channel blockers* because they work by blocking the influx of potassium during the cardiac action potential. Both class I and class III antiarrhythmic medications have serious potential side effects and, therefore, require careful nursing assessment and patient education. The term *antiarrhythmic medication* or *antiarrhythmic therapy* refers to medications in class I or III of this system. Table 11-1 outlines antiarrhythmics used in the management of atrial fibrillation.

One of the dangerous side effects of the class I and III medications used in the treatment of atrial fibrillation is development of ventricular arrhythmias, such as torsades de pointes, polymorphic or monomorphic ventricular tachycardia, or ventricular fibrillation. Medications with this potential are called *proarrhythmic*.

Torsades de pointes is a particular type of ventricular arrhythmia that can occur in the presence of a long QT interval. (Figure 11-1 points out the QT interval in a normal beat.) Class Ia and III agents place the patient at particular risk for torsades de pointes due to their potential for increasing the QT interval. For this reason, most of these medications are initiated only in a hospital setting, where the patient can be monitored with a cardiac monitor. Some antiarrhythmic medications also have atrial proarrhythmic effects and increase the recurrence of atrial fibrillation or promote conversion of the atrial arrhythmia to atrial flutter. Because of the high side effect profile of all antiarrhythmic medications, any reversible causes of atrial fibrillation should be eliminated before medications are initiated.

Amiodarone is a class III antiarrhythmic with unique considerations. Although effective, it has the potential to cause the development of extracardiac organ toxicity, including thyroid dysfunction, polyneuropathy, and liver and pulmonary toxicity (Clinical Pharmacology Database, 2004). One of the most dangerous side effects is a potentially lethal interstial pneumonitis that results in irreversible pulmonary fibrosis (Clinical Pharmacology Database, 2004). Patients should have a baseline pulmonary function study and chest radiographs every 3 to 6 months. Liver function studies are also monitored on a regular basis. Because the toxic effects are cumulative, the use of amiodarone is reserved for carefully selected patients who are not suited for other treatments.

Patients with heart failure are sensitive to the proarrhythmic effects of drugs; therefore, not all antiarrhythmic drugs are safe in patients with heart failure. Amiodarone is a safer medication in the presence of heart failure or considerable left ventricular hypertrophy because, although it does increase the QT interval, it rarely causes torsades de pointes.

TABLE 11-1: ANTIARRHYTHMICS (BY VAUGHAN WILLIAMS CLASSIFICATION) USED IN ATRIAL FIBRILLATION

Class	Specific Medications	Purpose of Medication	Major Cardiac Side Effects
Class Ia	Disopyramide	Rhythm control	Torsades de pointes, heart failure
	Procainamide	Rhythm control	Torsades de pointes
	Quinidine	Rhythm control	Torsades de pointes
Class Ib	Not used in atrial fibrillation		
Class Ic	Flecainide	Rhythm control	Ventricular tachycardia, heart failure, atrial flutter
	Propafenone	Rhythm control	Ventricular tachycardia, heart failure, atrial flutter
Class II	Beta-blockers	Rate control	
Class III	Amiodarone	Rhythm control (also controls rate)	Torsades de pointes (rare) Extracardiac organ toxicity
	Dofetilide	Rhythm control	Torsades de pointes
	Ibutilide	Rhythm control	Torsades de pointes
	Sotalol (also contains beta-blocker)	Rhythm control (also controls rate)	Torsades de pointes, heart failure, beta-blocker side effects
Class IV	Calcium channel blockers	Rate control	

(Fuster, Ryden, et al., 2001)

Clinical Application

Amiodarone is generally not used in young patients because the risk of toxicity is cumulative and increases with the length of therapy.

Cardioversion

Most cardioversions are performed electively. (Special considerations for emergency cardioversions are discussed at the end of this chapter.) When the decision is made to restore a patient's rhythm to sinus rhythm, the choice between electrical and pharmacological cardioversion must be made. Pharmacological cardioversion is most effective in patients presenting with their first episode of atrial fibrillation that has lasted 7 days or less. Whether pharmacological or electrical cardioversion is chosen, the patient's heart rate should be controlled prior to elective cardioversion. Patients who are in atrial fibrillation longer than 48 hours require anticoagula-

tion prior to cardioversion to decrease the risk of stroke. If a patient presents with atrial fibrillation of an onset less than 48 hours, then the decision to anticoagulate prior to cardioversion is based on the patient's other risk factors for thrombus formation.

The risk of thrombotic stroke is the same for electrical and pharmacological cardioversion (Dresing & Schweikert, 2002). Two approaches to anticoagulation can be taken prior to cardioversion. Patients can be started on warfarin and wait until INR is between 2 and 3, usually at least 3 to 4 weeks. If waiting for a therapeutic INR for this period of time is not desirable, patients can be anticoagulated with heparin and have a transesophageal echocardiogram (TEE) to rule out thrombi in the left atrium or left atrial appendage. Once thrombi are ruled out by TEE, then cardioversion can be performed.

TEE is used to assess for atrial thrombi because the left atrial appendage, a common site for thrombi formation, is not well visualized using transthoracic echocardiography. Patients anticoagulated with heparin prior to cardioversion should remain on heparin until INR is therapeutic. Anticoagulation with warfarin should continue after cardioversion and until sinus rhythm is maintained for at least 4 weeks.

After cardioversion, the left atrium experiences a period of mechanical dysfunction (spontaneous, electrical, or pharmacological) that lasts for several weeks. Thrombi can still form during this period of mechanical dysfunction, and emboli can be released when mechanical function returns to normal (Fuster, Ryden, et al., 2001). Patients need to continue on anticoagulation for some time after cardioversion to prevent thrombus formation. Even patients with no thrombi on TEE prior to cardioversion have the possibility of developing thrombi and emboli after cardioversion.

Direct Current Cardioversion

In direct current (DC) cardioversion, the electrical shock is synchronized with the intrinsic activity of the heart. DC cardioversion is different from the delivery of a desynchronized shock (defibrillation) in the treatment of pulseless ventricular tachycardia or ventricular fibrillation. Most cardioversions are performed with the two paddles in the anterior (sternum) and posterior (left scapular area) positions. If using a monophasic waveform to perform cardioversion, an initial shock of 200 J or greater is generally used. New biphasic defibrillators allow the cardioversion of atrial fibrillation with less energy. The success rate of cardioversion with biphasic defibrillators is higher than with monophasic defibrillators.

DC cardioversion is performed with the use of short-acting anesthetic agents; therefore the patient must be given nothing by mouth prior to the procedure. Skilled personnel in airway management must be present and the patient should be monitored with a cardiac monitor and pulse oximetry. Emergency equipment must be readily available, including oxygen, suction, intubation supplies, and other emergency medications and equipment. Short-term cardiac arrhythmias are a potential complication of cardioversion. Patients are monitored on a cardiac monitor for a period of time after cardioversion to observe for arrhythmias. Patients with hypokalemia or digoxin toxicity are at increased risk for developing serious ventricular arrhythmias after cardioversion.

Clinical Application
Potassium levels and digoxin levels (for patients on digoxin) should be assessed prior to elective cardioversion.

The initial success rate of cardioversion is much higher than the long-term success rate. If the patient has an early relapse into atrial fibrillation, then repeat cardioversion using preprocedure antiarrhythmic drug therapy can help reduce the rate of recurrent atrial fibrillation. Patients with permanent pacemakers or implantable cardioverter-defibrillators (ICDs) can safely be cardioverted out of atrial fibrillation. The paddles should be placed away from the device to avoid damage, and the device is interrogated before and after the procedure to assure correct functioning.

Pharmacological Cardioversion

The advantage of pharmacological cardioversion is there is no need for sedation of the patient. In addition, some patients are not comfortable with DC cardioversion and prefer pharmacological cardioversion. Medications proven effective in pharmacological cardioversion are listed in Box 11-1. Not all of these medications are approved or labeled for this use in the United States (Fuster, Ryden, et al., 2001). Many other antiarrhythmic agents can be used to maintain sinus rhythm after successful cardioversion has occurred.

Use of Pharmacological Agents to Maintain Sinus Rhythm

Pharmacology is used to maintain sinus rhythm in patients with recurrent paroxysmal atrial fibrillation or after cardioversion in patients with persistent atrial fibrillation. Because of the chronic nature of atrial fibrillation, most patients are likely to have a recurrence if

BOX 11-1: DRUGS PROVEN MOST EFFECTIVE FOR PHARMACOLOGICAL CARDIOVERSION OF ATRIAL FIBRILLATION

Dofetilide

Flecainide

Ibutilide

Propafenone

Note: All of these drugs have a class 1 recommendation for the cardioversion of arterial fibrillation with a duration of less than or equal to 7 days. Dofetilide also has a class 1 recommendation for the cardioversion of atrial fibrillation with a duration greater than 7 days.

(Fuster, Ryden, et al., 2001)

BOX 11-2: MEDICATIONS USED TO MAINTAIN SINUS RHYTHM IN PATIENTS WITH ATRIAL FIBRILLATION

Amiodarone

Disopyramide

Dofetilide

Flecainide

Procainamide

Propafenone

Quinidine

Sotalol

(Fuster, Ryden, et al., 2001)

not treated with antiarrhythmic therapy. Patients who are older, have been in atrial fibrillation longer, and who have underlying heart disease are at risk for increased recurrent episodes. Even with antiarrhythmic therapy, many patients experience a relapse. A relapse does not necessarily indicate treatment failure. Antiarrhythmic therapy that controls the frequency and severity of occurrences may be considered a success.

Before antiarrhythmic drug therapy is used to maintain sinus rhythm, it is important to identify and treat any reversible causes. Due to potential toxic side effects, antiarrhythmic therapy is typically not used in treating the first episode of atrial fibrillation or in treating infrequent episodes of paroxysmal atrial fibrillation that produce tolerable symptoms. Box 11-2 lists medications used to maintain sinus rhythm.

Listed in Table 11-2 are first-line medications for maintenance of sinus rhythm in special patient populations. Second- and third-line agents are not discussed. All medication decisions should be based on individual patient characteristics. In addition, if a single drug therapy fails, combination therapy may be used.

Permanent Pacemaker Insertion

Permanent pacemaker insertion is required after any ablation of the AV node. Implantation of a permanent pacemaker may also be used for more aggressive medication administration for rate control. Pacemakers inserted in patients with atrial fibrillation have only mode-switching capability to change modes when the patient enters into atrial fibrillation. The purpose of a mode-switching pacemaker is to avoid a rapid pacing response to the sensing of rapid atrial activity. Ventricular pacing during atrial fibrillation can also provide symptomatic relief by providing a regular ventricular response.

In patients who receive permanent pacemakers for reasons other than atrial fibrillation, atrial pacing, as opposed to ventricular pacing, has reduced the occurrence of atrial fibrillation (Fuster, Ryden, et al., 2001). Atrial pacing was thus thought to be a potential primary strategy for atrial fibrillation prevention. Atrial pacing, however, has not been proven to prevent the development of atrial fibrillation when used as a primary strategy. Pacemaker devices can also be programmed to perform overdrive pacing in response to episodes of atrial fibrillation. The goal of therapy is to override the atrial fibrillation with a paced rhythm.

Atrial Defibrillators

Atrial defibrillators are approved but not widely used. Unlike with ICDs, which shock patients out of life-threatening ventricular arrhythmias, most patients are not willing to receive a cardioversion shock for non-life-threatening atrial fibrillation. Attempts have

TABLE 11-2: MEDICATIONS USED TO MAINTAIN SINUS RHYTHM IN SPECIAL PATIENT POPULATIONS

Special Patient Population Description	Medication Used to Maintain Sinus Rhythm
Lone atrial fibrillation	Flecainide Propafenone Sotalol Beta-blockers
Neurogenic atrial fibrillation	Disopyramide or flecainide (for vagal induced) Beta-blockers or sotalol (for adrenergic induced)
Atrial fibrillation in heart failure	Amiodarone (less proarrhythmic effects) Dofetilide
Atrial fibrillation in CHD	Sotalol (beta-blocking properties)
Atrial fibrillation in hypertensive heart disease with left ventricular hypertrophy	Propafenone (class Ic - does not prolong QT interval) Flecainide (class Ic - does not prolong QT interval) Amiodarone (with significant hypertrophy)

(Fuster, Ryden, et al., 2001)

been made to find a shock waveform that can successfully cardiovert atrial fibrillation yet be tolerated by a conscious patient. Limitations of this technology still prevent it from being frequently used.

Maze Surgical Procedure

The Maze surgical procedure is commonly performed in patients with symptomatic atrial fibrillation undergoing open heart surgery for another reason. The addition of the Maze procedure to another open heart surgical procedure increases the risk of surgery. The Maze procedure involves making a series of incisions in the atria using radiofrequency or some other form of energy. Incisions are made to block reentrant pathways within the atrial tissue and to channel conduction in a more normal fashion. The barriers created by the incisions limit the amount of myocardium available to sustain the reentrant circuits. The pulmonary veins can also be electrically isolated during the Maze procedure. Because the procedure is so invasive, it is seldom done as a stand-alone surgery. If done alone, the complications of the Maze procedure are similar to

other procedures involving a median sternotomy and cardiopulmonary bypass. Less-invasive techniques not requiring a sternotomy are being developed to make this procedure a more attractive option in the treatment of atrial fibrillation.

Catheter Ablation Techniques

Linear Ablation

Linear catheter ablation techniques were developed to achieve the same effect as with the surgical Maze procedure. Linear ablation is not as effective when limited to the right atrium. Effectiveness increases when the left atrium is involved; however, access to the left atrium increases procedure risk. Procedure time is lengthy, and linear ablation is still not yet widely used (Fuster, Ryden, et al., 2001).

Pulmonary Vein Ectopic Foci Ablation

New developments in ablation techniques have led to ablation of the trigger points for atrial fibrillation from the pulmonary veins. The pulmonary veins have been identified as the source of origination of atrial fibrillation in many cases of paroxysmal atrial fibrillation. During focal ablation, the areas around the four pulmonary veins are isolated with radiofrequency energy to create a block and eliminate the ability of the foci to enter the left atrium (Blancher, 2005). The procedure requires the septum to be punctured to gain access to the left atrium and pulmonary veins. The patient is anticoagulated during the procedure. This procedure places the patient at risk for stroke, pulmonary vein stenosis, pericardial effusion, tamponade, esophageal perforation, and phrenic nerve paralysis (Blancher, 2005; Fuster, Ryden, et al., 2001).

Because of the risk of the serious complication of pulmonary vein stenosis, this procedure is usually reserved for symptomatic patients who have failed to respond successfully to at least two antiarrhythmic drugs. However, in some young patients who desire a curative approach, it may be considered as initial therapy. Ablation of the foci eliminates or reduces the recurrence of atrial fibrillation in the majority of patients; however, many patients still require antiarrhythmic drug therapy. Newer technology is being investigated to make ablation of the pulmonary vein trigger points safer. These newer technologies include the use of ultrasonic energy and use of cryothermy (Fuster, Ryden, et al., 2001). Although promising, ablation treatment for atrial fibrillation is not used in the majority of patients. Ablation therapy is more effective and used more often in the treatment of atrial flutter.

AV Node Ablation

Ablation of the AV node does not cure atrial fibrillation but rather permanently prevents any rapid ventricular response. Patients who require AV nodal ablation due to uncontrolled rapid ventricular response also need permanent pacemaker implantation.

Percutaneous left atrial appendage transcatheter occlusion (PLAATO) is performed to prevent thromboembolic stroke in patients with nonvalvular atrial fibrillation. This procedure is done in a cardiac catheterization laboratory. Right cardiac catheterization is done with a transseptal puncture. An occlusive device is placed in the left atrial appendage to prevent embolization of a thrombus (Jacobson, 2005). The atrial appendage can also be sutured during open heart surgery in patients with a history of atrial fibrillation. The goal is to prevent embolization of a thrombus from the left atrial appendage into systemic circulation.

ATRIAL FIBRILLATION IN SPECIAL CIRCUMSTANCES

Atrial Fibrillation in Acute Myocardial Infarction

Atrial fibrillation can be the complication of an acute MI. If a patient develops atrial fibrillation as a complication of acute MI, then the patient is at higher risk for other adverse outcomes (Antman et al., 2004). Immediate cardioversion is commonly indicated. Intravenous (IV) beta-blockers can be used to slow heart rate if acute heart failure and significant left ventricular dysfunction are absent. IV digoxin or amiodarone can also be used to slow heart rate. Class Ic antiarrhythmics are contraindicated in acute MI.

Atrial Fibrillation with Hypertrophic Cardiomyopathy

Atrial fibrillation is a common complication of HCM. Patients with HCM are also among the patients most dependent on atrial kick to maintain adequate cardiac output. These patients can experience considerable loss of cardiac output and potential syncope with the development of atrial fibrillation. Disopyramide and amiodarone are the two preferred antiarrhythmics in maintaining sinus rhythm.

Atrial Fibrillation in Wolff-Parkinson-White Syndrome

Patients with WPW syndrome have an accessory pathway that connects the atria to the ventricles. During atrial fibrillation, conduction from the rapidly firing atria can travel over the accessory pathway and cause a faster ventricular response than conduction through the AV node. If this rapidly conducted atrial fibrillation is treated with the typical agents that slow conduction over the AV node, there can be increased conduction over the accessory pathway. The ventricular response can be so rapid that the rhythm can deteriorate to ventricular fibrillation. Long-term treatment involves ablation of the accessory pathway to eliminate conduction over it. If the patient is hemodynamically unstable, then electrical cardioversion is indicated. If the patient is hemodynamically stable, then IV procainamide or ibutilide may be used to slow conduction over the accessory pathway (Fuster, Ryden, et al., 2001).

Clinical Application

It is important to know the history of WPW syndrome in patients with atrial fibrillation. If an accessory pathway is present, patients are at risk for a rapid ventricular response. Patients on atrial fibrillation with known WPW syndrome are treated differently than those without WPW syndrome. Medications that slow conduction through the AV node (including beta-blockers and calcium channel blockers) are not indicated in the treatment of atrial fibrillation in the presence of WPW syndrome.

Acute Hemodynamically Unstable Atrial Fibrillation

If a patient presents emergently with new-onset atrial fibrillation, a rapid ventricular rate, and hemodynamic instability, then emergency cardioversion is indicated. Patients should be given unfractionated heparin or low-molecular-weight heparin prior to cardioversion. Immediate cardioversion should happen in situations in which atrial fibrillation rate control cannot be achieved with pharmacological treatment, including presence of acute MI or angina, symptomatic hypotension, and heart failure (Clark, 2004; Fuster, Ryden, et al., 2001).

CONCLUSION

Atrial fibrillation is a common, chronic cardiac arrhythmia with no definitive cure. It can be caused by or can complicate many other cardiac disorders. Patients with atrial fibrillation are at risk for acute decompensation from rapid ventricular response and are also at risk for long-term hemodynamic and thromboembolic complications. The increased risk of stroke is one of the most important potential complications. Long-term anticoagulation is required in most patients with atrial fibrillation to reduce the risk of stroke.

Rate control is an important aspect of treatment for all patients with atrial fibrillation. Patients who are symptomatic also have the option of rhythm control through pharmacological or electrical cardioversion. Most patients require ongoing antiarrhythmic medications to maintain sinus rhythm.

Nurses outside the cardiac arena are likely to care for patients with atrial fibrillation and play a crucial role in the management of these patients. Assessment of the initial and ongoing rhythm, patient symptoms, and potential complications are key nursing considerations. Patient education regarding high-risk antiarrhythmic and anticoagulation medications is critical to the patient in persistent or permanent atrial fibrillation.

EXAM QUESTIONS

CHAPTER 11
Questions 86-93

86. Atrial fibrillation can be described as an arrhythmia that

    a. looks the same as sinus rhythm but has an impulse that initiates in the atria instead of the SA node.

    b. is characterized by rapid, irregular atrial activity that produces atrial fibrillatory waves on an ECG and a very variable ventricular response.

    c. is characterized by rapid, irregular atrial activity that produces atrial fibrillatory waves on an ECG and a very predictable ventricular response.

    d. produces atrial and ventricular fibrillation waves on an ECG.

87. Known causes or triggers of atrial fibrillation include

    a. alcohol use and cardiomyopathy.

    b. osteoarthritis and myocarditis.

    c. adolescence and thoracic surgery.

    d. hypertension and hyperglycemia.

88. Paroxysmal atrial fibrillation can be defined as atrial fibrillation that

    a. lasts longer than 7 days.

    b. has only occurred one time.

    c. occurs in patients younger than age 40.

    d. comes on spontaneously and self-terminates.

89. The pathophysiology associated with permanent atrial fibrillation is

    a. focal trigger points at the pulmonary veins.

    b. structural disease of the atria with reentrant circuits.

    c. ventricular septal defect.

    d. congenital small atria.

90. Common complications of atrial fibrillation include

    a. MI and sudden death.

    b. aortic valve stenosis and outflow tract obstruction.

    c. hemodynamic compromise and thromboembolic complications.

    d. endocarditis and pericarditis.

91. Rhythm control is necessary in the management of atrial fibrillation when

    a. the rate is well controlled.

    b. the patient is asymptomatic.

    c. paroxysmal episodes are very infrequent.

    d. the patient is symptomatic despite rate control.

92. Potential toxicities associated with amiodarone therapy include

    a. liver and pulmonary toxicity.

    b. frequent torsades de pointes.

    c. allergy reaction to aspirin.

    d. development of diabetes mellitus.

93. A true statement about anticoagulation prior to cardioversion is

    a. anticoagulation is more important for electrical cardioversion.

    b. anticoagulation is more important for pharmacological cardioversion.

    c. anticoagulation can only be achieved by use of IV heparin.

    d. anticoagulation is important prior to electrical or pharmacological cardioversion.

CHAPTER 12

CARDIAC PACEMAKERS AND IMPLANTABLE DEFIBRILLATORS

CHAPTER OBJECTIVE

After completing this chapter, the reader will recognize the indications for cardiac pacemakers and defibrillators and understand the impact of these devices on a patient.

OBJECTIVES

After studying this chapter, the reader will be able to

1. list three indications for the insertion of a cardiac pacemaker.

2. differentiate between single- and dual-chamber cardiac pacing.

3. identify two potential pacemaker complications.

4. cite two key education topics for the recipient of a permanent cardiac pacemaker.

5. identify the benefit of biventricular cardiac pacing.

6. describe the effect of magnets on an ICD.

7. recall the appropriate patient response to a defibrillation received from an implantable cardioverter-defibrillator (ICD).

INTRODUCTION

Physicians have been experimenting with electrical stimulation of muscles for many years. In 1788 in London, Charles Kite, wrote a paper titled *An Essay Upon the Recovery of the Apparently Dead,* in which he described how he used electrical stimulation to the heart to revive a 3-year-old child (Bakkan Library and Museum, 2004). Many devices have been developed over the years in an attempt to stimulate the electrical system of the heart. In the mid-1950s, the first pacemakers were used (Bakkan Library and Museum, 2004). Initially, a small wire was placed in the heart. The wire was then connected to an external pacemaker that was the size of a microwave oven. The patient could only travel as far as the power cord could stretch. This drawback was desirable to the alternative, which was death. In 1957, the first battery-powered pacemaker was developed. This device, still an external device, was small enough to be strapped to the patient (Bakkan Library and Museum, 2004). In 1960, the first totally implantable human cardiac pacemaker was implanted (Medtronic, Inc., n.d.).

During the past 40 years, the science of cardiac pacing has grown and changed dramatically. Today, 250,000 pacemakers are implanted annually (Lowy & Freedman, 2004). Technology has advanced from a device that was external and the size of a microwave oven to a device that is totally implantable and the size of a half dollar.

Additionally, the field of electrophysiology has become a specialty of its own. As time goes on, the search for a device that mimics the heart's natural electrical system continues. For health care professionals, the devices become more complex and intricate. For patients, the implantation and impact on their lives becomes less obtrusive.

CARDIAC PACEMAKERS

Temporary versus Permanent Cardiac Pacemakers

Pacemakers can be inserted on a temporary or permanent basis. Temporary cardiac pacing is utilized in acute care settings. If a patient presents with a slow rhythm and is symptomatic, a temporary pacemaker wire is inserted into the patient's heart. This wire is connected to an external pacemaker that functions similarly to a permanent pacemaker. If the cause of the slow rhythm is then determined to be permanent, a permanent pacemaker is implanted. Temporary pacemakers are also implanted during cardiac surgery because some patients experience cardiac arrhythmias after surgery that require cardiac pacing. In most cases, there is no need for permanent cardiac pacing after cardiac surgery.

The development of a totally external temporary cardiac pacing system has decreased the number of temporary pacemakers wires that are inserted. An external temporary cardiac pacing system involves the placement of two pads on the chest wall at specific locations. These pads adhere to the chest wall as an electrode used for cardiac monitoring would adhere to the chest wall. These pads are connected to a machine, usually a defibrillator, with pacemaker capabilities. The external pacemaker is turned on and an impulse is delivered that stimulates the heart to beat at a rate established by the attached machine. The totally external pacemaker has eliminated the need for a temporary pacemaker in situations when the patient has a slow rhythm with no symptoms. The patient is observed and a determination is made

regarding the need for a permanent pacemaker. The external pacemaker eliminates the need to subject the patient to the risks associated with inserting a temporary pacemaker wire, which is an invasive procedure. However, this device is not appropriate for patients who require continuous temporary pacing because the delivery of the impulse is uncomfortable and at times painful. The totally external system is best utilized during a cardiac arrest. This chapter focuses only on permanent cardiac pacemakers and does not cover temporary cardiac pacemakers.

Review of the Conduction System

In order to understand how cardiac pacemakers work, one must understand the cardiac conduction system (see Figure 12-1).

Sinoatrial Node

The sinoatrial (SA) node is the natural pacemaker of the heart. In an adult, this natural pacemaker fires at a rate of 60 to 100 beats per minute. As the natural pacemaker, the SA node begins the electrical cascade of events that results in organized depolarization and contraction of the heart. Once the SA node initiates this cascade, the impulse travels through the right atrium via internodal pathways and the left atrium via Bachmann's bundle. In normal circumstances, this impulse results in contraction of the atria.

Atrioventricular Node

From the internodal pathways, the impulse travels to the atrioventricular (AV) node. The AV node slows conduction from the atria to the ventricles. Conduction is slowed to assure that the ventricles are relaxed at the time of atrial contraction and have time to fill completely before contracting. The AV node is located in the right atrium just above the insertion of the tricuspid valve.

Bundle of His

From the AV node, the electrical impulse travels along the bundle of His. The AV node and the bundle of His are surrounded by tissue known as the *AV junction*. In an adult, the AV junction contains pace-

FIGURE 12-1: NORMAL CARDIAC CONDUCTION SYSTEM

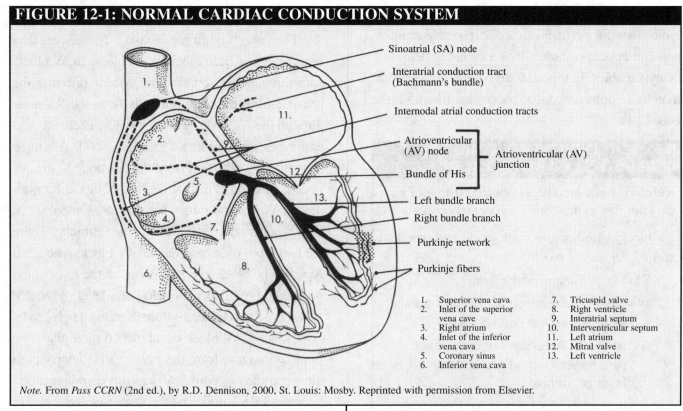

Sinoatrial (SA) node

Interatrial conduction tract (Bachmann's bundle)

Internodal atrial conduction tracts

Atrioventricular (AV) node

Bundle of His

Atrioventricular (AV) junction

Left bundle branch

Right bundle branch

Purkinje network

Purkinje fibers

1.	Superior vena cava	7.	Tricuspid valve
2.	Inlet of the superior vena cave	8.	Right ventricle
		9.	Interatrial septum
3.	Right atrium	10.	Interventricular septum
4.	Inlet of the inferior vena cava	11.	Left atrium
		12.	Mitral valve
5.	Coronary sinus	13.	Left ventricle
6.	Inferior vena cava		

Note. From *Pass CCRN* (2nd ed.), by R.D. Dennison, 2000, St. Louis: Mosby. Reprinted with permission from Elsevier.

maker cells and initiates a heart rate of 40 to 60 beats per minute if no impulse is received from the SA node.

Bundle Branches

The bundle of His divides into the right and left bundles branches. The right bundle branch carries the impulse to the right ventricular myocardium. The left bundle branch divides into the left posterior bundle branch and the left anterior bundle branch. The left posterior bundle branch carries the impulse to the posterior and inferior left ventricle, and the left anterior bundle branch carries the impulse to the anterior and superior left ventricle.

Purkinje Fibers

From the ventricles, the impulse travels to the Purkinje fibers, where the depolarization is carried through to the endocardial layers of the heart. The Purkinje network is the location for the heart's third group of pacemaker cells. In an adult, if no impulse has been received through the normal conduction patterns, the Purkinje system initiates a heart rate of 20 to 40 beats per minute.

Indications for Cardiac Pacing

As pacemakers continue to improve over the years, the indications continue to change. The decision to insert a pacemaker draws the attention of not only the medical community but also the insurance industry. These devices, especially implantable defibrillators, can be expensive and many people scrutinize the need for their insertion. The American College of Cardiology (ACC) and American Heart Association (AHA) have worked jointly for more than 20 years to develop guidelines for a variety of disease processes and procedures related to cardiology. In the late 1990s, these two groups, in conjunction with the North American Society of Pacing and Electrophysiology (NASPE), developed a committee on pacemaker implantation (Gregoratos et al., 2002). As a result, the ACC/AHA/NASPE Guidelines for Implantation of Cardiac Pacemakers and Antiarrhythmia Devices were developed. These guidelines were most recently updated in 2002. The guidelines have become the gold standard for this procedure. It is important to remember that the field of electrophysiology is rapidly changing. Practitioners should make decisions based on each patient. Indications for permanent cardiac pacemaker insertion can appear complex. It is a complex field with many variables. In this text, we cover the most common indications for cardiac pacemaker insertion (see Box 12-1).

BOX 12-1: INDICATION FOR PERMANENT CARDIAC PACING

Note: This is a greatly abbreviated listing of all the complex indications for pacemakers.

AV blocks (third-degree, high-grade, and type II second-degree AV blocks)

> With symptomatic bradycardia

> With heart rate less than 40 beats per minute in awake, asymptomatic patients

> As the result of necessary drug therapy in patients with a heart rate less than 40 beats per minute

> Asymptomatic third-degree AV block with awake heart rates of 40 or more, especially if left ventricular dysfunction is present

Bifascicular block

> With third-degree block

> With type II second-degree block

> With alternating bundle branch blocks

SA node dysfunction

> With symptomatic bradycardia, including pauses in heart beat

> As the result of necessary drug therapy with a heart rate less than 40 beats per minute

> With chronotropic incompetence

Hypersensitive carotid sinus and neurocardiogenic syncope

> With recurrent syncope caused by carotid sinus stimulation resulting in more than 3 seconds of ventricular asystole (cardiac standstill)

> Significantly symptomatic and recurrent neurocardiogenic syncope associated with bradycardia documented spontaneously or at the time of tilt-table testing

(Gregoratos et al., 2002)

Atrioventricular Block

The most common reason for pacemaker implantation is heart block, or AV block. In AV block, something in the conduction system prevents the impulse from traveling normally from the SA node through the AV node to the ventricles. There are several types of AV block (see Box 12-2). A simple slowing of conduction from the SA node to the AV node is referred to as first-degree AV block. Second-degree AV block occurs when one atrial impulse at a time is not conducted through to the ventricles. There are two types of second-degree AV block: type I and type II. The block in type I occurs at the level of the AV node; type II occurs below the level of the AV node. Type II is generally more serious. High-grade, or advanced, AV block occurs when more than one impulse in a row from the atrium fails to conduct to the ventricle. A complete loss of communication between the SA node and the ventricles is referred to as *complete heart block,* or third-degree AV block. Patients are generally unaware of first-degree block; second-degree block can cause symptoms; and high-grade blocks and third-degree heart blocks usually result in symptoms, ranging from dizziness to complete unresponsiveness.

BOX 12-2: TYPES OF AV BLOCK

First-degree AV block

Second-degree AV block

> Type I (Wenckebach) block

> Type II block

Advanced (high-grade) block

Third-degree AV block

Any type of AV block with symptomatic bradycardia is an indication for cardiac pacing. If patients do not have symptoms but have documented heart rates of less than 40 beats per minute, they too are candidates for cardiac pacing. Occasionally, aggressive disease treatment with medications may result in AV blocks and low heart rates. Because many of the medications that lower rates or cause blocks are important to patient welfare, a pacemaker may be implanted instead of stopping the medication. Finally, any patient with third-degree AV block may be a candidate for pacing, even if no symptoms are present. Studies show that placing pacemakers in patients with third-degree AV block with or without symptoms can decrease mortality rates (Gregoratos et al., 2002). The presence of left ventricular dysfunction with AV block further supports the need for a pacemaker.

Bifascicular Block

The next group of patients requiring pacemakers is those with bifascicular blocks, or bundle branch blocks. The right bundle branch has one fascicle, and the left bundle branch has two fascicles: the anterior and posterior fascicles. One or more of these fascicles can become blocked. When the right bundle branch and one of the left bundle branch fascicles become blocked, the patient has a bifasicular block. Many people with bundle branch blocks do not require cardiac pacemakers; however, several situations require pacing. The bundle branches supply the impulse to the ventricles. If the right fascicle and both fascicles of the left bundle branch become blocked, no message is sent to the ventricles to contract. The ACC/AHA/NASPE guidelines have identified that patients with bifascicular block and intermittent third-degree AV block or type II second-degree AV block are at high risk for death and require permanent pacing.

Sinoatrial Node Dysfunction

When the SA node fails, a variety of arrhythmias may result. SA node dysfunction is referred to as sick sinus syndrome (SSS). These arrhythmias include bradycardia (slow heart beat), sinus arrest (no heart beat), SA block (no impulse initiated in the SA node), and paroxysmal supraventricular tachycardias (very fast heart rates alternating with very slow heart rates). Patients with SSS experience very fast and very slow heart rates and are commonly symptomatic. They may actually have a pause in the heartbeat and experience momentary dizziness. All of these arrhythmias occur intermit-

tently, and 24-hour monitoring is very helpful in documenting rhythm irregularities.

SA node dysfunction may also be demonstrated as chronotropic incompetence. During exercise, heart rate increases as a normal response to meet the body's increased needs. This rate increase is referred to as a chronotropic response. In some patients with SA node dysfunction, this response is no longer present, resulting in symptoms of activity intolerance. Although this response is essential for exercise, it is also important for any increase in activity.

Hypersensitive Carotid Sinus and Neurocardiogenic Syncope

Syncope that is the result of carotid sinus stimulation can be caused by hypersensitive carotid sinus or neurocardiogenic syncope. All other causes of syncope should be ruled out prior to implanting a permanent pacemaker. Hypersensitive carotid sinus reflex is the result of increased parasympathetic (vagal) response, resulting in a variety of types of slowing of the heart rate when pressure is applied to the carotid sinus. The normal vagal response can produce a normal pause of the heartbeat for up to 3 seconds. In patients with hypersensitive carotid sinus, the pause is longer, resulting in syncope.

The reflex response in neurocardiogenic syncope is caused by a reduction in sympathetic activity that results in hypotension. This type of syncope accounts for 10% to 40% of all syncopal episodes (Gregoratos et al., 2002). Situations that normally increase stimulation of the sympathetic nervous system may result in syncope in patients with this condition. Usually, such situations as extreme fright, emotional upset, crowded rooms, and pain normally result in increased heart rate and cause vasoconstriction to increase blood pressure. In this population, the normal sympathetic response is reduced, resulting in bradycardia and hypotension.

Concepts of Permanent Cardiac Pacing

As discussed in chapter 1, the action potential is a series of events that results in a change of the electrical charge inside the cell from negative (resting) to positive (stimulated) and back to negative. This action potential consists of depolarization (stimulation of cardiac muscle cells) and repolarization (return of cells to their resting state). Depolarization is conducted in a systematic method through the electrical system of the heart, as described earlier in this chapter. As depolarization occurs, healthy cardiac muscle cells respond by contracting the muscle. Patients requiring permanent pacemakers no longer have a systematic method for sending the message to the cardiac muscle. Rather, the implanted pacemaker takes over and stimulates the cardiac muscles to contract.

Components of a Permanent Cardiac Pacemaker

The standard cardiac pacemaker that is implanted to regulate heartbeat has several components: the pacemaker generator, the pacemaker lead wire, and the pacemaker electrode (see Figure 12-2).

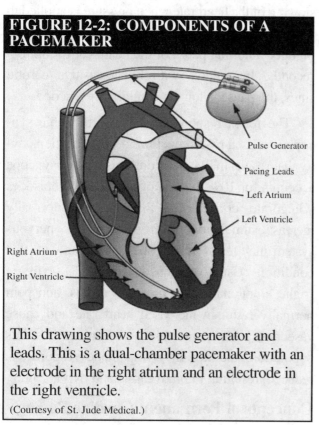

FIGURE 12-2: COMPONENTS OF A PACEMAKER

Pulse Generator

Pacing Leads

Left Atrium

Left Ventricle

Right Atrium

Right Ventricle

This drawing shows the pulse generator and leads. This is a dual-chamber pacemaker with an electrode in the right atrium and an electrode in the right ventricle.

(Courtesy of St. Jude Medical.)

The Pacemaker Generator

The pacemaker generator is also referred to as the *battery* or *can*. It usually consists of a lithium battery and electrical microcircuitry necessary for the cardiac pacemaker to function. The pacemaker generator is usually placed in a subcutaneous pocket in the chest wall. The preferred site is the shoulder (left shoulder of a right-handed person and the right shoulder of a left-handed person). The battery is the only part of a pacemaker system that is removed and replaced.

Clinical Application

It is important to take the patient's lifestyle into consideration prior to insertion. For example, if a patient is a hunter and uses a rifle, the pacemaker generator should be placed in the shoulder that is not used when aiming the gun.

The Pacemaker Lead

The pacemaker lead is an insulated wire that is connected to the pacemaker battery. For a ventricular pacemaker, the lead is threaded through a vein to the superior vena cava into the right atrium, then through the tricuspid valve and into the right ventricle. The end of the lead wire is left in contact with the wall of the right ventricle. The lead contains a conducting wire that carries the impulse from the pacemaker battery to the wall of the heart. It is insulated to protect against fracture. If the lead fractures, the electrical stimulus no longer reaches the heart and the pacemaker fails. If a lead fractures, a new lead is placed and the old lead is disconnected from the battery but left in place. When pacemaker batteries are replaced, the leads are left in place. It is not unusual to leave a nonfunctioning lead in place and simply add a new functional lead beside it. Removal of a lead may result in a tear in the myocardial wall. If a lead does need to be removed—for example, if it becomes infected—it should only be done by a physician well trained in lead removal.

The Pacemaker Electrode

At the end of the lead is an electrode. The electrode is the device that delivers the stimulus to the cardiac wall. The ability of the electrode to have good contact with healthy cardiac tissue is critical. Many types of "fixation" devices are available to assist with a good connection. Some leads naturally adhere to the wall over time, whereas others can be screwed into the myocardial wall. Different devices are utilized depending on the ease or difficulty of establishing a good connection. Over time, the electrode at the end of the lead in the heart becomes covered over with fibrous tissue, which helps keep the electrode in place.

Types of Permanent Cardiac Pacing

Single-chamber Pacing

With single-chamber pacemakers, one lead is placed in one chamber of the heart. When pacemakers were first developed, a single lead was placed in the right ventricle. These are called *right ventricular pacemakers*. However, now, a single lead can also be placed in the right atrium only, for example, when the SA node does not fire on its own. If an impulse is initiated by the pacemaker in the atrium, simulating the SA node, the rest of the conduction system responds normally.

Right ventricular pacemakers are programmed to stimulate the right ventricle if no other stimulus is received by the ventricle within a preset time frame. This system completely ignores atrial activity and there is loss of atrial kick. Atrial kick contributes 25% of cardiac output. Over time, patients with single-chamber right ventricular pacemakers developed what was referred to as "pacemaker syndrome," primarily as a result of the loss of atrial kick. Pacemaker syndrome is discussed in detail later in this chapter. As a result of the negative effects, or just less-than-optimal effects, of single chamber right ventricular pacemakers, researchers strived to develop a pacemaker that better mimicked the normal activities of the heart. As a result, dual-chamber pacemakers were developed.

Dual-chamber Pacing

Dual-chamber pacing involves two leads placed in the heart, one in the right atrium and one in the right ventricle. A dual-chamber pacing system is the typical pacemaker configuration that is implanted today. With a lead in the atrium and a lead in the ventricle, the pacemaker can sense the activity in both chambers and respond to activity that is present or not present. This configuration much better mimics the heart's normal conduction system and provides the patient with better cardiac output. As patients present for pacer battery replacement, dual-chamber systems may replace single-chamber pacemakers that were originally placed. Replacing a single-chamber pacemaker with a dual-chamber pacemaker is only done if a cardiologist determines that the patient would benefit from dual-chamber pacing.

Biventricular Pacemakers

Placing pacing leads in both the right and left ventricles is a newer technology that has been developed. This therapy is reserved for a very specific population of patients and will be discussed in more detail later in this chapter.

Cardiac Pacing Modes

Once implanted, cardiac pacemakers are programmed to function in a manner that is determined by a cardiologist to be best for that specific patient. Today, pacemakers can be programmed noninvasively and painlessly in a cardiologist's office. They can be reprogrammed and changed as the patient's needs dictate.

The Pacer Code

When referring to a pacemaker and its function, a series of letters are used to assist health care professionals in determining how the pacemaker should function. NASPE and the British Pacing and Electrophysiology Group (BPEG) developed the

NASPE/BPEG generic code (Bernstein et al., 2002) to establish a system for identifying pacemaker functioning that would be utilized and recognized internationally. The first four letters of this code are consistently utilized to identify pacing modes, while the fifth one is not yet used consistently (see Table 12-1). Discussion of the fifth position is beyond the scope of this text.

VVI Pacing Mode

The original pacemakers were ventricular pacemakers only and were designated as VVI pacemakers. Some patients continue to have pacemakers programmed in the VVI mode. In the VVI mode, the first position indicates that the pacemaker electrode in the right ventricle is sensing activity in the ventricle. The second position indicates that the electrode in the right ventricle paces the ventricle. The third position indicates that, upon sensing normal activity in the ventricle, the pacer will not fire (inhibits pacing activity). If there is no normal activity from the heart, the pacemaker will fire. The most common reason for the VVI mode is atrial fibrillation. In atrial fibrillation, communication between the atrium and the ventricle is not normal, and there is little ability to set up a communication system with a dual-chamber pacemaker. It is becoming more common to find patients with a dual-chamber pacemaker in atrial fibrillation to have a pacer mode

of DDI. This is a more technologically complex configuration that is beyond the scope of this text but is mentioned because it is one of the many configurations. A few patients also still have old single-chamber pacemakers that were placed many years ago; these systems only function in VVI mode (see Figure 12-3).

DDD Pacing Mode

The most common configuration seen is the DDD mode. When the pacemaker is programmed for DDD, an electrode in the right atrium and one in the right ventricle are both utilized for the pacing mode. The DDD mode is commonly referred to as *AV pacing* (see Figure 12-4). The D in the first position indicates that the device senses any activity (depolarization) in the atrium or ventricle. The D in the second position indicates that the electrode in the atrium and the electrode in the ventricle are programmed to pace the atrium or the ventricle. The D in the third and final position refers to the pacemaker's response as it senses the activity of the heart. The best situation in most patients is to allow the heart to function as normally as possible and only utilize the pacemaker if the heart is unable to do so. Therefore, the atrial electrode is set up to allow a preset period of time for the atrium to contract naturally. If normal contraction occurs, the atrial electrode is inhibited and does not fire. The atrial

TABLE 12-1: REVISED NASPE/BPEG GENERIC CODE FOR ANTIBRADYCARDIA PACING

Position I	Position II	Position III	Position IV	Position V
Chamber(s) paced	Chamber(s) sensed	Response to sensing	Rate modulation	Multisite pacing
O = None	O = None	O = None	O = None	O = None
A = Atrium	A = Atrium	T = Triggered	R = Rate modulation	A = Atrium
V = Ventricle	V = Ventricle	I = Inhibited		V = Ventricle
D = Dual (A+V)	D = Dual (A+V)	D = Dual (T+I)		D = Dual (A+V)

(Bernstein et al., 2002)

FIGURE 12-3: VVI PACING MODE

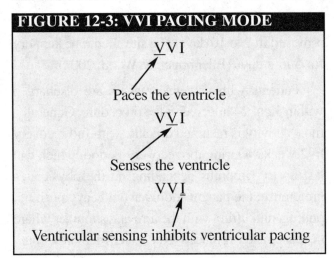

V<u>V</u>I

Paces the ventricle

V<u>V</u>I

Senses the ventricle

VV<u>I</u>

Ventricular sensing inhibits ventricular pacing

electrode then sends a message (trigger) to the ventricular electrode. The message to the ventricular electrode is the same as if a message was coming through the AV node to the ventricles via the bundle branches. This message sets up another cycle. The ventricular electrode, while triggered by the atrial system, waits a preset amount of time for the patient's own system to function, causing the ventricle to contract. If natural contraction occurs, then the ventricular electrode senses this and is inhibited and does not fire. Then the cycle repeats itself in the atrium. Any time that the atrium or ventricle does not depolarize naturally, the pacemaker sends an impulse to that part of the heart (see Figure 12-4).

FIGURE 12-4: DDD PACING MODE

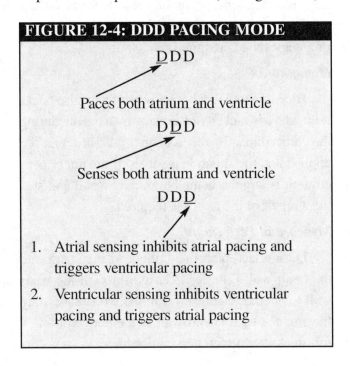

<u>D</u>DD

Paces both atrium and ventricle

D<u>D</u>D

Senses both atrium and ventricle

DD<u>D</u>

1. Atrial sensing inhibits atrial pacing and triggers ventricular pacing
2. Ventricular sensing inhibits ventricular pacing and triggers atrial pacing

Rate Responsiveness

The fourth position noted with pacemaker modes is an R. This stands for rate responsiveness. The body's natural ability to increase heart rate in response to physiologic needs is called a *chronotropic response*. Rate responsiveness provides the chronotropic response when the patient's body does not. A pacemaker with rate-responsive pacing increases the pacemaker rate based on the physiologic needs of the body. A wide variety of methods are available for detecting the physiologic needs of the body; however, a discussion of these methods is beyond the scope of this chapter.

Other Pacemaker Modes

Multiple combinations can be programmed into pacemakers. Pacemaker systems have become very complex, and a physician trained in the complex physiology of cardiac pacing is required to configure the pacemaker functions to best meet the physiologic needs of the patient. Those needs may change as the patient changes, and the pacemaker is reprogrammed to meet those needs.

Pacemaker Insertion

Pacemaker Insertion

Once inserted in the operating room by a thoracic surgeon, permanent pacemakers are now commonly inserted in cardiac catheterization laboratories or electrophysiology laboratories by cardiologists who specialize in the field of electrophysiology. The procedure itself is conducted in a room with the same physical requirements as an operating room. Patients are usually awake during the procedure, with light medication to keep them comfortable. A local anesthetic is used at the site of insertion. A small incision, 2" to 3" in length, is made for pacemaker generator insertion in the left or right shoulder area over the location of the subclavian vein. The leads are fed through the subclavian vein into the heart and connected to the pacemaker generator. The pacemaker is programmed and tested. Once accurate pacing is assured, the incision is closed. The procedure is relatively quick, usually less than 2 hours. If a patient is only having a generator or battery replaced, even less time is required because the leads remain in place. The old incision is opened, and the old generator is disconnected from the old leads and removed. The new generator is connected to the old leads and inserted into the pocket. The pacemaker is programmed and, once functioning is confirmed, the incision is closed. As stated earlier, if a new lead is required the old lead is usually left in place to avoid the possibility of a myocardial tear or bleeding that can be associated with removal of a lead.

Recovery After Insertion

Patients may go to a recovery room after pacemaker placement but most often return to a nursing unit that has cardiac monitoring capabilities. With a routine new pacemaker insertion, the patient is hospitalized over night. If only the generator has been replaced, the procedure may be done on an outpatient basis (Ellenbogen & Wood, 2002). It is important that the leads remain at the location of placement in the operating room. Over time, fibrous tissue grows around the electrode and keeps the lead in place. The patient initially has some limitation of movement, until there is assurance that the lead is secure. Specifically, the patient should avoid raising the arm above the head on the side where the pacemaker was inserted for approximately 2 weeks after implantation (Ellenbogen & Wood, 2002). These restrictions are only used when a new lead has been implanted – not for generator replacement only. The patient is also instructed to limit the movement of the effected shoulder and not to lie on the affected side for the first 12 to 24 hours.

As with any surgical procedure, it is not uncommon for patients to experience discomfort at the site for the first several days. Generally, over-the-counter pain relief medications ease the discomfort, and discomfort should lessen as the wound heals. The incision may also be discolored. The incision is often closed with internal sutures that do not require

removal. If external sutures are used, they are removed in 7 to 10 days. The site should be kept dry for 5 to 7 days (Ellenbogen & Wood, 2002).

Patients with new pacemakers are discharged within 12 to 24 hours after the procedure. Generally, most activity is resumed quickly, with full recovery in 2 weeks. During the recovery period, which can last up to 3 months depending on the physician's preference, the patient should avoid heavy pushing, pulling, and lifting with the arm and shoulder where the pacemaker is placed (Rochester Medical Center, n.d.). Driving is also limited for a period of 1 to 4 weeks, again according to the physician's preference (Rochester Medical Center, n.d).

Pacemaker Complications

Pneumothorax

Pacemaker implantation is not without complications. During the procedure, the physician may puncture the lung while attempting to obtain vein access. A punctured lung may not be initially evident and all pacemaker implant patients should have a chest X-ray after the procedure to assess for pneumothorax. Respiratory distress during or after the procedure should raise the suspicion of pneumothorax. Treatment of pneumothorax depends on the size and symptoms. In more severe cases, insertion of a chest tube is required.

Hemothorax

Bleeding into the thoracic cavity may also occur if an artery is nicked or lacerated by a needle during the procedure. If this occurs, pressure can be applied and the situation resolves. If the artery penetration is large, a hemothorax may result and surgical repair of the artery is required.

Myocardial Perforation

During lead placement, the lead may perforate the heart wall. The lead can go through the heart wall to another chamber or, in the worst case, may traverse the entire heart wall to the pericardium. A full-thickness perforation can occur when myocardial tissue is old, steroid therapy has been used, or there was recent infarction of the right ventricular wall (Ellenbogen & Wood, 2002). Cardiac tamponade (bleeding into the pericardial sac) may occur quickly, requiring pericardiocentesis to remove the fluid in the pericardial sac or surgery to repair the damage. Perforation of the tissue may occur without this severe complication in healthier cardiac muscle tissue. Anticoagulated patients should have anticoagulants held for 8 to 12 hours after the procedure until there is an assurance of no bleeding (Ellenbogen & Wood, 2002).

Infection

Pacemaker infection can occur in the early postoperative stage or months to years after implantation. *Staphylococcus aureus* is typically the infecting organism in early infections, whereas *S. epidermis* is found with late-developing infections (Weinberger & Brilliant, 2001). Patients with diabetes mellitus and patients who develop postoperative hematomas tend to have a higher incidence of pacemaker site infection (Ellenbogen & Wood, 2002). Bacteria actually adhere to the pacing generator and leads. It is difficult to eliminate the infection; therefore, the pacemaker system must be removed (Lowy & Freedman, 2004). Once an infection is noted, intravenous antibiotic therapy is initiated. The pacemaker generator and leads are then removed and a new system is placed if the antibiotic therapy has successfully sterilized the blood (Ellenbogen & Wood, 2002). The new pacemaker system will usually be placed in a new location to avoid any possible reinfection of the new system. If antibiotics were not initiated early enough, a temporary pacing system is placed until a permanent implantation is appropriate.

Twiddler's Syndrome

Twiddler's syndrome results from a patient manipulating the pacer generator under the skin. The 'twiddler' actually turns the device over and over and over again under the skin. As the device is turned, the leads twist to the point of actual damage to the lead. Usually, the damage is discovered after the pacemaker fails to function properly. On chest X-ray film, the twisted wires are readily seen. Surgical intervention is required to open the incision and replace the leads. It is only early after the implantation of a device that one can turn it over. Over time, the device becomes attached to its surroundings, making twiddling difficult.

Clinical Application
Instruct patients to ignore the urge to touch their pacemaker in the early, postoperative setting to avoid the possibility of twiddler's syndrome.

Other Complications

Other complications include pacemaker generator migration, which involves actual movement of the pacemaker generator from its original location to a new location in the chest wall. This migration may be of little consequence if there is no malfunction of the pacemaker due to lead displacement or if there is no patient discomfort from the new location of the device. The pacemaker may also erode through the skin, usually due to pressure on the site. Early recognition of pressure on the pacemaker generator by tight skin allows the physician to intervene before the skin is penetrated. Once the skin is penetrated, the entire system is considered contaminated and requires replacement (Ellenbogen & Wood, 2002).

Postoperative Follow-Up

Most patients with new implants return to their physicians' offices within the first 4 weeks after insertion. This follow-up appointment allows the physician to observe the insertion site and assess pacemaker function. After this initial visit, patients can have pacemaker function assessed over the telephone.

Telephone Electrocardiogram Transmission

Pacemaker function should be assessed on a regular basis, depending on physician preference. Telephone assessment allows the physician to determine if the pacemaker is functioning as it should be and if the pacemaker battery is ready for replacement. Pacemaker patients are given a transmitting device that allows them to transmit the needed information. There is usually a prescheduled time for the patient to make the phone call to the office. Once the call is made, the patient is given instructions on how to transmit. This transmission involves utilizing the phone with the transmitting device over the pacemaker. If the patient is not pacemaker dependent (not utilizing the pacemaker all of the time for a heart rate), the patient needs to transmit using a magnet. A magnet placed over the pacemaker generator causes the pacemaker to function without sensing any of the heart's normal activity. The office receives the transmittal in the form of an electrocardiogram (ECG). The ECG allows the physician to determine if the pacemaker is functioning normally and determines battery life. After the office has received the information, the "appointment" is over. The physician reviews the information and calls the patient if there are any concerns regarding pacemaker function.

Many patients can successfully transmit over the phone without any difficulty. Some patients may require some help from a second person. It is usually during the first office visit after insertion that transmission instructions are reviewed and an assessment of the patient's ability to use this method is made.

The need for battery replacement is usually discovered during one of these transmittals. The lithium-iodine pacemaker batteries have a "staged" level of functioning. Staged functioning means that the battery functions at full level of voltage for a period of time. At the end of its life, usually around 90% depletion, the battery decreases the voltage to a lower level (Ellenbogen & Wood, 2002). This change is detected with the phone transmission. When a transmission indicates that the battery is at the end of its life, the patient is notified that a replacement will be necessary in the near future. This replacement is not an emergent situation but should be done soon after end-of-life is reached. The procedure is usually scheduled as an outpatient procedure.

Clinical Application

It is important to assure patients that by completing pacemaker checks over the phone and following up with the physician according to the scheduled time frames , there will be plenty of warning regarding battery end-of-life. Patients who are not well informed about battery end-of-life and battery replacement may think that they will die when the battery is depleted.

Pacemaker Reprogramming

Occasionally, the original settings on a pacemaker may require adjusting to better meet the physiologic needs of the patient or to optimize the pacemaker function and preserve the battery. During an office visit, a pacemaker programmer is used to assess all the functions of the pacemaker. Pacemakers have multiple parameters that may be adjusted at any time with the programmer. Reprogramming a pacemaker involves placing a programmer device over the pacemaker generator. The size and shape of the device varies from one manufacturer to another, but most devices are no larger than the size of a man's hand. The device is a hand-held device that is connected to a computer. Once over the pacemaker, the device transmits information to the computer. Large amounts of information can be obtained from the pacemaker. Once the information is obtained, the physician can make adjustments on the computer that are transmitted back to the pacemaker. After all of the necessary changes have been made, the reprogramming is over. Reprogramming is a painless, short procedure that should result in improved functioning of the pacemaker.

Patient Education

As pacemakers become more sophisticated, the restrictions for the patient decrease. However, patients should be aware of some specific instructions after they have had a pacemaker inserted. A variety of patient education materials are available. The AHA has a pamphlet on permanent pacing. The patient education information listed below is adapted from the AHA patient education information:

1. Patients should receive a pacemaker card identifying the type of pacemaker, leads, and date of insertion. Patients should always carry this card.

2. Patients should always inform any physician or dentist that they have a pacemaker prior to receiving care. Dental equipment should not negatively affect pacemakers.

3. A pacemakers may trigger airport metal detectors, but the metal detectors will not harm the pacemaker. Even so, patients should not linger around metal detectors. Patients should inform security personnel of the pacemaker and ask them not to hold metal detectors near their pacemakers longer than necessary.

4. Microwave ovens no longer affect pacemakers. Neither do most typical household electrical appliances, including CB radios, HAM radios, power tools, television remote controls, heating pads, or home metal detectors.

5. Cellular phones less than 3 watts (most typically used in the United States) have not been shown to interfere with pacemaker function. However, as phone technology continues to change, patients should be instructed to keep cell phones 6" away from their pacemaker. This allows patients to use cell phones with the ear on the side opposite the pacemaker.

6. Patients with pacemakers should not undergo magnetic resonance imaging (MRI) because it can damage the pacemaker. In some instances, some reprogramming may be done to allow for MRI. However, this is limited to very specific instances. Other radiology procedures have not been show to affect pacemakers.

7. Radiation equipment used for treating cancer can damage pacemakers. Patients with pacemakers should not have radiation treatments until arrangements have been made with the physician managing the pacemaker. The pacemaker should be shielded as much as possible because as radiation dosing increases, so does the risk to the pacemaker. In some situations, the pacemaker may be moved to another location in the body to avoid direct radiation. The pacemaker should be checked after each radiation treatment. If the patient is pacemaker dependent (fully dependent on the pacemaker for a heart rate), a temporary pacemaker may be inserted during treatment to assure there is no loss of heart rate. The temporary pacemaker battery can be placed away from the body and shielded during the procedure.

8. Lithotripsy (hydraulic shocks to dissolve kidney stones) may cause changes in the pacemaker. Patients with pacemakers may have lithotripsy, but they require close follow-up after the procedure, and some reprogramming may be necessary.

9. Power-generating equipment, arc welding equipment, and powerful magnets (such as those found in some medical equipment and motors) can inhibit a pacemaker from functioning properly. Patients should avoid being near this type of equipment. If a patient becomes dizzy around questionable equipment, such as a power station, or while working on a running engine, he or she should back away from the equipment and the pacemaker should resume normal functioning.

10. After the initial recovery period, no restrictions to arm movement are necessary.

11. Patients should report any dizziness or syncope to their physicians. If they are able to learn to take their own pulse, they can be instructed to notify the physician if their pulse is less than the programmed low rate on the pacemaker. This may be difficult for some patients. The best indicator for patients with pacemakers is how they are feeling.

12. Patients should be reminded of the importance of keeping appointments for routine pacemaker checks.

CARDIAC RESYNCHRONIZATION THERAPY

Cardiac resynchronization therapy (CRT) is a relatively new strategy for the treatment of heart failure. As researchers searched for treatment strategies for patients with heart failure, they found that dyssynchrony of contraction of the right and left ventricles contributed to a poor prognosis in patients with dilated cardiomyopathy (DCM) (Albert, 2003). This dyssynchrony occurs with left bundle branch block. Cardiac dyssynchrony in patients with DCM results in poor hemodynamic functioning. These patients have decreased ejection fractions, decreased cardiac output, decreased arterial pressure, increased volume in the ventricle at the end of systole, and decreased cardiac relaxation (Albert, 2003). Research shows that QRS duration on an ECG wider than 120 ms (normal is 100 ms or less) is associated with a 46% increase in mortality in patients with heart failure and 10 or more ventricular contractions per minute (Albert, 2003). As QRS width increases, so does mortality rate. In left bundle branch block, the right ventricle contracts first, followed by the left ventricle. Generally, the lateral wall of the left ventricle is the last wall to contract in left bundle branch block. CRT is a therapy aimed at eliminating the dyssynchrony and involves the utilization of a pacemaker lead in each ventricle (biventricular pacing) to resynchronize the ventricles.

Indications

CRT can be costly, so the guidelines for device implantation are strict. Currently, the Food and Drug Administration (FDA) has approved CRT for a specific group of patients (see Table 12-2). This population includes patients who are symptomatic on full medical therapy for their heart failure. They must also fall into New York Heart Association (NYHA) class III or IV (Table 12-3). They must also meet strict criteria for ejection fraction and QRS duration on an ECG.

TABLE 12-2: INDICATIONS FOR CARDIAC RESYNCHRONIZATION THERAPY

Severity of illness	Moderate to severe heart failure Symptomatic on full medical therapy
NYHA functional class	Class III or class IV
Ejection fraction	$\leq 35\%$
QRS duration	≥ 130 ms
Left ventricular size	Diameter at end of diastole > 55 mm

(Gregaratos et al., 2002)

TABLE 12-3: NEW YORK HEART ASSOCIATION CLASSIFICATION OF HEART FAILURE

Class I	Patients with no limitation of activities who suffer no symptoms from ordinary activities
Class II	Patients with slight, mild limitation of activity who are comfortable with rest or with mild exertion
Class III	Patients with marked limitation of activity who are comfortable only at rest
Class IV	Patients who should be at complete rest and confined to a bed or chair; any physical activity brings on discomfort and symptoms occur at rest

(The Criteria Committee of the New York Heart Association, 1994)

Biventricular Pacemaker Insertion

Like other pacemakers, the biventricular pacemaker generator is placed in a pocket in the chest wall. Pacemaker leads are placed in the right atrium and right ventricle in the normal method. A third lead is attached to the left ventricle in the location of the left lateral ventricular wall. The right atrial and ventricular leads are placed inside the chambers, whereas the left ventricular lead is threaded through the coronary sinus and into the left ventricular cardiac vein. This approach results in a lead that is pacing from the outer surface of the heart. The left lateral wall placement of the lead is effective because the left lateral wall of the left ventricle is the part of the heart that contracts last. Implantation of this lead may be difficult because the ventricle is typically quite dilated. Occasionally, the lead cannot be placed percutaneously and must be placed in the operating room through a surgical incision in the chest wall (see Figure 12-5).

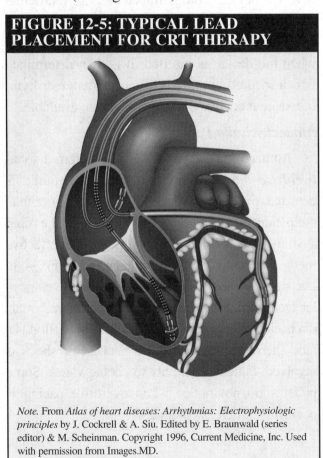

FIGURE 12-5: TYPICAL LEAD PLACEMENT FOR CRT THERAPY

Note. From *Atlas of heart diseases: Arrhythmias: Electrophysiologic principles* by J. Cockrell & A. Siu. Edited by E. Braunwald (series editor) & M. Scheinman. Copyright 1996, Current Medicine, Inc. Used with permission from Images.MD.

Once the leads are in place, the goal of therapy is to have both ventricular pacemaker leads stimulating the respective ventricles at the same time. This is achieved though extensive programming efforts. Then the procedure is over. Today, almost all patients who are candidates for biventricular pacing are also candidates for ICDs, which are placed at the same time as biventricular pacing leads.

Postoperative Care

Postoperative care differs little from that for standard pacemaker implantation. However, patients with CRT are likely to require more frequent follow-up as the pacemaker is adjusted and reprogrammed to best meet the physiologic needs of the patient.

Patient Education

The standard education that was reviewed for traditional pacemaker insertion is the same for CRT. It is, however, important for CRT patients to realize that this therapy does not eliminate the need for continued medical therapy. In fact, medications may actually be increased to higher levels, that the patient was unable to tolerate without biventricular pacing.

Outcomes

Many studies continue to evaluate the long-term effectiveness of CRT. The preliminary studies are positive. For example, in the Comparing Medical Therapy, Pacing and Defibrillation in Chronic Heart Failure study, preliminary reports demonstrated a reduction in death and hospitalizations in those who received CRT (Albert, 2003). Patients also report increased activity ability and tolerance and an improvement in quality of life (Albert, 2003).

IMPLANTABLE CARDIOVERTER-DEFIBRILLATORS

In 1980, the first implantable defibrillator was implanted in a human being (Ganz, 2004). In 1985, the FDA approved their use in a limited population

(Ganz, 2004). Over the past 20 years, the technology for ICDs has changed dramatically. The initial devices were large and bulky, requiring thoracic surgery for implantation. The generators were implanted in the abdomen, with patches applied to the heart. Currently, implantation of the device is similar to that of a pacemaker, with the generator, (which is slightly larger than that of a pacemaker), implanted in the shoulder.

Indications

The indications for implantation of an ICD are very specific. However, these devices are very expensive and have quite an impact on the patient, which is discussed later. As technology and research continue, the indications for ICDs increase. Originally developed to prevent sudden cardiac death from ventricular tachycardia and ventricular fibrillation, these devices now also treat bradycardia and atrial tachycardias (Gregoratos et al., 2002).

Initially, ICDs were indicated, with few exceptions, in patients who had sustained ventricular tachycardia or resuscitated cardiac arrest (Ganz, 2004). The indications have now expanded to include patients with prior myocardial infarction (MI), ejection fractions less than 40%, and spontaneous nonsustained ventricular tachycardia if the arrhythmia can be induced in the electrophysiology laboratory (Ganz, 2004). This means that patients who meet the criteria undergo electrophysiology studies. During these studies, the electrophysiologist stimulates the heart in an attempt to cause ventricular tachycardia. If the arrhythmia occurs, then the patient is considered "inducible" and an ICD in indicated.

Most recently, the Multicenter Automatic Defibrillator Implantation Trail II opened the door for further utilization of ICDs. This trial demonstrated a measurable decrease in mortality for patients with prior MI and ejection fractions less than 35%. These patients are not required to have the ventricular tachycardia component to qualify for an ICD (Ganz, 2004).

Functions

Like pacemakers, ICDs are multiprogrammable, with a large variety of technical options for treating arrhythmias. The ultimate goal of therapy is to avoid the arrhythmias completely. Appropriate administration of antiarrhythmic medications controls the arrhythmias. It is preferred that the ICD never fires but firing is available in the event that medications do not totally suppress the arrhythmia.

Clinical Application
Patients with ICSd should be instructed to continue taking their medications. ICDs do not eliminate the development of arrhythmias; they only terminate the arrhythmias once they have occurred. Antiarrhythmic medications control the development of arrhythmias.

The ICD generator includes technology for permanent cardiac pacing as well as cardiac defibrillation. The device is programmed to sense ventricular tachycardia through a variety of sophisticated methods that are programmed to the specific patient when the device is inserted. It is then determined which method is utilized to terminate the arrhythmia once it occurs. Several options are available.

Antitachycardia Pacing

Antitachycardia pacing is also referred to as *overdrive pacing*. Once the rapid arrhythmia is detected, the pacemaker paces at a rate higher than the patient's rate in an attempt to override the rapid rhythm. This method has proven to be an effective method to control some ventricular tachycardias. In one study, 96% of all detected episodes of ventricular tachycardia were terminated with antitachycardia pacing (Gregoratos et al., 2002). This option is a nice alternative for the patient because no shock is involved. Patient sensitivity to pacing varies. Some patients do not notice when overdrive pacing is occurring, whereas others do.

Defibrillation

Defibrillation is utilized as needed to terminate arrhythmias. The shock administered can be either a cardioversion shock or a full defibrillation shock. The cardioversion shock uses less energy than the defibrillation shock. If the cardioversion shock is programmed into the device as a therapy, it is attempted before the defibrillation shock. If cardioversion does not terminate the arrhythmia, a defibrillation shock is administered. The administration of a shock to the heart is not as strong as those seen with external defibrillators. However, they are most definitely felt by patients and are painful. The lowest amount of energy needed to terminate the arrhythmia is determined when the device is implanted. The shock administered should be strong enough to take control of the heart and eliminate the arrhythmia as the controlling rhythm.

Implantation

An electrophysiologist who is trained in ICD insertion should implant the device. Occasionally, an ICD is placed in the operating room by a heart surgeon in conjunction with open-heart surgery, but this occurs only in unusual situations. The defibrillator is located on the lead that is placed in the right ventricle. The pacemaker functions as a normal pacemaker. In many cases, the pacemaker is only needed after a shock is delivered and a brief pause in the patient's own rhythm occurs as the heart resets itself after the shock. During implantation of the device, the patient is awake. However, after implantation, it is necessary to test the device to assure it will fire. During this portion of the procedure, conscious sedation or anesthesia is utilized to protect the patient from discomfort associated with defibrillation. The electrophysiologist programs the device to the most effective settings. After the procedure, the patient is returned to a recovery room or a nursing unit capable of cardiac monitoring. Patients are commonly discharged the next day if no complications occur and ventricular arrhythmias are under control.

Postoperative Follow-Up

Postoperative care is similar to the postoperative care necessary for patients with pacemakers. However, ICD patients are generally restricted from driving. These limitations vary somewhat by physician. The ACC/AHA/NASPE guidelines recommend no driving for 6 months after the last symptomatic arrhythmia (Gregoratos et al., 2002). Many electrophysiologists also require the patient to be shock-free for 6 months (Ganz, 2004). The most current literature supports varied driving restrictions based on the reason for the implant (Gimbel, 2004). The goal is to prevent the possibility of developing an arrhythmia that incapacitates the driver while behind the wheel. Many patients find this restriction very difficult to adhere to.

Office Visits

Follow-up visits after ICD implantation are usually more frequent than with permanent pacemaker insertion. Patients have office visits rather than phone transmissions because electrophysiologists want to assess the function of the device. With a programmer similar to the one used for pacemakers, electrophysiologists can determine the number of therapies that have been delivered by the device, including the success of the therapy. During this time, the battery level is also checked. Battery life depends on the frequency of the therapy as well as the energy utilized with those therapies. As with pacemakers, it is predetermined when battery end-of-life is near so replacement of the battery can be scheduled. These office visits are essential in maintaining good function of the ICD.

Magnet Function with an ICD

As noted earlier in the text, a magnet placed over the pulse generator in a normal pacemaker causes the pacemaker to pace without sensing any of the heart's normal activity. An ICD does not function in the same manner. A magnet placed over an ICD disables the device while the magnet is in place. Once the magnet is away from the device, the device functions in the normal manner. If the magnet is placed over the device for an extended period (20 to 30 seconds), the device is turned off. The magnet can then be removed and the device remains off. Different manufacturers have different systems programmed into their devices for activation and deactivation. It is important for health care workers to be aware that a magnet over an ICD disables the device and no treatment will occur if the patient develops arrhythmias. The best practice is not to utilize magnets near these devices unless instructed to do so by a qualified physician.

Patient Education

Emotional Impact

Patient education for the recipient of an ICD involves technical aspects of care as well as emotional aspects. Implantation of an ICD is generally emotionally difficult because the patient realizes that his or her life may depend on the device. The emotional impact extends beyond the patient to the family. There is a fear of death as well as a fear that the device may not function. Patients have reported sleeplessness due to fear and anxiety. Families may also become overprotective because they worry about the device. Good patient education is essential to help patients and families understand the device. ICD support groups are available in some areas. The patient's electrophysiologist should be aware of this opportunity.

Device Activation Education

As stated earlier, the goal of therapy is to have a medication regime that prevents arrhythmias from occurring. However, arrhythmias may occur, so the patient and family should be aware of the proper response. Physicians may vary in preference regarding notification of a shock, but the following is basic information regarding patient response to device activation:

1. All patients with ICDs should have a well-thought-out plan for obtaining emergency medical assistance. Close family and friends should be aware of the plan in the event that the device

does not work properly. Close family and friends should all be trained in cardiopulmonary resuscitation (CPR).

2. Patients describe the feeling of a full defibrillation shock as being "kicked in the chest". A cardioversion shock is less intense. The patient should not notice normal cardiac pacing, but may or may not notice antitachycardia pacing (Guidant Corporation, n.d.).

3. Family and friends should be aware they are in no danger if they come in contact with the patient when the defibrillator discharges (Yeo & Berg, 2004). If a shock occurs during sexual intercourse, the partner may experience a tingle or buzz. This shock is not harmful to the partner (Guidant Corporation, n.d.).

4. Once shock has occurred, the patient should notify the physician who is handling the ICD that the shock occurred. The physician does not need to be called immediately but should be notified when the office is next open. The physician needs to be aware of device firing so adjustments can be made as needed.

5. If the device fires multiple times and the patient returns to normal, the physician should be called at that time.

6. If the device continues to fire without success, the family should place a call to the emergency medical system (EMS) and begin CPR if the patient becomes unconscious.

7. If at any time the ICD fires and the patient does not return to normal (awake and appropriate) after the shock, even if only one shock was delivered, the patient should be taken to the nearest emergency department via EMS.

Electromagnetic Interference

On rare occasions (less than 1% per patient per year), electromagnetic interference may cause an ICD to fire (Yeo & Berg, 2004). All precautions noted with pacemakers apply to ICDs. It is important for patients to notify security personnel of the

ICD. Patients should not allow handheld metal detector wands near the pacemaker site. These contain magnets that can reset the device if left in place too long (Yeo & Berg, 2004). Again, carrying the manufacturer's identification card is a must.

ICDs should be turned off prior to any surgery requiring electrocautery because electrocautery interferes with the device. Generally, arrangements are made to turn the device back on immediately after surgery.

Clinical Application

If a beeping tone is heard coming from the device, the patient is most likely in the area of a strong magnetic field. He or she should immediately move away from the object that may be causing the device to beep and should also notify the physician.

CONCLUSION

The field of cardiac pacemakers has grown dramatically over the past 40 years. Research allows for devices that more closely mimic the heart's natural pacemaker. The development of biventricular pacing to resynchronize the ventricles is proving to be a life-prolonging strategy that improves quality of life for many patients with heart failure. Most patients who undergo CRT are also candidates for ICDs. As technology becomes more complex, the costs of these therapies continues to rise. Many decisions are made as to the appropriate candidates for these expensive therapies. Ethical dilemmas come into play, and determinations need to be made about replacement of defibrillators in elderly patients who are reaching the end of life. These defibrillators may prevent what is the natural progression to death as someone ages.

EXAM QUESTIONS

CHAPTER 12
Questions 94-100

94. The most common reason for pacemaker implantation is
    a. hypersensitive carotid sinus syncope.
    b. bifascicular block.
    c. sinoatrial (SA) node dysfunction.
    d. atrioventricular block (AV block).

95. A true statement about dual-chamber cardiac pacemakers is
    a. dual-chamber pacemakers eliminate atrial kick by controlling the atrium and ventricle.
    b. dual-chamber pacemakers most closely mimic the heart's normal conduction system.
    c. dual-chamber pacemakers are the best therapy for patients with heart failure.
    d. dual-chamber pacemakers can cause pacemaker syndrome.

96. A patient with a permanent cardiac pacemaker implanted 1 year ago presents to the office with a temperature of 99.4° F and concerns about his pacemaker site. Upon examination, the nurse notes a small open area at the pacemaker site and the pacemaker can be seen through the opening. The skin surrounding the open area is red and swollen with some pus noted. The nurse anticipates treatment with
    a. antibiotics, removal of the entire pacemaker system (leads and generator), and implantation of a new pacemaker system in a different location.
    b. antibiotics, removal of the entire pacemaker system (leads and generator), and implantation of a new pacemaker system in the same location.
    c. antibiotics and aggressive wound care.
    d. antibiotics and removal of the pacemaker generator, with placement of a new generator in a new location.

97. Devices that can affect the function of permanent cardiac pacemakers include
    a. microwave ovens.
    b. cellular phones more than 6" away from the pacemaker.
    c. MRI and lithotripsy.
    d. television remote controls and home metal detectors.

98. The benefits of biventricular pacing include

    a. increased cardiac output due to strong ventricular contraction.

    b. control of atrial fibrillation.

    c. increased cardiac output due to resynchronization of the contraction of the ventricles.

    d. the ability to pace and shock the heart at the same time.

99. Any patient with an ICD should know that a magnet placed over the ICD will

    a. make the ICD defibrillate.

    b. make the ICD revert to antitachycardia mode.

    c. deactivate the ICD.

    d. transmit information to the programmer so the device can be evaluated.

100. A 64-year-old man with an ICD is watching TV at home Sunday evening. His ICD suddenly discharges delivering one defibrillation shock. After the shock, the 64-year-old feels fine. At this point the patient knows he should

    a. call his physician at the next most convenient time during normal office hours to let the physician know the ICD has delivered a shock.

    b. call the physician immediately for further instructions and to have the ICD reset.

    c. drive to the hospital to have the ICD checked with the programmer.

    d. call 911 for immediate transport to the hospital.

This concludes the final examination.

GLOSSARY

abdominal obesity: Obesity with a distribution of fat around the abdomen that produces an abnormal waist-to-hip ratio.

acetylcholine: The neurotransmitter of the parasympathetic nervous system.

acidosis: Condition characterized by an arterial blood pH less than 7.35.

activated clotting time (ACT): A test to evaluate coagulation status that can be evaluated at the bedside.

activated partial thromboplastin time (aPTT): Coagulation test used to monitor the therapeutic effectiveness and safety range of heparin.

acute coronary syndrome (ACS): The presentation of coronary artery disease in the form of unstable angina, non-ST segment-elevation MI, or ST-segment elevation MI.

acute respiratory distress syndrome (ARDS): A complex clinical syndrome resulting in acute respiratory failure from hypoxic lung injury.

adenosine: Coronary vasodilator used in chemical stress testing. Also used as an antiarrhythmic to slow conduction through the atrioventricular node during some forms of tachycardia.

adenosine diphosphate (ADP): Substance responsible for activation of glycoprotein IIb/IIIa receptors.

adenosine diphosphate (ADP) inhibitors: Medications that prevent ADP-mediated activation of platelets.

adenosine triphosphate (ATP): An enzyme in muscle cells that stores energy and produces energy when split.

adrenal cortex: Outer layer of the adrenal gland.

adrenergic receptor: Receptor of the sympathetic nervous system.

adventitia: Fibrous outer layer of an artery that is designed to protect the vessel and provide connection to other internal structures.

afterload: Pressure the ventricle must overcome to eject its contents.

aggregation: Clustering or coming together.

albumin: A simple protein widely distributed in tissues that circulates in the blood as serum albumin.

alkalosis: Condition characterized by a pH more than 7.45.

aldosterone: A mineralocorticoid hormone that increases sodium and water reabsorption.

aldosterone antagonist: Medication that blocks the effects of aldosterone.

alpha$_1$ adrenergic receptor: Sympathetic nervous system receptor located in the vessels of vascular smooth muscle.

alveolar membrane: Membrane of the alveoli in the lungs and the site of gas exchange.

aminophylline: Pulmonary vasodilator used as an antidote for adenosine or dipyridamole during chemical stress testing.

amiodarone: A class III antiarrhythmic with vasodilative properties that is generally well tolerated in patients with left ventricular dysfunction; used to treat atrial and ventricular arrhythmias.

amyloidosis: Disease in which protein fibrils (amyloid) collect in body tissues and impair organ function.

anaphylactic shock: Shock caused by an allergic reaction.

androgen: Hormone that produces male characteristics.

anemia: Reduced hemoglobin level or red blood cell count.

angina pectoris: The clinical symptom resulting from decreased blood flow to the myocardium.

angioedema: Allergic response in which the skin, mucous membranes, and viscera become edematous. Commonly occurs around the eyes or lips. Swelling is deep, extending beneath the skin, and can involve the airways.

angiography: Procedure in which serial radiographs of a blood vessel are taken in rapid sequence after the injection of a radiopaque substance. Used to determine the size and shape of vessels. Coronary angiography is also called *cardiac catheterization.*

angiojet thrombectomy: Atherectomy procedure used for the extraction of visible thrombi within the coronary artery.

angiotensin converting enzyme: A proteolytic enzyme that converts angiotensin I to angiotensin II.

angiotensin-converting enzyme (ACE) inhibitor: Medication that prevents the conversion of angiotensin I to angiotensin II.

angiotensin I: Precursor to angiotensin II.

angiotensin II: Potent vasoconstrictor and stimulator of aldosterone secretion.

angiotensin II receptor blocker (ARB): Medication that blocks the effects of angiotensin II.

ankle-brachial index (ABI): Blood pressure in the ankle divided by blood pressure in the arm. A decrease in ABI during exercise is an indication that peripheral arterial disease is present.

annulus: Fibrous ring that forms the opening of the valve and joins the valve cusps (leaflets) together.

anorexia: Loss of appetite.

antagonize: To counteract.

anterior myocardial infarction: Myocardial infarction involving the anterior, or front wall, of the left ventricle.

anterolateral myocardial infarction: Myocardial infarction involving the anterior and lateral walls of the left ventricle.

anteroseptal myocardial infarction: Myocardial infarction involving the anterior wall of the left ventricle and the septum.

antianginal: Medication effective in preventing or decreasing angina.

antibody: A protein substance developed in response to an antigen.

anticoagulant: Medication that interferes with clot formation by disrupting the intrinsic, extrinsic, or common pathway of the coagulation cascade.

antioxidant: An agent that protects against oxidation.

antiplatelet: An agent or medication interfering with the action of platelets in clot formation.

antiproliferative: Blocking of rapid cell reproduction.

antitachycardia pacing: Pacemaker therapy that utilizes the pacemaker to override a fast rhythm with a higher pacemaker rate. Once the pacemaker has control of the rhythm, the pacemaker slows the rate to a normal range. Also known as *overdrive pacing.*

antithrombin III: An agent that opposes the action of thrombin, inhibits the coagulation of blood, and inactivates several clotting factors.

antithrombotic: Agent that counteracts clot formation.

anxiolytic: Medication given to reduce anxiety.

aorta: Main trunk of the arterial system, which originates from the left ventricle.

aortic dissection: Separation of the layers of the aorta.

aortic regurgitation: Abnormal aortic valve function in which valve cusps do not close tightly, causing retrograde movement of blood through the valve during ventricular systole.

aortic root: Beginning of the aorta, where the aorta attaches to the aortic valve.

aortic stenosis: Abnormal aortic valve function resulting in obstruction of flow from the left ventricle to incorrect or incomplete valve opening.

aortic valve: Valve between the left ventricle and the aorta.

apex: The bottom of the heart. Located approximately at the fifth intercostal space, at the midclavicular line.

apical impulse: The area normally near the apex of the heart where the contraction of the heart can be palpated.

apoptosis: Programmed cell death.

aprotinin: A serine protease inhibitor and hemostatic agent used to prevent bleeding in high-risk patients undergoing coronary artery bypass graft surgery. Also an anti-inflammatory agent.

arginine vasopressin: Antidiuretic hormone that can also be used as a vasopressor.

arrhythmia: Abnormal heart rhythm.

arrhythmogenic right ventricular cardiomyopathy: A genetic disorder characterized by right ventricular cardiomyopathy caused by an electrical disturbance that produces arrhythmias.

arterioles: Small arteries with thick muscular walls.

ascites: Accumulation of serous fluid in the peritoneal cavity.

atelectasis: A condition in which a portion of the lung is unexpanded or collapsed.

atherectomy: Interventional procedure utilizing a cutting tool to cut atherosclerotic plaque away from the wall of the coronary artery.

atheroma: Extracellular lipid core of atherosclerotic plaque.

atheromatous: Pertaining to atheroma.

atherosclerosis: The deposit of lipids, calcium, fibrin, and other cellular substances within the lining of the arteries and the progressive inflammatory response that results from the effort to heal the endothelium.

atherosclerotic plaque: A buildup of the deposits of lipids, calcium, fibrin, and other cellular substances that occur with atherosclerosis.

atrial defibrillator: Implantable defibrillator programmed to shock and cardiovert the rhythm of atrial fibrillation.

atrial fibrillation: Rapid chaotic activity of the atria that results in the deterioration of atrial mechanical activity and produces irregular atrial fibrillation waves with an atrial rate greater than 350 beats per minute. Variable ventricular conduction resulting in an irregularly irregular ventricular rhythm.

atrial kick: Atrial contraction, or systole.

atrial myxoma: A benign tumor located in the upper chamber of the heart on the wall that separates the left chamber from the right (the atrial septum).

atrial natriuretic peptide (ANP): Hormone released by the atria during periods of volume overload. Increased production causes vasodilatation and diuresis.

atrioventricular (AV) block: Block of the impulse that normally travels from the sinoatrial node to the AV node, disrupting the normal heart rhythm and conduction of impulses through the heart.

atrioventricular (AV) junction: Tissue surrounding the AV node and bundle of His that contains pacemaker cells capable of firing at a rate of 40 to 60 beats per minute.

atrioventricular (AV) node: A small mass of tissue that slows conduction from the atria to the ventricles and is located in the right atrium, just above the insertion of the tricuspid valve.

atrioventricular (AV) node ablation: Ablation of the AV node that permanently prevents any rapid ventricular response. Patients who require AV node ablation also need permanent pacemaker implantation.

atrioventricular (AV) valves: Valves located between the atria and ventricles.

autoimmune response: Process by which the body produces an immunological response against itself.

autologous transfusion: Transfusion of blood donated by the patient himself or herself.

automated external defibrillator (AED): Defibrillator designed to be used by trained laypeople in the event of cardiac arrest due to ventricular fibrillation. Rhythm recognition and defibrillation are done automatically via a hands-off approach.

automaticity: Intrinsic ability to depolarize spontaneously.

autonomic dysfunction: Dysfunction of the autonomic nervous system.

autonomic nervous system: Nervous system that controls involuntary bodily functions. Consists of the sympathetic and parasympathetic nervous systems.

Bachmann's bundle: Conduction pathway that allows depolarization of the left atrial tissue as conduction travels from the sinoatrial node to the atrioventricular node.

baroreceptors: Specialized nerve tissues functioning as sensors that are located in the aortic arch and carotid sinus (the origin of the internal carotid artery).

base: Top of the heart, which is located at approximately the second intercostal space.

beta$_1$ adrenergic receptor: Sympathetic nervous system receptor located in the heart.

beta$_2$ adrenergic receptor: Sympathetic nervous system receptor located in the lungs and periphery.

beta-blocker: Medication that blocks either beta$_1$ or beta$_2$ adrenergic receptors.

beta radiation: Type of radiation used for in-stent restenosis with less dwell time and less scatter that gamma radiation.

Bezold-Jarisch reflex: Cardiovascular reflex that causes a vasovagal response when triggered.

bifascicular block: A block of the normal conduction system involving simultaneous blockage of the right bundle branch and blockage of one of the two fascicles of the left bundle branch.

bile acid sequestrant: Also called a *resin*, a lipid-lowering drug that combines with bile acids in the intestine to form an insoluble complex that is excreted in feces.

bioprosthetic valve: Tissue valve from a human or animal donor.

biphasic waveform defibrillator: Newer generation of defibrillators that use energy more efficiently, therefore requiring lower amounts of energy for a defibrillation or cardioversion shock.

bisferiens carotid pulse: Characteristic of a patient with hypertrophic obstructive cardiomyopathy in which the initial upstroke of the carotid pulse is brisk; however, as systole progresses, left ventricular outflow tract obstruction can occur. This obstruction results in a collapse of the pulse and then a secondary rise.

biventricular pacing: See *cardiac resynchronization therapy.*

body mass index (BMI): An index used to define overweight and obesity. Calculated by using height, weight, and a constant.

brachial plexus: Network of nerves supplying the arm, forearm, and hand.

brachiocephalic artery: Also called the *innominate artery*, the largest branch off the aortic arch that divides into the right common carotid and right subclavian arteries.

bradyarrhythmia: Arrhythmias characterized by a ventricular rate less than 50 beats per minute.

bradycardia: Heart rate below 50 beats per minute.

brain natriuretic peptide (BNP): A hormone released from myocytes during heart failure that produces vasodilation. Serum BNP levels are used in the diagnosis of heart failure.

bruit: An adventitious sound heard on auscultation of a vessel.

bundle branch block: Block of either the right or left bundle branch.

bundle of His: Conduction pathway that divides and gives rise to the right and left bundles.

bupropion: Oral antidepressant used for smoking cessation.

calcium channel blocker: Medication that decreases the flux of calcium across the cell membrane.

cannulation: The placement of a tube inside a vessel to allow the escape of blood and other fluids from the body. Used in cardiopulmonary bypass surgery.

capillary: The very smallest vessel that connects the smallest arteries and veins. Also the location of oxygen and nutrient exchange.

carbon monoxide: A poisonous gas that is colorless, odorless, and tasteless.

cardiac biomarker: Substance released into the blood when necrosis occurs as a result of myocyte membrane rupture.

cardiac catheterization: An invasive diagnostic procedure used to identify blockage of coronary arteries whereby a catheter is threaded through an artery into the heart, a contrast agent (dye) is injected into the coronary arteries, and angiography is performed.

cardiac myoplasty: Surgery that involves wrapping a muscle from the patient's back around the heart and stimulating it to contract via a pacemaker wire.

cardiac output: The amount of blood ejected by the left ventricle every minute.

cardiac resynchronization therapy (CRT): Pacemaker therapy aimed at eliminating dyssynchrony of the contraction of the right and left ventricles that occurs in severe heart failure. Utilizes a pacemaker lead for each ventricle (biventricular pacing).

cardiac tamponade: Accumulation of excess fluid in the pericardium that prevents ventricular filling.

cardiogenic shock: Failure of tissues to receive an adequate blood supply due to severely decreased cardiac output caused by left ventricular failure.

cardiomyopathy: A disorder caused by dysfunction of the myocardium; heart muscle disease.

cardioplegia: Paralysis of the heart.

cardiopulmonary bypass: Process by which the normal circulation of blood bypasses the heart and lungs during the administration of cardioplegia for coronary artery bypass graft surgery. This is accomplished by rerouting the blood through a cardiopulmonary bypass machine that functions in place of the heart and lungs.

cardioversion: Restoration of a tachyarrhythmia (atrial fibrillation, supraventricular tachycardia, ventricular tachycardia) to a normal sinus rhythm using electrical stimulation or pharmacotherapy.

carotid endarterectomy: A surgical procedure whereby the fatty buildup of plaque is removed from the carotid artery.

catalyze: To speed up the rate of a reaction.

catecholamines: The sympathetic nervous system neurotransmitters epinephrine and norepinephrine.

cerebral vascular accident (CVA): Also known as *stroke*. Injury to the brain caused by inadequate oxygenated blood supply. Can be caused by thrombus or embolus (ischemic stroke), or by hemorrhage (hemorrhagic stroke).

cephalosporin: Class of antibiotics most frequently used to prevent postoperative infection in coronary artery bypass graft surgery.

chemoreceptors: Receptors located in the aortic arch and carotid arteries that respond to changes in blood chemistry, including arterial oxygen content, arterial carbon dioxide levels, and arterial pH.

cholinergic: Name of response of the parasympathetic nervous system.

chordae tendineae: Delicate strands of fibrous material that attach atrioventricular valve leaflets to the papillary muscles.

chronic obstructive pulmonary disease (COPD): A chronic lung disease characterized by a limitation in airflow during normal breathing.

chronotropic: Affecting the heart rate.

cirrhosis: Chronic disease of the liver involving connective tissue, fatty infiltrates, and degenerative changes.

coagulopathy: Pathology of the coagulation system.

coarctation of the aorta: Malformation resulting in narrowing of the aorta.

collagen: Fibrous protein found in connective tissue.

commissure: Point where the cardiac valve leaflets connect.

commissurotomy: Procedure during which the valve commissures are cut apart to allow for increased movement of the leaflets.

common pathway: Final pathway in clotting cascade in which a fibrinogen is converted to fibrin and a fibrin stable clot is formed.

complete heart block: Complete failure of the atrial impulses to be conducted to the ventricles.

concentric hypertrophy: A change in the walls of the ventricle resulting in thickened walls that are stiff and noncompliant but do not increase the overall size of the ventricle.

conduit: Term used to describe a blood vessels used as a bypass graft during coronary artery bypass graft surgery.

contractility: Ability of the ventricle to pump independent of preload or afterload.

contrast-induced nephropathy: Renal dysfunction caused by the administration of contrast agents during invasive or interventional cardiac procedures.

coronary artery bypass graft (CABG) surgery : Surgery during which blood flow through a coronary artery is rerouted around a blockage or narrowing in the coronary artery utilizing a bypass graft. A variety of veins or arteries from the patient or a donor can be utilized as bypass grafts.

coronary artery disease (CAD): Disease process that results in narrowing or occlusion of the coronary artery.

coronary heart disease (CHD): Term used interchangeably with CAD.

coronary sinus: The vessel that receives blood from the cardiac veins and empties into the right atrium.

creatine kinase (CK): Biomarker present in the heart, brain, and skeletal muscle.

creatine kinase-MB: Biomarker specific to the heart that rapidly rises in the presence of myocardial damage.

cryopreservation: Preservation by subjection to very low temperatures.

cryotherapy: Therapy using cold.

crystalloid solution: Clear intravenous solution with dissolved substances that can diffuse across cell membranes. For example, normal saline solution.

cutting balloon: A device used to make incisions into the plaque prior to dilation during percutaneous transluminal coronary angioplasty.

cyclooxygenase: Chemical substance that performs the first step in the creation of prostaglandins.

cyclosporin: Medication used to suppress the immune system.

cytokine: Protein secreted by cells of the immune system that helps to regulate the immune system.

DDD pacemaker: Dual chamber pacemaker that senses and paces in both the right atrium and right ventricle. Responds to any sensed activity by either triggering an action or inhibiting one.

debridement: Removal of dead or damaged tissue from a wound.

defibrillation: Desynchronized shock delivered to patients in ventricular fibrillation.

depolarization: Stimulation of cardiac muscle cells.

diabetes mellitus: Insulin deficit (type I) or inappropriate response to insulin (type II), resulting in a random glucose level more than 200 mg/dl or a fasting glucose level more than 126 mg/dl.

diastole: Relaxation of the heart muscle that permits filling of the chamber.

diastolic dysfunction: Left ventricular dysfunction whereby the ventricle has impaired relaxation and does not fill properly.

Dietary Approaches to Stop Hypertension (DASH) diet: A diet that manipulates potassium, calcium, and magnesium while holding sodium constant.

dilatation: Expansion of an organ or a vessel.

dilated cardiomyopathy (DCM): Cardiomyopathy caused by an enlarged, dilated cardiac chamber that affects the ability of the ventricle to contract, resulting in systolic dysfunction.

dipyridamole: A coronary vasodilator used in chemical stress testing.

direct current cardioversion: Procedure in which an electrical shock is synchronized with the intrinsic activity of the heart to convert an abnormal rhythm back into a normal sinus rhythm.

directional atherectomy: Procedure used to cut and remove plaque in native vessels or in saphenous vein grafts by directing a rotating cutter toward the plaque to be removed.

distensibility: Ability to stretch.

dobutamine: Inotropic agent used for chemical stress testing. Also used in critically ill patients in cardiogenic shock or end-stage heart failure.

dopaminergic receptor: Sympathetic nervous system receptor located in the renal, mesenteric, and coronary blood vessels.

Dressler's syndrome: Pericarditis occurring several weeks after an infarction.

dromotropic: Affecting cardiac conduction.

drug-eluting stent: Stent coated with a pharmacological agent aimed at decreasing restenosis.

dual-chamber pacemaker: Pacemaker that has an electrode for pacing in two chambers of the heart, traditionally, the right atrium and the right ventricle.

Duroziez's sign: Systolic murmur heard over the femoral artery when compressed proximally or diastolic murmur heard over the femoral artery when compressed distally.

dyslipidemia: An abnormal amount of lipids in the blood.

eccentric hypertrophy: Hypertrophy caused by volume overload and resulting in ventricular dilation. Wall thickness is in proportion to chamber size.

echocardiogram: Cardiac ultrasound.

ectopic beat: Beat originating outside the sinus node.

ejection: The second phase of systole, during which blood is ejected.

ejection fraction: The percent of volume ejected with each beat.

electrocautery: Cauterization (destruction of tissue) by means of a device heated by a current of electricity.

electromechanical interference: Electrical signals external to a pacemaker that may be sensed by the pacemaker, making it difficult for the pacemaker to sense the heart's activity in the normal manner. This can lead to a dysfunctional pacemaker.

electrophysiology: Field of cardiology dedicated to the study and treatment of disorders of the heart's rhythm.

embolus: A particle of undissolved matter in the blood (can be solid, liquid, or gas; for example, a piece of a clot or fat, or an air bubble).

emergency medical system (EMS): Community response system where paramedics and other trained personnel respond to medical emergencies. Activated by dialing "911" in most parts of the country.

endocarditis: Inflammation of the endocardium (the inner lining of heart), including the heart valves.

endocardium: The inner surface of the heart chambers and valves that also covers the walls of the vessels of the entire vascular system.

endomyocardial biopsy: Tissue biopsy obtained from the septal wall of the right ventricle using an invasive catheter-based approach. Used in the diagnosis of restrictive cardiomyopathy.

endomyocardial fibrosis: Fibrosis of the ventricular endocardium and subendocardium that extends to the mitral and tricuspid valves and greatly decreases the functioning of the ventricular chambers.

endothelin: Endogenous hormonal vasoconstrictor released by the endothelium.

endothelium: Layer of epithelial cells that lines the heart, blood vessels, and other body cavities.

endovascular: Minimally invasive techniques using catheter-based treatments as opposed to full, open surgeries.

epiaortic imaging: Ultrasound imaging directly over the aorta that is used in coronary artery bypass graft surgery.

epicardium: The smooth outer layer of the heart that contains the network of coronary arteries and veins, the autonomic nerves, the lymphatic system, and fat tissue.

epigastric: Referring to the area over the pit of the stomach.

epinephrine: Also called *adrenaline*, a neurotransmitter of the sympathetic nervous system.

epistaxis: Bleeding from the nose.

ergonovine maleate: Arterial vasoconstrictor that can be given during cardiac catheterization to assist in the diagnosis of vasospastic angina.

erythropoietin: A hormone that regulates red blood cell production.

estrogen: Female sex hormone.

external counterpulsation: Nonpharmacological treatment option for debilitating angina in which a series of cuffs are wrapped around the patient's legs and compressed air is used to apply pressure in the cuffs in synchronization with the cardiac cycle, resulting in increased arterial pressure that increases retrograde aortic blood flow into the coronary arteries during diastole.

extrinsic pathway: Pathway in the clotting cascade activated by injured tissue.

extubation: Removal of an endotracheal tube.

Fabry's disease: A lipid storage disorder caused by the deficiency of an enzyme involved in the biodegradation of fats.

fibric acids: A group of lipid-lowering medications most noted for their ability to lower triglycerides. Also called *fibrates*.

fibrin: Fine protein filaments formed by the action of thrombin on fibrinogen that entangle red and white blood cells and platelets and form a clot.

fibrinogen: A protein that is converted to fibrin through the action of thrombin in the presence of calcium ions.

fibrinolytic: Fibrin-specific medication used to break down clots.

fibrous atheroma: Atheroma characterized by the accumulation of fibrous connective tissue within the intima.

fibrous cap: Fibrous tissue, mainly collagen, that covers the lipid core.

fibrous pericardium: External cover of the pericardium.

foam cell: Macrophage (scavenger cell) that is engorged with lipids.

free graft: Graft where both ends of the vessel are removed from their original locations and reattached elsewhere.

gamma radiation: Type of radiation used to treat in-stent restenosis. Has a longer dwell time than beta radiation and is used to treat more difficult lesions.

glomerular filtration rate (GFR): A calculation to determine how well the blood is filtered by the kidneys that is calculated using a mathematical formula that compares a person's age, sex, and race to serum creatinine, albumin, and blood urea nitrogen levels. Normal GFR in adults is 120 to 125 ml/min.

glycoprotein (GP) IIb/IIIa receptor: Receptor site on platelet surface where platelets and fibrinogen bind to form a fibrin mesh.

graft: A portion of a vessel taken from another part of the body that is used to bypass a coronary artery blockage during coronary artery bypass graft surgery.

great vessels: The aorta, the pulmonary artery, the inferior vena cava, and the superior vena cava.

gynecomastia: Enlarged mammary glands in a male.

glutaraldehyde: Chemical that is used as a cold sterilant and a tissue fixative.

heart block: Condition that arises due to a cardiac conduction system disturbance resulting in the lack of coordination of the atrial and ventricular activity of the heart.

heart failure: Disorder in which the heart is unable to pump enough oxygenated blood to meet the metabolic needs of the body.

heart rate: Number of times the heart beats in a minute.

hematoma: Mass of blood within the tissue caused by bleeding from a blood vessel.

hemochromatosis: Condition in which the body stores excess iron, causing organ damage.

hemodynamics: Forces influencing the circulation of blood throughout the body.

hemoglobin A_{1c} (HbA_{1c}): Glycosylated hemoglobin, a refelection of the average blood sugar level for 2 to 3 months prior to the test.

hemoptysis: Coughing or spitting up blood that is the result of bleeding from the respiratory system.

hemostasis: Cessation of bleeding.

hemothorax: Collection of blood in the pleural cavity.

hepatojugular reflux: Response of jugular venous pressure when firm pressure is applied to the midepigastric region. This response is exaggerated in right-sided heart failure.

hepatomegaly: Enlargement of the liver.

high-degree atrioventricular (AV) block: The true block of two or more atrial impulses (not in atrial flutter). Also called *advanced AV block.*

high-density lipoprotein cholesterol (HDL-C): A high-density lipoprotein that contains small amounts of cholesterol and triglycerides. Usually associated with a decreased risk of heart disease.

hirudin: Direct thrombin inhibitor.

HMG-CoA reductase: Key enzyme in the synthesis of cholesterol.

HMG-CoA reductase inhibitor: Also called a *statin,* the most widely used lipid-lowering medication in the treatment of cardiovascular disease. Inhibits HMG-CoA reductase during cholesterol synthesis.

holosystolic murmur: A murmur that can be heard throughout systole.

homocysteine: An amino acid that has toxic effects on the endothelium when elevated.

homologous: Similar in both structure and source.

high sensitivity C-reactive protein (hs-CRP): A marker of inflammation. Elevated levels increase cardiovascular risk.

hydrogenated oil: Oil that has hydrogen added to it to make it solid at room temperature.

hydrostatic pressure: Pushing pressure inside a vessel that forces fluids and nutrients across a membrane.

hypercholesterolemia: Elevated serum cholesterol.

hyperdynamic: Increased contractility and ejection fraction (when referring to the left ventricle).

hyperhomocysteinemia: Elevated serum homocysteine.

hyperkalemia: Elevated serum potassium.

hyperlipidemia: Condition characterized by elevated total cholesterol (hypercholesterolemia), elevated low-density lipoprotein cholesterol, or elevated triglycerides.

hyperplasia: Excessive proliferation of normal cells.

hypersensitive carotid sinus: A reflex caused by increased parasympathetic tone when pressure is applied to the carotid sinus, resulting in a slowing of the heart rate.

hypertension: Condition characterized by a systolic or diastolic blood pressure above the normal range.

hyperthyroidism: Excessive secretion from the thyroid gland, resulting in increased basal metabolic rate.

hypertriglyceridemia: Elevated serum triglycerides.

hypertrophic cardiomyopathy (HCM): Cardiomyopathy characterized by hypertrophy of the myocardium, resulting in a decrease in ventricular filling and a decrease in cardiac output.

hypertrophic obstructive cardiomyopathy (HOCM): Hypertrophic cardiomyopathy with obstruction.

hypertrophy: Increased size.

hypokalemia: Low serum potassium.

hypomagnesemia: Low serum magnesium.

hypoperfusion: Decreased perfusion.

hypotension: A systolic or diastolic blood pressure below the normal range.

hypoventilation: Decreased ventilation (amount of inhaled oxygen).

hypovolemia: Diminished blood volume.

hypoxemia: Low level of oxygen in the blood.

hypoxia: Decreased oxygenation of the tissues.

idiopathic: Having no known cause.

idiopathic hypertrophic subaortic stenosis (IHSS): Previous name for hypertrophic cardiomyopathy.

implantable cardioverter-defibrillator (ICD): Device inserted into the heart that provides a defibrillation shock and other therapies to treat rapid heart rates in a variety of patients.

incentive spirometry: Procedure designed to mimic natural sighing by encouraging the patient to take long, slow, deep breaths using a device that provides visual or other positive feedback upon inhalation of a predetermined volume and sustained inflation for a minimum of 3 seconds.

inferior myocardial infarction: Myocardial infarction involving the inferior or bottom wall of the left ventricle.

inferior posterior myocardial infarction: Myocardial infarction involving the inferior and posterior walls of the left ventricle.

inferior vena cava: Principal vein that receives blood from below the level of the diaphragm, including the abdomen, pelvis, and lower extremities. The inferior vena cava empties into the right atrium.

innervation: Distribution of the nervous system.

inotrope: Medication used to increase heart rate.

inotropic: Influencing the force of contractility.

interatrial septum: A mass of connective tissue that separates the right and left atria.

intercalated disks: Disks that form a tight junction, allowing cardiac muscle cells to function as integrated units.

intermittent claudication: Severe pain in calf muscles with walking that is relieved by rest.

internal mammary artery graft: Most common arterial graft used in coronary artery bypass grafting. Has better long-term patency rates than vein grafts.

internal iliac arteries: Arteries that arise from the abdominal aorta and supply blood to the lower trunk, including the reproductive organs and the legs.

International Normalized Ratio (INR): A value that relates prothrombin time to the intensity of actual coagulation. Developed to correct problems with standardization of prothrombin time.

internodal pathways: Conduction pathways in the right atrium that allow conduction between the sinoatrial and atrioventricular nodes.

interstitial pneumonitis: Lung disease characterized by marked interstitial fibrosis. Has an insidious onset with slow but severe progression and a poor prognosis, with most patients dying from the disease.

interventricular septum: A mass of connective tissue that separates the right and left ventricles.

intima: The innermost wall of all arteries, which consists of a thin layer of endothelium.

intra-aortic balloon pump (IABP): An invasive catheter-based assistive device that uses counter-pulsation therapy. The balloon, located in the descending aorta, inflates during diastole and deflates during systole. The timing of balloon deflation just before systole reduces cardiac afterload, and balloon inflation during diastole increases myocardial perfusion.

intracoronary stent: Metal scaffold-type structure that is inserted into a coronary artery to help prevent elastic recoil and keep open the lumen of the vessel.

intracoronary (intravascular) ultrasound: A tiny ultrasound device that is threaded into an artery inside a millimeter-thick catheter. Ultrasound waves measure changes in wall thickness, providing a detailed cross section of the coronary artery.

intracranial hemorrhage: Bleeding inside the skull that encloses the brain.

intrinsic pathway (coagulation cascade): Pathway in the clotting cascade that is activated by damage to the red blood cells or the platelets. The intrinsic pathway can be assessed by monitoring activated partial thromboplastin time.

intubation: Placement of an endotracheal tube.

ischemia: Temporary lack of oxygen to the myocardium.

isolated systolic hypertension: A systolic blood pressure greater than 160 mm Hg that is accompanied by a normal diastolic blood pressure.

isovolumetric contraction: Contraction of the ventricle, occurring during the first phase of cardiac systole, when all cardiac valves are closed and the volume of blood in the ventricle remains constant. Also know as *isovolumic contraction.*

jugular venous pressure: Pressure in the jugular vein that increases or decreases in response to fluid status.

kinin: Substance that produces vasodilative effects.

lateral myocardial infarction: Myocardial infarction involving the lateral wall of the left ventricle.

left anterior descending artery (LAD): Coronary artery arising from the left main coronary artery that is responsible for supplying oxygenated blood to the anterior wall of the left ventricle.

left anterior hemiblock: Block of the anterior fascicle of the left bundle.

left atrial appendage: Appendage off the left atrium that is frequently the source of clot formation in atrial fibrillation.

left atrium: Chamber of the heart that receives oxygenated blood from the pulmonary veins.

left bundle branch: Conduction pathway that divides into the left posterior bundle branch and the left anterior bundle branch and carries impulses to the posterior, inferior, and anterior walls of the left ventricle.

left circumflex (LCX) artery: Coronary artery arising from the left main coronary artery that is responsible for supplying blood to the lateral wall of the left ventricle.

left common carotid artery: Artery that branches directly off the thoracic aorta and is one of two common carotid arteries that supply blood to the neck and head.

left main coronary artery: Major coronary artery arising from the left side of the aorta that supplies oxygenated blood to a major portion of the myocardium via the left anterior descending and left circumflex coronary arteries.

left subclavian artery: Artery that arises from the end of the aortic arch and is one of two subclavian arteries that supply blood to the upper extremities.

left ventricle: A thick-walled, high-pressure pump that receives oxygenated blood from the left atrium and pumps blood into the aorta.

left ventricular reduction surgery: Surgery in which a part of the left ventricle is cut out and the remaining walls are sewn together to decrease the size of the ventricle. Also called the *Batista procedure*.

leukocyte: White blood cell.

low-density lipoprotein cholesterol (LDL-C): This lipoprotein is commonly referred to as the "bad" cholesterol because of its role in the development of atherosclerosis. LDL lipoprotein deposits cholesterol on the artery walls.

linear ablation: Catheter-based technique developed to achieve the same effect as with the surgical Maze procedure.

lipid: Fat or fat-like substance that is insoluble in water.

lipoprotein a: A lipoprotein similar to low-density lipoprotein cholesterol.

Löffler's endocarditis: Endomyocardial disease characterized by endomyocardial fibrosis, an unusually large number of eosinophils in the blood with infiltration of the heart.

lone atrial fibrillation: Atrial fibrillation in patients with normal cardiac and pulmonary function and with no known predisposing factors.

loop diuretic: An agent that works at the loop of Henle to increase sodium and water excretion.

low-molecular-weight heparin (LMWH): Heparin that is lower in molecular weight and smaller in size than unfractionated heparin.

lysis: Dissolution or decomposition (as in clot lysis).

Marfan's syndrome: Disorder characterized by abnormal length of the extremities, congenital anomalies of the heart, and other associated deformities.

mast cells: Connective tissue cell that plays a key role in the initiation of inflammation.

Maze procedure: Surgical procedure in which a series of incisions are made in the atria using radiofrequency or another form of energy in order to block reentrant pathways within the atrial tissue and to channel conduction in a more normal fashion.

media: The middle layer of an artery, which consists of smooth muscle and elastic connective tissue.

mediastinitis: Inflammation of the tissue of the mediastinum.

mediastinum: The space near the midline of the chest between the pleural sacs of the lungs that extends from the sternum to the spine. This space contains all the organs and tissues of the chest except the lungs.

medulla: The vasomotor center of the brain that interprets all information received from the baroreceptors.

metabolic syndrome: A grouping of lipid and nonlipid risk factors of metabolic origin.

metastatic cancer: Cancer that has spread beyond the site of origin.

metformin: Oral hypoglycemic agent that can potentially cause nephrotoxicity.

MET level: Metabolic equivalent unit used to estimate the amount of oxygen utilized by the body during physical activity.

mevalonic acid: A precursor to cholesterol.

microvascular: Related to very small vessels.

microvascular complications (of diabetes): Vision loss, nephropathy, neuropathy, and amputation.

minimally invasive coronary artery bypass (MIDCAB): Procedure performed on a beating heart without cardiopulmonary bypass and without the use of a median sternotomy.

mitral facies: Pinkish purple discoloration of the cheeks that is common in patients with severe mitral stenosis.

mitral regurgitation: Inadequate closure of the mitral valve that results in backward flow of blood from the left ventricle to the left atrium during ventricular systole. Also called *mitral insufficiency.*

mitral stenosis: Condition in which the mitral valve is unable to open normally, causing an obstruction of blood flow from the left atrium to the left ventricle during ventricular diastole.

mitral valve: Valve located between the left atrium and left ventricle.

mitral valve prolapse: Condition in which one or both of the mitral valve leaflets collapse into the atrium, sometimes allowing small amounts of blood to flow back into the atrium.

monophasic waveform defibrillators: Early generation defibrillators that use energy inefficiently and require higher amounts of energy for defibrillation or cardioversion shock.

monounsaturated fat: Beneficial fat in a heart-healthy diet that derives from a plant source and is liquid at room temperature. Examples include canola oil and olive oil.

murmur: An atypical sound produced by vibrations caused by turbulent blood flow. A cardiac murmur is typically associated with cardiac valve disease that creates turbulent blood flow through a valve that does not open or close properly.

muscarinic receptor: Type of parasympathetic, or cholinergic, receptor located in the heart and smooth muscle.

Musset's sign: Bobbing of the head with each heart beat.

myocardial imaging: Noninvasive studies utilized to assess various functions of the heart. These studies include cardiac echocardiography and radionuclide imaging and can be done individually or in combination with a stress test.

myocardial infarction (MI): Death or necrosis of myocardial tissue.

myocarditis: Inflammation of the myocardium.

myocardium: Thick middle layer of heart that contains cardiac muscle fibers.

myocyte: Contractile cardiac muscle cell.

myofibril: Small fiber that is the contractile element of muscle cells.

myoglobin: Sensitive cardiac biomarker that rises the earliest with myocardial damage.

natriuretic peptide: Hormones released by the heart during periods of volume overload. Increased production of these hormones causes vasodilatation, both pulmonary and systemic, as well as diuresis. The release of these hormones is beneficial during periods of acute decompensated heart failure. Types of natriuretic peptides include atrial natriuretic peptide and brain natriuretic peptide.

necrosis: Accidental death of a portion of tissue.

nephrotoxic: Toxic to the kidneys.

nesiritide (Natrecor): A synthetic form of brain natriuretic peptide that is administered intravenously for patients in acute heart failure.

neurogenic atrial fibrillation: Atrial fibrillation caused by either increased vagal tone or increased adrenergic tone.

neurocardiogenic syncope: A loss of consciousness caused by overstimulation of the vagus nerve and a reduction in normal sympathetic activity resulting in hypotension, bradycardia, and peripheral vasodilatation.

neurohormonal responses: Various hormonal and neurological responses that occur in heart failure to attempt to compensate for decreased cardiac output.

niacin: A B complex vitamin with additional dose-related pharmacological positive effects on lipid levels. Also called *nicotinic acid.*

nicotine: The physically addictive substance in tobacco.

nicotinic receptor: Type of parasympathetic, or cholinergic, receptor.

noncompliant ventricle: A ventricle that is unable to relax and fill properly during diastole.

nonvalvular atrial fibrillation: Atrial fibrillation in the absence of rheumatic heart disease that causes mitral stenosis or the absence of a prosthetic heart valve.

nonhomologous graft: Grafts from another species.

norepinephrine: A neurotransmitter of the sympathetic nervous system. Also called *nonadrenaline.*

nosocomial pneumonia: Pneumonia acquired in the hospital.

NPO: Nothing by mouth.

non-ST-segment elevation myocardial infarction (non-STEMI): A myocardial infarction made by the diagnosis of elevated cardiac biomarkers or enzymes. This type of myocardial infarction does not present with ST segment elevation on the 12 lead ECG.

omega-3 fatty acid: Nonessential fatty acid contained in oily fish, such as salmon, lake trout, tuna, and herring.

oncotic pressure: The pulling pressure inside a vessel that draws fluid and other substances into the vessel.

off-pump coronary artery bypass (OPCAB): Coronary artery bypass surgery done without the use of cardiopulmonary bypass machine. This approach to surgery does require an open chest procedure with a midline sternal incision.

opening snap: Abnormal sound made by the opening of a stenotic mitral or tricuspid valve.

opioid: Drug derived from an opium alkaloid. Examples include morphine.

orthopnea: Shortness of breath when in a supine position.

orthostatic: Concerning an upright position.

ostium: Small opening in the aorta that gives rise to the right and left coronary artery systems.

oxidation: The process of a substance combining with oxygen.

pacemaker electrode: Electrode located at the end of a pacemaker lead wire that delivers the stimulus to the heart muscle to make it contract.

pacemaker generator: Lithium battery and the electrical microcircuitry necessary to operate a pacemaker. Also referred to as the *battery* or *can.*

pacemaker lead: Wire that travels from the pacemaker generator to the wall of the heart that carries the message to contract from the generator to the heart. Houses the pacemaker electrode at the end of the wire.

pacemaker pacing: The ability of a pacemaker to send an impulse through a lead wire to an electrode and stimulate the heart to contract.

pacemaker sensing: The ability of a cardiac pacemaker to recognize native cardiac activity that is occurring in a cardiac chamber that has a cardiac pacing electrode.

paclitaxel: An antiproliferative or antineoplastic agent used on drug-eluting stents that is also used as a chemotherapeutic agent.

papillary muscles: Muscle projections from the inner surface of the ventricles that attach to the chordae tendineae of the atrioventricular valves.

parasympathetic nervous system: Branch of the autonomic nervous system that helps the body conserve and restore resources.

parasympatholytic: Medication that lyses the parasympathetic nervous system.

parietal pericardium: Inner lining of the fibrous pericardium.

paroxysmal: Coming on suddenly and terminating without intervention. Used to describe tachyarrhythmias.

paroxysmal atrial fibrillation: Atrial fibrillation that comes on spontaneously and terminates itself. Cannot last longer than 7 days and usually lasts less than 24 hours.

paroxysmal nocturnal dyspnea: Awakening from a sleep state with sudden and intense shortness of breath.

pathological Q wave: Abnormally deep or wide Q wave that indicates necrosis of myocardial tissue.

percutaneous alcohol septal ablation (PASA): Procedure performed in a cardiac catheterization lab during which a catheter is inserted into a septal perforator branch (provides blood flow to the septum). Ethyl alcohol is then injected to produce a controlled septal myocardial infarction.

pedicle graft: Graft in which one end of an artery is left in its original position. Examples include internal mammary artery graft.

percutaneous left atrial appendage transcatheter occlusion (PLAATO): Procedure using a right cardiac catheterization in which a transseptal puncture is made and an occlusive device is placed in the left atrial appendage to prevent embolization of a thrombus.

percutaneous transluminal coronary angioplasty (PTCA): Catheter-based procedure in which a balloon is inflated at the site of coronary stenosis to increase the vessel lumen diameter.

pericardial knock: High-frequency heart sound heard in patients with restrictive pericarditis.

pericardiocentesis: Perforation of the pericardium via a needle for the purpose of removal of fluid from the pericardial space.

pericarditis: Inflammation of the pericardium.

pericardium: Thin fibrous sac that surrounds the heart.

perioperative: Period around surgery, which can include the preoperative, intraoperative, and postoperative periods.

peripartum cardiomyopathy: Cardiomyopathy associated with the last trimester of pregnancy or the postpartum period.

peritoneum: Membrane that lines the abdominal cavity.

permanent atrial fibrillation: Atrial fibrillation that is accepted as permanent or lasts longer than 1 year.

permanent pacemaker: Artificial device implanted in the heart that consists of a battery or generator, a lead wire, and an electrode that delivers a stimulus to the heart to maintain a normal heart beat.

persistent atrial fibrillation: Atrial fibrillation that lasts longer than 7 days.

pheochromocytoma: A tumor that produces catecholamines.

phrenic nerve: A motor and sensory nerve that provides innervation to the diaphragm, pericardium, and pleura.

plasmin: Fibrinolytic enzyme derived from plasminogen.

plasminogen: A protein important in preventing fibrin clot formation. The precursor to plasmin.

pleura: Membrane surrounding the lungs.

pneumothorax: Collection of air in the pleural cavity from a perforation through the chest wall or visceral pleura covering the lung.

plain old balloon angioplasty (POBA): Percutaneous transluminal coronary angioplasty (PTCA) done without the placement of an intracoronary stent.

polyneuropathy: Noninflammatory disorder that affects the peripheral nerves.

portal hypertension: Increased pressure in the portal vein (vein providing blood flow to the liver) caused by obstruction of blood flow through the liver.

posterior descending artery (PDA): Coronary artery arising from the right coronary artery in most people that supplies oxygenated blood to the posterior wall of the left ventricle.

posterior myocardial infarction: Myocardial infarction involving the posterior wall of the left ventricle.

postpericardiotomy syndrome: Inflammation of the pericardium late after coronary artery bypass graft surgery due to autoimmune response.

precordial leads: Chest leads on a 12-lead electrocardiogram; V_1 to V_6 or V_{1R} to V_{6R}.

preload: Stretch on the ventricular myocardial fibers caused by the volume in the ventricle at the end of ventricular diastole.

pressure gradient: Difference in pressure from one side of a valve to the other side of that valve.

prevalence: The number of cases of a disease in a specified population at a given time.

primary aldosteronism: Excessive excretion of aldosterone by the adrenal cortex.

primary coronary intervention (PCI): A procedure that treats coronary artery disease without the use of surgery. Most commonly, balloon angioplasty with or without stent placement. Also referred to as *percutaneous coronary intervention*.

primary prevention: Reducing risk in people without known coronary heart disease to prevent the development of disease.

proarrhythmic: Causing arrhythmias.

procainamide: A potent class Ia antiarrhythmic agent used in the treatment of several cardiac arrhythmias, including atrial fibrillation and ventricular tachycardia. A derivative of the local anesthetic procaine.

progesterone: A steroid hormone responsible for changes in the endometrium during the second half of the menstrual cycle, development of the maternal placenta, and development of the mammary glands.

progestin: Hormone that prepares the endometrium to receive a fertilized egg. Also a synthetic drug that has a progesterone-like effect on the uterus.

prolonged QT syndrome: A condition characterized by a prolonged QT interval on an electrocardiogram that predisposes a person to torsades de pointes.

prostaglandin I2: A chemical substance that produces vasodilation and inhibits platelet aggregation.

prothrombin: A circulating chemical substance that interacts with calcium salts to produce thrombin.

prothrombin time (PT): Coagulation test used to monitor the safety and effectiveness of warfarin.

protease: A protein-splitting enzyme.

pruritus: Severe itching.

pseudo: False.

pulmonary artery catheter: Catheter that is threaded through right heart and placed in the pulmonary artery. Has various ports that allow for measurement of various heart pressures and cardiac output.

pulmonary edema: Fluid in the pulmonary alveoli that interferes with gas exchange.

pulmonary embolus: Embolus in the pulmonary artery system that increases pulmonary pressure that can cause pulmonary infarction.

pulmonary vascular resistance: Resistance in the pulmonary system that the right ventricle must pump against. Also called *right-sided afterload.*

pulmonary vein ectopic foci ablation: Catheter-based procedure in which areas around the four pulmonary veins are isolated with radiofrequency energy to create a block and eliminate the ability of the foci to enter the left atrium.

pulmonary veins: Veins that carry oxygenated blood from the lungs to the left atrium.

pulmonic valve: Valve between the right ventricle and the pulmonary artery.

pulse pressure: Difference between systolic and diastolic blood pressure.

pulsus alternans: An alternation between weak and strong heart beats, with weak beats occurring every other beat.

Purkinje fibers: Conduction fibers located in the ventricles. Serve as the third option as a pacemaker for the heart, with the ability to pace at a rate of 20 to 40 beats per minute.

P wave: Wave on an electrocardiogram that represents atrial depolarization.

QRS complex: Complex on an electrocardiogram that represents ventricular depolarization.

Q wave: First negative deflection of the QRS complex.

radial artery: Artery along the thumb side of the wrist, which is used as a conduit for coronary artery bypass graft surgery.

recombinant deoxyribonucleic acid (DNA): DNA that has been artificially manipulated to combine DNA from one organism with DNA of another organism.

reentrant mechanism: Mechanism of an arrhythmia whereby a wave of depolarization turns upon itself and reenters the tissue it just activated.

reflex tachycardia: Increased heart rate that occurs in response to a lowered blood pressure.

remodeling: A process of pathological growth whereby a ventricle hypertrophies and then dilates.

renin: An enzyme produced by the kidneys that, when released, stimulates activation of the renin-angiotensin-aldosterone system.

renin-angiotensin-aldosterone system (RAAS): Neurohormonal system that is activated in response to low cardiac output or low blood pressure. The end result is angiotensin II, a potent vasoconstrictor, and aldosterone, which causes sodium and water reabsorption.

renovascular disease: Disease of the renal arteries.

reperfusion: Restoration of oxygen to ischemic tissue.

repolarization: Return of a cardiac cell to a resting state.

resistant hypertension: Continued hypertension on full-dose therapy, including a diuretic.

restenosis: Renarrowing of the vessel lumen after a primary coronary intervention.

restrictive cardiomyopathy (RCM): Cardiomyopathy characterized by rigidity of the myocardial wall with decreased ability of the chamber walls to expand during cardiac filling.

retroperitoneal bleed: Bleeding into the space behind the peritoneum.

revascularization: Restoration, to the extent possible, of normal blood flow to the myocardium by surgical or percutaneous means.

rhabdomyolysis: Breakdown of muscle fibers with leakage of potentially toxic cellular contents into the systemic circulation.

rheumatic fever: A hemolytic streptococcal infection.

rheumatic heart disease: Damage to the heart that is the result of rheumatic fever. Normal cardiac complications include bacterial endocarditis with damage to the cardiac valves.

right atrium: Chamber of the heart that receives deoxygenated blood from the venous system.

right bundle branch: Conduction pathway that carries impulses to the right ventricle.

right coronary artery (RCA): Major coronary artery arising from the right side of the aorta that supplies blood to the inferior wall of the left ventricle.

right gastroepiploic artery: Artery that supplies blood to the greater curvature of the stomach and can be used as a conduit in coronary artery bypass graft surgery.

right ventricle: A thin-walled, low-pressure pump that receives deoxygenated blood from the right atrium and pumps blood into the pulmonary artery.

risk equivalent: Same risk as someone diagnosed with a disease, such as coronary heart disease.

risk factor: A characteristic found in a healthy person that is independently related to the future development of a disease, such as coronary heart disease.

Ross procedure: Procedure in which the pulmonic valve is placed in the aortic valve position and a tissue valve is placed in the pulmonic valve location.

rotational atherectomy: Use of high-speed rotating blades or burs to remove components of atherosclerotic plaque.

S_3: Third heart sound; heard immediately after the second heart sound; an indication of fluid overload.

S_4: Fourth heart sound; heard just before the first heart sound; an indication of a noncompliant ventricle.

saphenous vein graft: Vein graft taken from the greater saphenous vein of the leg. Most common vein graft material used in coronary artery bypass graft surgery.

sarcoidosis: Disease that causes inflammation or small lumps (also called *nodules* or *granulomas*) in the tissues.

sarcomere: A portion of the myofibril that contains protein units.

saturated fats: Fats that are usually solid at room temperature and typically come from animals.

secondary prevention: Method of reducing risk in people with known coronary heart disease to prevent future events.

second-degree heart block: A cardiac arrhythmia that results when atrial impulses are not conducted normally through the AV node to the ventricle. Also referred to as *second-degree AV block.*

selective serotonin reuptake inhibitors (SSRIs): Class of antidepressant medications commonly used to treat depression in cardiac patients.

semilunar valves: The valves located between the ventricles and great vessels.

senile degenerative calcification: Progressive calcification of the valve leaflets.

serine: An amino acid found in many proteins.

sheath: Small, flexible catheter in a vascular access site. Guidewires and diagnostic and interventional devices are thread through the sheath during invasive and interventional procedures.

shoulder: Edge of a fibrous cap. A particularly vulnerable area that is frequently the location of ruptured plaque.

sick sinus syndrome (SSS): Rhythm marked by sinus node dysfunction (bradycardia or sinus arrest) alternating with periods of rapid atrial arrhythmias. Also called *tachy-brady syndrome.*

single chamber pacemaker: A pacemaker that has an electrode for pacing in one chamber of the heart; traditionally, a ventricular pacemaker.

sinoatrial (SA) node: Natural pacemaker of the heart, which is located in the right atrium near the junction of the superior vena cava.

sirolimus: An immunosuppressive agent used on drug-eluting stents that is also used to prevent organ rejection during kidney transplantation.

ST-segment elevation myocardial infarction (STEMI): A myocardial infarction that produces ST-segment elevation on an electrocardiogram.

stable angina pectoris: Angina with a stable pattern that is brought on by exertion and relieved by rest or sublingual nitroglycerin.

stanol: A sterol that has been saturated.

statins (HMG-CoA reductase inhibitors): Another name for HMG-Co A reductase inhibitors; all drugs in this class end with the letters "statin."

stenosis: Narrowing of a passage.

sternotomy: The act of cutting through the sternum.

sterol: Compound found in the cell membrane of plants and animals. Plant sterols are used in the treatment of high cholesterol.

sternum: Flat bone in the middle of the thorax, or chest.

stress testing: Noninvasive assessment tool for coronary artery diseases that uses exercise or chemicals to stress the heart. May be done with or without myocardial imaging.

stroke volume: Volume of blood ejected by the left ventricle with each beat.

subendocardium: Middle myocardium.

substernal: Below the sternum.

superior vena cava: A principal vein that receives venous blood returning from the head, neck, upper extremities, and thorax and empties into the right atrium.

supraventricular arrhythmia: Arrhythmia originating above the ventricles. Called *supraventricular tachycardia* when the heart rate is more than 100 beats per minute.

sympathetic nervous system (SNS): Branch of the autonomic nervous system that allows the body to function under stress.

sympathomimetic: A medication that mimics the sympathetic nervous system.

syncope: Transient lack of consciousness due to inadequate blood flow to the brain.

systemic lupus erythematosus (SLE): An autoimmune disease characterized by fever, skin rash, and arthritis, often with small hemorrhages in the skin and mucous membranes and inflammation of the pericardium.

systole: Contraction of the heart muscle that results in ejection of blood from the chamber.

systolic dysfunction: Left ventricular dysfunction involving a problem with ejection.

systolic ejection murmur: A murmur that occurs as blood is ejected through a stenotic aortic or pulmonic valve during early systole.

tachyarrhythmia: Cardiac arrhythmias with a ventricular rate more than 100 beats per minute.

tachycardia: Heart rate greater than 100 beats per minute.

tachypnea: Increased respiratory rate.

tacrolimus: A potent immunosuppressant medication used to prevent and treat organ rejection.

thiazide diuretic: Diuretic that inhibits sodium and water reabsorption. Works in the ascending loop of Henle and the early distal tubule.

thiocyanate: Cyanide ions released into the system are converted to thiocyanate in the liver. Thiocyanate level should be monitored during infusions of nitroprusside because nitroprusside releases cyanide ions into the system.

thoracic aorta: Portion of aorta located in the thoracic cavity that contains the ascending aorta, the aortic arch, and the descending thoracic aorta.

thoracotomy: Surgical incision of the chest wall.

thrombin: A enzyme formed from prothrombin that converts fibrinogen to fibrin.

thrombocytopenia: Abnormal decrease in platelet number.

thromboembolus: Embolus that has broken away from a thrombus.

thrombolytic: Nonfibrin medication used to break down clots.

thrombophlebitis: Inflammation of a vein in conjunction with the formation of a thrombus.

thrombosis: Formation or existence of a blood clot.

thrombotic stroke: Ischemic stroke caused by a thrombus or an embolus from a thrombus.

thromboxane A2: Substance released with vascular injury that is a potent vasoconstrictor and platelet agonist.

thrombus: A blood clot that causes obstruction.

T lymphocyte: Lymphocyte cell that differentiates in the thymus and is responsible for cellular immunity.

torsades de pointes: A special ventricular tachycardia associated with a prolonged QT interval.

Traube's sign: Booming systolic and diastolic sounds heard over the femoral artery. Also called *pistol-shot sounds*.

transesophageal echocardiography (TEE): Placement of an ultrasound probe into the esophagus to view the aorta and cardiac structures. Eliminates the need to image through the chest wall.

transluminal extraction atherectomy: Procedure used for the extraction of visible thrombi within the coronary artery.

transmural: Full thickness of myocardium.

transmyocardial laser revascularization (TMLR): Form of revascularization whereby a series of transmural endomyocardial channels are created with lasers to improve myocardial blood supply.

transverse (T) tubules: Extensions of cell membranes in the cardiac muscle that allows calcium to enter the cells.

tricuspid valve: Valve located between the right atrium and right ventricle.

trifascicular block: A block of the normal conduction system involving simultaneous blockage of the right bundle branch, one of the two fascicles of the left bundle branch, and AV block.

triglyceride: Chemical compound of glycerol and three fatty acids that is a component of most animal and vegetable fats.

troponin I: Biomarker found only in cardiac muscle. The most sensitive indicator of myocardial damage.

T wave: Wave on an electrocardiogram that represents ventricular repolarization.

ulnar artery: Artery alongside the wrist, opposite the thumb.

unfractionated heparin (UFH): A commercially available anticoagulant produced from porcine or bovine tissue. Heparin prevents the extension of thrombus but does not lyse clots.

unstable angina pectoris: Angina at rest or with minimal exertion or an increased need for nitroglycerin.

urticaria: A vascular skin that produces papules or wheals and causes severe itching.

vagal: Response related to the stimulation of the parasympathetic nervous system, specifically the vagus nerve. A vagal response is characterized by a low heart rate, low blood pressure, light-headedness, and nausea.

Valsalva's maneuver: A maneuver that increases intrathoracic pressure, elicits the parasympathetic response, and decreases venous return to the heart.

valvuloplasty: Procedure in which a balloon is inflated in the cardiac valve orifice to fracture calcium deposits in the leaflets and stretch the annulus to return the valve to normal functioning.

vasoconstriction: Constriction of vessels.

vasodilation: Dilation of vessels.

vasopressor: Medication used to increase blood pressure and afterload.

vasospastic angina: Angina caused by spasm of a coronary artery. Also called *Prizmetal's angina.*

vasovagal response: Response of the parasympathetic nervous system that produces hypotension, bradycardia, diaphoresis, nausea, and vomiting.

Vaughan Williams classification system: Classification system for antiarrhythmic pharmacology that contains four classes.

venous oxygen saturation: The percent of oxygen saturation of venous blood after the tissues have extracted oxygen from the arterial blood. Normal range is 60% to 80%.

ventricular aneurysm: Localized dilatation of the left ventricle at the site of infarction.

ventricular arrhythmia: Arrhythmia originating from the ventricles. Called *ventricular tachycardia* when the heart rate is more than 100 beats per minute.

ventricular ectopy: Abnormal heart beats that originate from a ventricle rather than from the sinus node.

ventricular fibrillation: A quivering of the ventricles that results in a pulseless rhythm and cardiac arrest and is treated with immediate defibrillation.

ventricular outflow tract: The path the blood in a ventricle must follow when ejected from the ventricle.

ventricular pacemaker: Pacemaker that has a lead in the right ventricle and paces only the right ventricle.

ventricular septal myectomy: Surgical removal of a portion of a hypertrophied septum that is contributing to outflow obstruction.

viable: Capable of living.

visceral pericardium: Inner lining of the pericardium and outer lining of the heart and great vessels. Also called the *epicardium.*

vulnerable plaque: Atherosclerotic plaque that is prone to ulceration and rupture.

VVI pacemaker: Single chamber pacemaker with an electrode in the right ventricle that paces the right ventricle, senses normal activity in the left ventricle, and inhibits the pacemaker when the electrode senses normal cardiac activity.

wall motion abnormality: Abnormal movement of a wall of the left ventricle. Can be seen on echocardiogram.

warfarin: An oral anticoagulant agent that works indirectly through the liver by altering vitamin K–dependent clotting factors.

water-hammer pulse: A rapid rise and collapse of the pulse that can be felt upon palpation. Also called *Corrigan's pulse.*

Wolff-Parkinson-White (WPW) syndrome: Syndrome in which one or more accessory pathways connect the atria to the ventricles. Conduction over the accessory pathways causes preexcitation of the ventricles, predisposing the patient to tachyarrhythmias.

BIBLIOGRAPHY

Adair Albert, N.M. (2003). Cardiac resynchronization therapy through biventricular pacing in patients with heart failure and ventricular dyssynchrony. *Critical Care Nurse, 23*(Suppl. 3), S2.

Adair, O.V., & Fuenzalida, C.E. (2001). Beta-adrenergic receptor blockers. In O.V. Adair (Ed.,) *Cardiology secrets* (2nd ed., pp. 257-263). Philadelphia: Hanley & Belfus, Inc.

Antman, E.M., Anbe, D.T., Armstrong, P.W., Bates, E.R., Green, L.A., Hand, M., et al. (2004). ACC/AHA guidelines for the management of patients with ST-elevation myocardial infarction – Executive summary: A report of the Task Force on Practice Guidelines (American College of Cardiology/American Heart Association Committee to Revise the 1999 Guidelines for the Management of Patients with Acute Myocardial Infarction). *Journal of the American College of Cardiology, 44*(3), 671-719.

Aouizerat, B. (2005). Atherosclerosis. In S.L. Woods, E.S. Froelicher, S.A. Motzer, & E.J. Bridges (Eds.), *Cardiac nursing* (5th ed., pp. 139-149). Philadelphia: Lippincott Williams & Wilkins.

Apstein, C. (2004). *Atlas of heart diseases: Heart failure.* Current Medicine, Inc. Retrieved July 5, 2005, from http://www.imagesMD.com

Bakken Library and Museum. (2004). Pacemakers: A brief history. Retrieved December 1, 2004, from http://www.thebakken.org/artifacts/pacemakers.htm

Balentine, J., & Eisenhart, A. (2005). Aortic stenosis. Retrieved March 3, 2005, from http://www.emedicine.com/emerg/topic40.htm

Bene, S., & Vaughan, A. (2005). Acute coronary syndromes. In S.L. Woods, E.S. Froelicher, S.A. Motzer, & E.J. Bridges (Eds.), *Cardiac nursing* (5th ed., pp. 550-584). Philadelphia: Lippincott Williams & Wilkins.

Bernstein, A.D., Daubert, J.C., Fletcher, R.D., Hayes, D.L., Luderitz, B., Reynolds, D.W., et al. (2002). The revised NASPE/BPEG generic code for antibradycardia, adaptive-rate, and multisite pacing [Electronic version]. *Pacing and Clinical Electrophysiology, 25*(2), 260-264.

Blancher, S. (2005). Cardiac electrophysiology procedures. In S.L. Woods, E.S. Froelicher, S.A. Motzer, & E.J. Bridges (Eds.) *Cardiac nursing* (5th ed., pp. 425-438). Philadelphia: Lippincott Williams & Wilkins.

Bond, E.F. (2005). Cardiac anatomy and physiology. In S.L. Woods, E.S. Froelicher, S.A. Motzer, & E.J. Bridges (Eds.), *Cardiac nursing* (5th ed., pp. 3-48). Philadelphia: Lippincott Williams & Wilkins.

Bonow, R.O., Carabello, B., de Leon, A.C., Edmunds, L.H., Jr., Fedderly, B.J., Freed, M.D., et al. (1998). ACC/AHA guidelines for the management of patients with valvular heart disease. Executive summary. A report of the American College of Cardiology/American Heart Association Task Force on Practice Guidelines (Committee on Management of Patients with Valvular Heart Disease). *Journal of the American College of Cardiology, 32*, 1486-1588.

Botz, G., & Mark, J. (1997). *Atlas of anesthesia: Scientific principles of anesthesia.* Current Medicine, Inc. Retrieved July 5, 2005, from http://www.imagesMD.com

Bozkurt, B., & Mann, D.L. (2000). Dilated cardiomyopathy. In J.T. Willerson & J.N. Cohn, (Eds.), *Cardiovascular medicine* (2nd ed., pp. 1034-1053). New York: Churchill Livingstone.

Braunwald, E., Antman, E.M., Beasley, J.W., Califf, R.M., Cheitlin, M.D., Hochman, J.S., et al. (2002). ACC/AHA 2002 guideline update for the management of patients with unstable angina and non-ST-segment elevation myocardial infarction: A report of the American College of Cardiology/American Heart Association Task Force on Practice Guidelines (Committee on the Management of Patients with Unstable Angina). Retrieved November 12, 2004, from http://www.acc.org/clinical/guidelines/unstable/unstable.pdf

Bridges, C.R., Horvath, K.A., Nugent, W.C., Shahian, D.M., Haan, C.K., Shemin, R.J., et al. (2004). The Society of Thoracic Surgeons practice guideline series: Transmyocardial laser revascularization [Electronic version]. *Annals of Thoracic Surgery, 77*, 1494-1502.

Bridges, E.J. (2005a). Regulation of cardiac output and blood pressure. In S.L. Woods, E.S. Froelicher, S.A. Motzer, & E.J. Bridges (Eds.), *Cardiac nursing* (5th ed., pp. 81-108). Philadelphia: Lippincott Williams & Wilkins.

Bridges, E.J. (2005b). Systemic circulation. In S.L. Woods, E.S. Froelicher, S.A. Motzer, & E.J. Bridges (Eds.), *Cardiac nursing* (5th ed., pp. 49-70). Philadelphia: Lippincott Williams & Wilkins.

Butany, J., & Gotlieb, A. (2000). *Atlas of cardiovascular pathology for the clinician.* Current Medicine, Inc. Retrieved July 5, 2005, from http://www.imagesMD.com

Butany J., & Schoen, F. (1998). *Atlas of heart diseases: Cardiomyopathies, myocarditis, and pericardial disease.* Current Medicine, Inc. Retrieved July 5, 2005, from http://www.imagesMD.com

Calagan, J.L., Schachter, D.T., Kruger, M., Cameron, R.W., & Loghin, C. (2001). Diuretics and nitrates. In O.V. Adair (Ed.), *Cardiology secrets* (2nd ed., pp. 270-274). Philadelphia: Hanley & Belfus, Inc.

Calclasure, T.F., Kozlowski, C.M., Highfill, W.T., & Loghin, C. (2001). Angiotensin-converting enzyme inhibitors and other vasodilators. In O.V. Adair (Ed.), *Cardiology secrets* (2nd ed., pp. 275-279). Philadelphia: Hanley & Belfus, Inc.

Califf, R. (2001). *Atlas of heart diseases: Acute myocardial infarction and other acute ischemic syndromes.* Current Medicine, Inc. Retrieved July 5, 2005, from http://www.imagesMD.com

Carabello, B.A., & Crawford, M.H. (2003). Aortic stenosis. In M.H. Crawford (Ed.), *Current diagnosis and treatment in cardiology* (2nd ed., pp. 108-120). New York: McGraw-Hill.

Carroll, J.D., & Crawford, M.H. (2003). Restrictive cardiomyopathy. In M.H. Crawford (Ed.), *Current diagnosis and treatment in cardiology* (2nd ed., pp. 1188-1195). New York: McGraw-Hill.

Centers for Disease Control and Prevention. (2005). *Body mass index for adults.* Retrieved October 19, 2005, from http://www.cdc.gov/nccdphp/dnpa/bmi/bmi-adult-formula.htm

Chebaclo, M., & Loghin, C. (2001). Digoxin and other positive inotropic drugs. In O.V. Adair (Ed.), *Cardiology secrets* (2nd ed., pp. 280-284). Philadelphia: Hanley & Belfus, Inc.

Clark, A.D. (2004). Atrial fibrillation. Retrieved December 31, 2004, from http://www.emedicine.com/emerg/topic46.htm

Clinical Pharmacology Database. (2004). *Gold Standard Multimedia.* Retrieved September 13, 2005, from http://www.gsm.com

Cockrell, J., & Siu, A. (1996). *Atlas of heart diseases: Arrhythmias: Electrophysiologic principles.* Current Medicine, Inc. Retrieved July 5, 2005, from http://www.imagesMD.com

Crawford, M.H. (2003). Mitral regurgitation. In M.H. Crawford (Ed.), *Current diagnosis and treatment in cardiology* (2nd ed., pp. 142-150). New York: McGraw-Hill.

Cray, J.V., Kothare, V.S., & Weinstock, D. (Eds.). (1999). *Auscultation skills: Breath & heart sounds.* Springhouse, PA: Springhouse Corp.

Cummins, R.O. (Ed.). (2003). *ACLS provider manual.* Dallas: American Heart Association.

Cunningham, S. (2005). Hypertension. In S.L. Woods, E.S. Froelicher, S.A. Motzer, & E.J. Bridges (Eds.), *Cardiac nursing* (5th ed., pp. 856-896). Philadelphia: Lippincott Williams & Wilkins.

Darovic, G.O. (2002). *Hemodynamic monitoring: Invasive and noninvasive clinical application* (3rd ed.). Philadelphia: Saunders.

Deedy, M.G. (2002). Coronary artery disease. Retrieved September 26, 2004, from http://www.clevelandclinicmeded.com/diseasemanagement/cardiology/cad/cad.htm

Deelstra, M.H. (2005). Interventional cardiology techniques. In S.L. Woods, E.S. Froelicher, S.A. Motzer, & E.J. Bridges (Eds.), *Cardiac nursing* (5th ed., pp. 585-600). Philadelphia: Lippincott Williams & Wilkins.

Dennison, R.D. (2000). *Pass CCRN* (2nd ed.). St. Louis: Mosby.

Dorman, B. (1999). *Atlas of anesthesia: Cardiothoracic anesthesia.* Current Medicine, Inc. Retrieved July 5, 2005, from http://www.imagesMD.com

Dresing, T.J., & Schweikert, R.A. (2002). Atrial fibrillation. Retrieved November 18, 2004, from http://www.clevelandclinicmeded.com/diseasemanagement/cardiology/atrialfibrillation/atrialfibrillation.htm

Eagle, K.A., Guyton, R.A., Davidoff, R., Edwards, F.H., Ewy, G.A., Gardner, T.J., et al. (2004). ACC/AHA 2004 guideline update for coronary artery bypass graft surgery: A report to the American College of Cardiology/American Heart Association Task Force on Practice Guidelines (Committee to Update the 1999 Guidelines for Coronary Artery Bypass Graft Surgery). Retrieved September 13, 2005, from http://www.acc.org/clinical/guidelines/cabg/index.pdf

Ellenbogen, K.A., & Wood, M.A. (Eds.). (2002). *Cardiac pacing and ICDs* (3rd ed.). Malden, MA: Blackwell Science.

Falk, E., & Shah, P. (2001). *Atlas of heart diseases: Acute myocardial infarction and other acute ischemic syndromes.* Current Medicine, Inc. Retrieved July 5, 2005, from http://www.imagesMD.com

Fair, J.M., & Berra, K.A. (2005). Lipid management and coronary artery disease. In S.L. Woods, E.S. Froelicher, S.A. Motzer, & E.J. Bridges (Eds.), *Cardiac nursing* (5th ed., pp. 897-915). Philadelphia: Lippincott Williams & Wilkins.

Faxon, D. (1995). *Atlas of heart diseases: Chronic ischemic heart disease.* Current Medicine, Inc. Retrieved July 5, 2005, from http://www.imagesMD.com

Ferraris, V.A., Ferraris, S.P., Moliterno, D.J., Camp, P., Walenga, J.M., Messmore, H.L., et al. (2003). The Society of Thoracic Surgeons practice guideline series: Aspirin and other antiplatelet agents during operative coronary revascularization. Retrieved on December 22, 2004, from http://www.sts.org

Fiore, M.C., Bailey, W.C., Cohen, S.J., Dorfman, S.F., Goldstein, M.G., Gritz, E.R., et al. (2000). *Treating tobacco use and dependence.* Clinical practice guideline. Rockville, MD: U.S. Department of Health and Human Services.

Fischbach, F. (2004). *A manual of laboratory and diagnostic tests* (7th ed.). Philadelphia: Lippincott Williams & Wilkins.

Folkeringa, R.J., Tieleman, R.G., & Crijns, H.J. (2004). Non-antiarrhythmic drugs to prevent atrial fibrillation. *Heart Rhythm, 1*(4), 516-518.

Fonseca, V., Bakris, G.L., Benjamin, E.M., Blonde, L., Boucher, J., Brancati, F.L., et al. (2005). Summary of revisions for the 2005 clinical practice recommendations [Electronic version]. *Diabetes Care, 28*(1), S3.

Fuster, V., Alexander, R.W., O'Rourke, R.A., Roberts, R., King, S.B. III, & Wellens, H.J.J. (Eds.). (2001). *Hurst's the heart: Manual of cardiology* (Vols. 1-2) (10th ed.). New York: McGraw-Hill.

Fuster, V., Alexander, R.W., O'Rourke, R.A., Roberts, R., King, S.B. III, Nash, I.S., et al. (Eds.). (2004). *Hurst's the heart: Manual of cardiology* (Vols. 1-2) (11th ed.). New York: McGraw-Hill.

Fuster, V., Ryden, L.E., Asinger, R.W., Cannom, D.S., Crijns, H.J., Frye, R.L., et al. (2001). ACC/AHA/ESC guidelines for the management of patients with atrial fibrillation. Executive summary: A report of the American College of Cardiology/American Heart Association Task Force on Practice Guidelines and the European Society of Cardiology Committee for Practice Guidelines and Policy Conferences (Committee to Develop Guidelines for the Management of Patients with Atrial Fibrillation). *Journal of the American College of Cardiology, 38*(4), 1231-1266.

Ganz, L. (2004). Implantable cardioverter-defibrillators. Retrieved December 16, 2004, from http://www.emedicine.com/med/topic3386.htm

Gardner, P., & Altman, G. (2005). Pathophysiology of acute coronary syndrome. In S.L. Woods, E.S. Froelicher, S.A. Motzer, & E.J. Bridges (Eds.), *Cardiac nursing* (5th ed., pp. 541-549). Philadelphia: Lippincott Williams & Wilkins.

Gibbons, R.J., Abrams, J., Chatterjee, K., Daley, J., Deedwania, P.C., Douglas, J.S., et al. (2002). ACC/AHA 2002 guidelines update for the management of patients with chronic stable angina: A report of the American College of Cardiology/American Heart Association Task Force on Practice Guidelines (Committee to Update the 1999 Guidelines for the Management of Patients with Chronic Stable Angina). Available at www.acc.org/clinical/guidelines/stable/stable.pdf

Gimbel, J.R. (2004). When should patients be allowed to drive after ICD implantation? [Electronic version]. *Cleveland Clinic Journal of Medicine, 71*(2), 125-128. Retrieved February 2, 2005, from http://www.clevelandclinicmeded.com/ccjm/feb04/gimbel.htm

GlaxoSmithKline. (2005). *Argatroban Clinical Monograph.* Retrieved August 29, 2005, from http://www.argatroban.com/anticoagulant_clinic_01.htm

Goswami, G., & Reddy, S. (2003). Cardiomyopathy, restrictive. Retrieved December 19, 2004, from http://www.emedicine.com/med/topic291.htm

Gregoratos, G., Abrams, J., Epstein, A.E., Freedman, R.A., Hayes, D.L., Hlatky, M.A., et al. (2002). ACC/AHA/NASPE 2002 guideline update for implantation of cardiac pacemakers and antiarrhythmia devices: Summary article. A report of the American College of Cardiology/American Heart Association Task Force on Practice Guidelines (ACC/AHA/NASPE Committee to Update the 1998 Pacemaker Guidelines). Available from http://www.acc.org/clinical/guidelines/pacemaker/incorporated/index.htm

Greinacher, A., Lubenow, N., & Eichler, P. (2003). Anaphylactic and anaphylactoid reaction associated with lepirudin in patients with heparin induced thrombocytopenia. *Circulation, 108*(17), 2062-2065.

Griffin, B., & Hayek, E. (2004). *Mitral valve disease.* Retrieved September 9, 2004, from http://www.clevelandclinicmeded.com/disease management/cardiology/mitralvalve/mitral valve.htm

Grundy, S.M., Cleeman, J.I., Merz, C.N., Brewer, H.B., Jr., Clark, L.T., Hunninghake, D.B., et al. (2004). Implications of recent clinical trials for the National Cholesterol Education Program Adult Treatment Panel III Guidelines. *Circulation, 110*(2), 227-239.

Guidant Corporation. (n.d.). Living with your defibrillator (ICD). Retrieved February 3, 2005 from http://www.guidant.com/webapp/emarketing/compass/comp.jsp?lev1=living&lev2=icd

Havranek, E.P., & Adair, A.V. (2001). Aortic stenosis and regurgitation. In O.V. Adair (Ed.), *Cardiology secrets* (2nd ed., pp. 237-240). Philadelphia: Hanley & Belfus, Inc

Heart Failure Society of America. (2004). Implications of recent trials for heart failure performance measures. *Journal of Cardiac Failure, 10*(1), 4-5.

Hilkert, R.J., & Yoo, H. (2002). Aortic regurgitation. Retrieved May 5, 2003, from http://www.emedicine.com/med/topic156.htm

Hobbs, R., & Boyle, A. (2004). Heart failure. Retrieved September 25, 2004, from http://www.clevelandclinicmeded.com/disease management/cardiology/heartfailure/heart failure.htm

Hunt, S.A., Abraham, W.T., Chin, M.H., Feldman, A.M., Francis, G.S., Ganiats, T.G., et al. (2005). ACC/AHA 2005 guideline update for the diagnosis and management of chronic heart failure in the adult: A report of the American College of Cardiology/American Heart Association Task Force on Practice Guidelines (Writing Committee to Update the 2001 Guidelines for the Evaluation and Management of Heart Failure). [Electronic version]. Retrieved September 15, 2005, from http://www.acc.org/clinical/guidelines/failure//index.pdf

Jacobson, C. (2005). Arrhythmias and conduction disturbances. In S.L. Woods, E.S. Froelicher, S.A. Motzer, & E.J. Bridges (Eds.), *Cardiac nursing* (5th ed., pp. 361-424). Philadelphia: Lippincott Williams & Wilkins.

Jacobson, C., & Gerity, D. (2005). Pacemakers and implantable defibrillators. In S.L. Woods, E.S. Froelicher, S.A. Motzer, & E.J. Bridges (Eds.), *Cardiac nursing* (5th ed., pp. 709-755). Philadelphia: Lippincott Williams & Wilkins.

Jessup, M. (2004). Resynchronization therapy is an important advance in the management of congestive heart failure: View of an antagonist [Electronic version]. *Journal of Cardiovascular Electrophysiology, 14*(9 Suppl.), S30-S34.

Kavinsky, C.J., & Parrillo, J.E. (2000). Severe heart failure in cardiomyopathy: Pathogenesis and treatment. In A. Grenvik, S.M. Ayers, P.R. Holbrook, & W.C. Shoemaker (Eds.), *Textbook of critical care* (4th ed., pp. 1105-1116). Philadelphia: W.B. Saunders.

Kossick, M.A. (2000). *EKG interpretation: Simple – thorough – practical* (2nd ed.). Park Ridge, IL: American Association of Nurse Anesthetists.

Kumar, V., Abbas, A.K., & Fausto, N. (2005). *Robbins & Cotran pathologic basis of disease* (7th ed.). Philadelphia: W.B. Saunders.

Laurent, D. (2005). Heart failure. In S.L. Woods, E.S. Froelicher, S.A. Motzer, & E.J. Bridges (Eds.), *Cardiac nursing* (5th ed., pp. 601-627). Philadelphia: Lippincott Williams & Wilkins.

LeDoux, D. (2005). Acquired valve disease. In S.L. Woods, E.S. Froelicher, S.A. Motzer, & E.J. Bridges (Eds.), *Cardiac nursing* (5th ed., pp. 756-775). Philadelphia: Lippincott Williams & Wilkins.

LeDoux, D., & Luikart, H. (2005). Cardiac surgery. In S.L.Woods, E.S. Froelicher, S.A. Motzer, & E.J. Bridges (Eds.), *Cardiac nursing* (5th ed., pp. 628-658). Philadelphia: Lippincott Williams & Wilkins.

Levine, B.S. (2002). *Cardiac vascular nursing review and resource manual.* Washington D.C.: American Nurses Credentialing Center.

Lewis, S.M., Heitkemper, M.M., & Dirksen, S.R. (2004). *Medical-surgical nursing: Assessment and management of clinical problems* (6th ed.). St. Louis: Mosby.

Loghin, C. (2001). Dilated cardiomyopathy. In O.V. Adair (Ed.), *Cardiology secrets* (2nd ed., pp. 156-160). Philadelphia: Hanley & Belfus, Inc.

Lorenz, R.A., Lorenz, R.M., & Codd, J.E. (2005). Perioperative blood glucose control during adult coronary artery bypass surgery [Electronic version]. *AORN Journal, 81*(1), 126-144.

Lowy, H., & Freedman, R.A. (2004). Pacemaker therapy. Retrieved February 1, 2005, from http://www.medscape.com.

Maden, S.K., & Froelicher, E.S. (2005). Psychosocial risk factors: Assessment and management interventions. In S.L. Woods, E.S. Froelicher, S.A. Motzer, & E.J. Bridges (Eds.), *Cardiac nursing* (5th ed., pp. 825-837). Philadelphia: Lippincott Williams & Wilkins.

Maron, B.J., McKenna, W.J., Danielson, G.K., Kappenberger, L.J., Kuhn, H.J., Seidman, C.E., et al. (2003). ACC/ESC clinical expert consensus document on hypertrophic cardiomyopathy: A report of the American College of Cardiology Task Force on Clinical Expert Consensus Documents and the European Society of Cardiology Committee for Practice Guidelines (Committee to Develop an Expert Consensus Document on Hypertrophic Cardiomyopathy). *Journal of the American College of Cardiology, 42*(9), 1687-1713.

Martin, K., & Froelicher, E.S. (2005). Smoking cessation: A systematic approach to managing patients with heart disease. In S.L. Woods, E.S. Froelicher, S.A. Motzer, & E.J. Bridges (Eds.), *Cardiac nursing* (5th ed., pp. 838-855). Philadelphia: Lippincott Williams & Wilkins.

Massie, B.M., & Amiodon, T.M. (2004). Heart. In L.M. Tierney, Jr., S.J. McPhee, & M.A. Papadakis (Eds.), *Current medical diagnosis & treatment* (43rd ed., pp. 315-400). New York: McGraw-Hill.

MedlinePlus. (2005a). National Library of Medicine and National Institutes of Health. *Sirolimus.* Micromedex, Inc. Available at http://www.nlm.nih.gov/medlineplus /druginfo/uspdi/500028.h t m l

MedlinePlus. (2005b). National Library of Medicine and National Institutes of Health. *Paclitaxel.* Micromedex, Inc. Available at http://www.nlm.nih.gov/medlineplus /druginfo/uspdi/202682.html

Medtronic, Inc. (n.d.). History of pacemakers: Technology development through the decades. Retrieved January 5, 2005, from http://www .medtronic.com/brady/patient/pacemaker_ history.html

Mendoza, R., & Loghin, C. (2001). Calcium channel antagonists. In O.V. Adair (Ed.), *Cardiology secrets* (2nd ed., pp. 285-288). Philadelphia: Hanley & Belfus, Inc.

Moore, K.L., & Dalley, A.F. (1999). *Clinically oriented anatomy* (4th ed.). Philadelphia: Lippincott Williams & Wilkins.

Mosca, L., Appel, L.J., Benjamin, E.J., Berra, K., Chandra-Strobos, N., Fabunmi, R.P., et al. (2004). Evidence-based guidelines for cardiovascular disease prevention in women. *Journal of the American College of Cardiology, 43*(5), 900-921.

Myers, J. (2005). Exercise and activity. In S.L. Woods, E.S. Froelicher, S.A. Motzer, & E.J. Bridges (Eds.), *Cardiac nursing* (5th ed., pp. 916-936). Philadelphia: Lippincott Williams & Wilkins.

National Vital Statistics Reports, Vol. 53, No. 15, February 28, 2005. Retrieved March 21, 2005, from http://www.cdc.gov/nchs/data/nvsr/nvsr 53/nvsr53_15.pdf

Newton, K.M., & Froelicher, E.S. (2005). Coronary heart disease risk factors. In S.L. Woods, E.S. Froelicher, S.A. Motzer, & E.J. Bridges (Eds.), *Cardiac nursing* (5th ed., pp. 809-824). Philadelphia: Lippincott Williams & Wilkins.

Niinami, H., Ogasawara, H., Suda, Y., & Takeuchi, Y. (2005). Single-vessel revascularization with minimally invasive direct coronary artery bypass: Minithoracotomy or ministernotomy? *Chest, 127*(1), 47-52.

Nishimura, R.A., & Holmes, D.R., Jr. (2004). Hypertrophic obstructive cardiomyopathy. *New England Journal of Medicine, 350*(13), 1320-1327.

Novaro, G.M., & Mills, R.M. (2004). Aortic valve disease. Retrieved September 9, 2004, from http://www.clevelandclinicmeded.com/disease managment/cardiology/aortic_valve/aortic_ valve.htm.

O'Neill, J.O., & Bott-Silverman, C. (2003). Dilated and restrictive cardiomyopathies. Retrieved November 11, 2004, from http://www.cleveland clinicmeded.com/diseasemanagement/cardiolo gy/cardiomyopathy/cardiomyopathy.htm

Opie, L.H. (2004). *Heart physiology: From cell to circulation* (4th ed.). Philadelphia: Lippincott Williams & Wilkins.

Porth, C.M. (2004). *Essential pathophysiology: Concepts of altered health states* (7th ed.). Philadelphia: Lippincott Williams & Wilkins.

Racz, M.J., Hannan, E.L., Isom, O.W., Subramanian, V.A., Jones, R.H., Gold, J.P., et al. (2004). A comparison of short- and long-term outcomes after off-pump and on-pump coronary artery bypass graft surgery with sternotomy. *Journal of the American College of Cardiology, 43*(4), 557-564.

Raghavan, M., & Marik, P.E. (2005). Anemia, allogenic blood transfusion, and immunomodulation in the critically ill [Electronic version]. *Chest, 127*(1), 295-307.

Rochester Medical Center. (n.d.). Permanent pacemakers. Retrieved February 1, 2005, from http://www.rochestermedicalcenter.com/ permanent_pacemakers.htm

St. Jude Medical. (n.d.). Pacemaker implantation. Retrieved February 1, 2005, from http://www .sjm.com/procedures/procedure.aspx?name= pacemaker+implantation

Salberg, L. (2004). How to choose a septal reduction method. From the Hypertrophic Cardiomyopathy Association. Retrieved December 31, 2004, from http://www.enews builder.net/hypertrophic/e_article000222719.cfm

Shah, P. (2003). Hypertrophic cardiomyopathies. In M.H. Crawford (Ed.), *Current diagnosis and treatment in cardiology* (2nd ed., pp. 179-187). New York: McGraw-Hill.

Smith, S.C., Jr., Dove, J.T., Jacobs, A.K., Kennedy, J.W., Kereiakes, D., Kern, M.J., et al. (2001). ACC/AHA guidelines for percutaneous coronary interventions: Executive summary. A report of the American College of Cardiology/American Heart Association Task Force on Practice Guidelines (Committee to Revise the 1993 Guidelines for Percutaneous Transluminal Coronary Angioplasty). *Journal of the American College of Cardiology, 37*(8), 2215-2238.

Smith, S.W., Zvosec, D.L., Sharkey, S.W., & Henry, T.D. (2002). *The ECG in acute MI: An evidence-based manual of reperfusion therapy.* Philadelphia: Lippincott Williams & Wilkins.

Stoltz, C., & Bryg, R.J. (2003). Mitral stenosis. In M.H. Crawford (Ed.), *Current diagnosis and treatment in cardiology* (2nd ed., pp. 131-141). New York: McGraw-Hill.

Stuenkel, C. & Wenger, N.K. (1999, March). In D. Herrington & N.K. Wenger (Co-chairs), *Completed and Ongoing Trails of Women and Heart Disease: PEPI and HERS.* Presented at the meeting of the American College of Cardiology 48th Annual Scientific Session, New Orleans, LA. Retrieved on October 20, 2005, from http://www.medscape.com/viewarticle/439518

Swain, D.K. (2001). Mitral stenosis. Retrieved May 5, 2003, from http://www.emedicine.com/emerg/top315.htm

The Criteria Committee of the New York Heart Association. (1994). *Nomenclature and Criteria for Diagnosis of Diseases of the Heart and Great Vessels* (9th ed., pp. 253-256). Boston, MA: Little, Brown & Co.

The Medicines Company. (2004). *Bivalirudin Product Monograph.* Retrieved August 29, 2005, from http://www.themedicinescompany.com/~products_content/Angiomax%20monogr%20Feb%202004.pdf

Thelan, L.A., Davie, J.K., Urden, L.D., & Lough, M.E. (1994). *Critical care nursing: Diagnosis and management* (2nd ed.). St. Louis: Mosby.

Theobald, K., & McMurray, A. (2004). Coronary artery bypass graft surgery: Discharge planning for successful recovery [Electronic version]. *Journal of Advanced Nursing, 47*(5), 483-491.

Thibodeau, G.A., & Patton, K.T. (2003). *Anatomy & physiology* (5th ed.). St. Louis: Mosby.

U.S. Department of Health and Human Services. (2001). *Third report of the National Cholesterol Education Program (NCEP) Expert Panel on detection, evaluation, and treatment of high blood cholesterol in adults (Adult Treatment Panel III)* (NIH publication No. 01-3670). Washington, DC: U.S. Government Printing Office.

U.S. Department of Health and Human Services. (2003). *The seventh report of the Joint National Committee on prevention, detection, evaluation, and treatment of high blood pressure* (NIH publication No. 03-5233). Washington, DC: U.S. Government Printing Office.

Virmani, R., Burke, A., & Farb, A. (1997). *Atlas of heart diseases: Valvular heart disease.* Current Medicine, Inc. Retrieved July 5, 2005, from http://www.imagesMD.com

Wallhagen, M.I., & Nolte, M.S. (2005). Diabetes mellitus. In S.L. Woods, E.S. Froelicher, S.A. Motzer, & E.J. Bridges (Eds.), *Cardiac nursing* (5th ed., pp. 948-960). Philadelphia: Lippincott Williams & Wilkins.

Weinberger, B.M., & Brilliant, L.C. (2001). Pacemaker and automatic internal cardiac defibrillator. Retrieved February 1, 2005, from http://www.emedicine.com/emerg/topic805.htm

Woods, S.E., Smith, J.M., Sohail, S., Sarah, A., & Engle, A. (2004). The influence of type 2 diabetes mellitus in patients undergoing coronary artery bypass graft surgery: An 8-year prospective cohort study [Electronic version]. *Chest, 126*(6), 1789-1795.

Wyse, D.G., Waldo, A.L., DiMarco, J.P., Domanski, M.J., Rosenberg, Y., Schron, E.B., et al. (2002). A comparison of rate control and rhythm control in patients with atrial fibrillation [Electronic version]. *New England Journal of Medicine, 347*(23), 1825-1833.

Yeo, T.P., & Berg, N.C. (2004). Counseling patients with implanted cardiac devices [Electronic version]. *The Nurse Practitioner, 29*(12), 58-65.

Zoghbi, W.A., & Afridi, I. (2003). Aortic regurgitation. In M.H. Crawford (Ed.), *Current diagnosis and treatment in cardiology* (2nd ed., pp. 121-130). New York: McGraw-Hill.

ADDITIONAL RESOURCES

Adams, K.F., Baughman, K.L., Konstam, M.A., Dec, W.G., Liu, P., Elkayam, U., et al. (1999). Heart Failure Society of America practice guidelines for management of patients with heart failure caused by left ventricular systolic dysfunction – Pharmacological approaches [Electronic version]. *Journal of Cardiac Failure, 5*(4), 357-382.

Agur, A.M., & Dalley, A.F. (2005). *Grant's atlas of anatomy* (11th ed.). Philadelphia: Lippincott Williams & Wilkins

American Heart Association. (n.d.). Women and coronary heart disease. Retrieved August 21, 2004, from http://www.americanheart.org/presenter.jhtml?identifier=2859

Arauz-Pacheco, C., Parrott, M.A., & Raskin, P. (2004). Hypertension management in adults with diabetes. *Diabetes Care, 27* (Suppl. 1), S65-S67.

Artificial Pacemaker. (n.d.). Retrieved January 3, 2005, from http://en.wikipedia.org

Bailey, W. (2001). Cardiac pacing in atrioventricular block. In O.V. Adair (Ed.), *Cardiology secrets* (2nd ed., pp. 92-93). Philadelphia: Hanley & Belfus, Inc.

Barold, S.S., Stroobandt, R.X., & Sinnaeve, A.F. (2004). *Cardiac pacemakers step by step: An illustrated guide.* Elmsford, NY: Futura Publishing.

Bhola, R., & Gill, E.A. (2001). Rheumatic heart disease and mitral stenosis. In O.V. Adair (Ed.), *Cardiology secrets* (2nd ed., pp. 226-235). Philadelphia: Hanley & Belfus, Inc.

Bloomquist, J., & Love, M.M. (2000). Cardiovascular assessment and diagnostic procedures. In L.D. Urden & K.M. Stacy (Eds.), *Priorities in critical care nursing* (3rd ed., pp. 99-145). St Louis: Mosby.

Bocka, J. (2002). External pacemakers. Retrieved December 5, 2004, from http://www.emedicine.com/emerg/topic699.htm

Bond, E.F., & Heitkemper, M.M. (2005). Complementary and alternative medicine in cardiac and vascular disease. In S.L. Woods, E.S. Froelicher, S.A. Motzer, & E.J. Bridges (Eds.), *Cardiac nursing* (5th ed., pp. 974-985). Philadelphia: Lippincott Williams & Wilkins.

Brennan, F.J. (2004). Ethical issues with implantable defibrillators [Electronic version]. *Pacing and Clinical Electrophysiology, 27*(7), 897-898.

Burke, L.E., & Cartwright, M.A. (2005). Obesity: An overview of assessment and treatment. In S.L. Woods, E.S. Froelicher, S.A. Motzer, & E.J. Bridges (Eds.), *Cardiac nursing* (5th ed., pp. 937-947). Philadelphia: Lippincott Williams & Wilkins.

Cabajal, E.V., & Deedwania, P.C. (2003). Congestive heart failure. In M.H. Crawford (Ed.), *Current diagnosis & treatment in cardiology* (2nd ed., pp. 1217-249). New York: McGraw-Hill.

Cardiology Channel. (n.d.). Pacemaker follow-up. Retrieved February 2, 2005, from http://www.cardiologychannel.com/pacemaker/followup.shtml

Carlson, M. (2004). Rate vs rhythm control and suppression algorithms for the management and prevention of atrial fibrillation. *Medscape Cardiology, 8*(2). Retrieved October 11, 2004, from http://www.medscape.com

Celebi, M., & Suleman, A. (2005). Cardiomyopathy, dilated. Retrieved December 19, 2004, from http://www.emedicine.com/med/topic289.htm

Chen, M.S., & Levere, H.M. (2003). *Hypertrophic cardiomyopathy*. Retrieved November 28, 2004, from http://www.clevelandclinicmeded.com/diseasemanagement/cardiology/hypertrophic/hypertrophic.htm

Crawford, M.H. (2004). *Essentials of diagnosis & treatment in cardiology* (2nd ed.). New York: McGraw-Hill.

Deelstra, M.H., & Jacobson, C. (2005). Cardiac catheterization. In S.L. Woods, E.S. Froelicher, S.A. Motzer, & E.J. Bridges (Eds.), *Cardiac nursing* (5th ed., pp. 459-477). Philadelphia: Lippincott Williams & Wilkins.

Del Bene, S., & Vaughan, A. (2005). Acute coronary syndrome. In S.L. Woods, E.S. Froelicher, S.A. Motzer, & E.J. Bridges (Eds.), *Cardiac nursing* (5th ed., pp. 550-584). Philadelphia: Lippincott Williams & Wilkins.

DiMarco, J.P. (2003). Implantable cardioverter-defibrillators [Electronic version]. *New England Journal of Medicine, 349*(19), 1836-1847.

Dirks, J. (2000). Cardiovascular therapeutic management. In L.D. Urden & K.M. Stacy (Eds.), *Priorities in critical care nursing* (pp. 183-209). St Louis: Mosby.

El Sakr, A., Clark, L.T, & Loghin, C. (2001). Hypertrophic cardiomyopathy. In O.V. Adair (Ed.), *Cardiology secrets* (2nd ed., pp. 161-165). Philadelphia: Hanley & Belfus, Inc.

Fenton, D.E., & Baumann, B.M. (2005). *Acute coronary syndrome*. Retrieved on December 31, 2004, from http://www.emedicine.com/emerg/topic31.htm

Flack, J.E., Cook, J.R., May, S.J., Lemeshow, S., Engelman, R.M., Rousou, J.A., et al. (2000). Does cardioplegia type affect outcome and survival in patients with advanced left ventricular dysfunction? [Electronic version]. *Circulation, 102*(10 Suppl. 3), III84-89.

Geiter, H.B., Jr. (2004a). Getting back to basics with permanent pacemakers, part I [Electronic version]. *Nursing 2004, 34*(10), 32cc1-32cc3.

Geiter, H.B., Jr. (2004b). Getting back to basics with permanent pacemakers, part II [Electronic version]. *Nursing 2004, 34*(11), 32cc1-32cc2.

Grady, D., McDonald, K., Bischoff, K., Cabou, A., Chaput, L., Hoerster, K., et al. (2003). *Results of systematic review of research on diagnosis and treatment of coronary heart disease in women*. (Publication No. 03-E035). Rockville, MD: Agency for Healthcare Research and Quality.

Haffner, S.M. (2004). Dyslipidemia management in adults with diabetes. *Diabetes Care, 27*(Suppl. 1), S68-S71.

Haire-Joshu, D., Glasgow, R.E., & Tibbs, T.L. (2004). Smoking and diabetes. *Diabetes Care, 27*(Suppl. 1), S74-S75.

Havranek, E.P., & Giuglian, G.R. (2001). Congestive heart failure. In O.V. Adair (Ed.), *Cardiology secrets* (2nd ed., pp. 124-128). Philadelphia: Hanley & Belfus, Inc.

Hayes, D.L., & Furman, S. (2004). Cardiac pacing: How it started, where we are, where we are going. *Pacing and Clinical Electrophysiology, 27*(5), 693-704.

Heidenreich, P.A., McDonald, K.M., Hastie, T., Fadel, B., Hagan, V., Lee, B.K., et al. (1999). *An evaluation of beta-blockers, calcium antagonists, nitrates and alternative therapies for stable angina* (Publication No. 00-E003). Rockville, MD: Agency for Healthcare Research and Quality.

Implantable cardioverter defibrillator. (n.d.). Retrieved February 3, 2005, from www.heart1 .com/care/procedure20.cfm/15

Implantable cardioverter defibrillators. (n.d.). Retrieved February 2, 2005, from http://www .hrspatients.org/patients/treatments/cardiac_ defibrillators/default.asp

Kass, D. (2004). Left ventricular versus biventricular pacing in cardiac resynchronization therapy: The plot in this tale of two modes [Electronic version]. *Journal of Cardiovascular Electrophysiology, 15*(12), 1348-1349.

Katchen, T.A., (2003). *American Heart Association dietary guidelines.* Retrieved June 22, 2004, from Medical College of Wisconsin web site: http://healthlink.mcw.edu/article/972602194 .html

Kaufman, E.S., Zimmermann, P.A., Wang, T., Dennish, G.W., III, Barrell, P.D., Chandler, M.L., et al. (2004). Risk of proarrhythmic events in the Atrial Fibrillation Follow-Up Investigation of Rhythm Management (AFFIRM) study: A multivariate analysis [Electronic version]. *Journal of the American College of Cardiology, 44*(6), 1276-1282.

Kaufman, E.S., Zimmermann, P.A., Wang, T., Dennish, G.W., III, Barrell, P.D., Chandler, M.L., et al. (2004). Risk of proarrhythmic events in the Atrial Fibrillation Follow-Up Investigation of Rhythm Management (AFFIRM) study: A multivariate analysis [Electronic version]. *Journal of the American College of Cardiology, 44*(6), 1276-1282.

Kowalak, J.P., Welsh, W., & Mills, E.J. (Eds.). (2003). *Critical care challenges: Disorders, treatments, and procedures.* Philadelphia: Lippincott Williams & Wilkins.

Kumar, S.P., & Sorrell, V.L. (2003). Renal-dose dopamine: Myth or ally in the treatment of acute renal failure? *Cardiovascular Reviews & Reports, 24*(8), 413-415.

Lilley, L.L., & Aucker, R.S. (2001). *Pharmacology and the nursing process* (3rd ed.). St. Louis: Mosby.

McComb, J.M., & Camm, A.J. (2002). Primary prevention of sudden cardiac death using implantable cardioverter defibrillators [Electronic version]. *British Medical Journal, 325*(7372), 1050-1051.

McKenry, L.M., & Salerno, E. (2001). *Mosby's pharmacology in nursing* (21st ed.). St. Louis: Mosby.

McNamara, R.L., Bass, E.B., Miller, M.R., Segal, J.B., Goodman, S.N., Kim, N.L., et al. (2001). *Management of new onset atrial fibrillation.* (Publication No. 01-E026). Rockville, MD: Agency for Healthcare Research and Quality.

Mauney, M.C., & Kron, I.L. (1995). The physiologic basis of warm cardioplegia [Electronic version]. *Annals of Thoracic Surgery, 60*(3), 819-823.

Mendoza, R., & Trujillo, N. (2001). Complications and care following myocardial infarction. In O.V. Adair (Ed.), *Cardiology secrets* (2nd ed., pp. 113-117). Philadelphia: Hanley & Belfus, Inc.

Miller, N.H., & Froelicher, E.S. (2005). Disease management models in cardiovascular care. In S.L. Woods, E.S. Froelicher, S.A. Motzer, & E.J. Bridges (Eds.), *Cardiac nursing* (5th ed., pp. 986-996). Philadelphia: Lippincott Williams & Wilkins.

Murphy-Lavoie, H., & Preston, C. (2005). Cardiomyopathy, dilated. Retrieved November 11, 2004, from http://www.emedicine.com/emerg/topic80.htm

New York Heart Association Classification. (n.d.). A functional and therapeutic classification for prescription of physical activity for cardiac patients. Retrieved February 2, 2005, from http://www.hcoa.org/hcoacme/chf-cme/chf00070.htm

O'Donnell, M., & Dirks, J. (2000). Cardiovascular disorders. In L.D. Urden & K.M. Stacy (Eds.), *Priorities in critical care nursing* (3rd ed., pp. 146-182). St. Louis: Mosby.

Olshansky, B., Rosenfeld, L.E., Warner, A.L., Solomon, A.J., O'Neill, G., Sharma, A., et al. (2004). The Atrial Fibrillation Follow-Up Investigation of Rhythm Management (AFFIRM) study: Approaches to control rate in atrial fibrillation [Electronic version]. *Journal of the American College of Cardiology, 43*(7), 1201-1208.

Ommen, S.R., & Nishimura, R.A. (2001). Treatment of patients with hypertrophic cardiomyopathy: a clinician's guide. Retrieved December 31, 2004, from http://www.mayoclinic.org/hypertrophic-cardiomyopathy/physiciansguide.html

Peck, P. (2003). Is the glass half empty? CMS expands ICD coverage, but decision falls short of MADIT II criteria. Retrieved January 15, 2005, from http://www.medscape.com/viewarticle/456960

Physicians' Desk Reference (57th ed.). (2003). Medical Economics Staff. Thomson Healthcare.

Porth, C.M. (1994). *Pathophysiology: Concepts of altered health states* (5th ed.). Philadelphia: J.B. Lippincott.

Powers, E. (1995). *Atlas of heart diseases: Chronic ischemic heart disease.* Current Medicine, Inc. Retrieved July 5, 2005, from http://www.imagesMD.com

Saxon, L.A., & De Marco, T. (n.d.). Resynchronization therapy for heart failure. Retrieved December 16, 2004, from www.hrsonline.org/positiondocs/crt_12_3.pdf

Scholten, M.F., Thornton, A.S., Theuns, D.A., Res, J., & Jordaens, L.J. (2004). Twiddler's syndrome detected by home monitoring device [Electronic version]. *Pacing and Clinical Electrophysiology, 25*, 1151-1152.

Shekelle, P., Morton, S., Atkinson, S., Suttorp, M., Tu, W., Heidenreich, P., et al. (2003). Pharmacologic management of heart failure and left ventricular systolic dysfunction: Effect in female, black, and diabetic patients, and cost-effectiveness (Publication No. 03-E045). Rockville, MD: Agency for Healthcare Research and Quality.

Sibbald, W.J. (2002). Use of vasopressors in critically ill patients. Retrieved September 4, 2004, from http://www.medscape.com/viewarticle/434220

Smith, S.C., Jr., Blair, S.N., Bonow, R.O., Brass, L.M., Cerqueira, M.D., Dracup, K., et al. (2001). AHA/ACC guidelines for preventing heart attack and death in patients with atherosclerotic cardiovascular disease: 2001 update. *Circulation, 104*(13), 1577-1579.

Staab, M., & Crowley, S.T. (2001). Angina. In O.V. Adair (Ed.), *Cardiology secrets* (2nd ed., pp. 100-104). Philadelphia: Hanley & Belfus, Inc.

Staab, M., & Krasnow, N. (2001). Prosthetic valves. In O.V. Adair (Ed.), *Cardiology secrets* (2nd ed., pp. 244-247). Philadelphia: Hanley & Belfus, Inc.

Stahmer, S., & Baumann, B.M. (2005). Myocardial infarction. Retrieved on December 31, 2004, from http://www.emedicine.com/emerg/topic327.htm

Steinberg, J.S., Sadaniantz, A., Kron, J., Krahn, A., Denny, D.M., Daubert, J., et al. (2004). Analysis of cause-specific morality in the Atrial Fibrillation Follow-Up Investigation of Rhythm Management (AFFIRM) study [Electronic version]. *Circulation, 109*(16), 1973-1980.

Straka, R.J., Swanson, A.L., & Parra, D. (1998). Calcium channel antagonists: Morbidity and mortality – What's the evidence? [Electronic version]. *American Family Physician, 57*(7). Retrieved January 18, 2005, from www.aafp.org/afp/980401ap/straka.html

Su, J.T., & Epstein, M.L. (2004). Mitral valve insufficiency. Retrieved May 5, 2004, from http://www.emedicine.com/ped/topic1464.htm

Sundt, T.M. (2004). Adult cardiac surgery: Coronary artery bypass grafting surgery. Society of Thoracic Surgeons. Retrieved on December 22, 2004, from http://www.sts.org/sections/patientinformation/adultcardiac surgery/cabg/index.html

Texas Heart Institute. (2005). Pacemakers. Retrieved February 2, 2005, from http://www.texasheartinstitute.org/pacemake.html

Trohman, R.G., Kim, M.H., & Pinski, S.L. (2004). Cardiac pacing: The state of the art [Electronic version]. *Lancet, 364*(9446), 1701-1719. Retrieved December 12, 2004, from www.the-lancet.com

Trujillo, N.P., & Lindenfeld, J. (2001). Myocardial infarction. In O.V. Adair (Ed.), *Cardiology secrets* (2nd ed., pp. 105-112). Philadelphia: Hanley & Belfus, Inc.

Trupp, R.J. (2004). Cardiac resynchronization therapy: Optimizing the device, optimizing the patient [Electronic version]. *Journal of Cardiovascular Nursing, 19*(4), 223-233.

Urden, L.D., & Stacy, K.M. (2000). *Priorities in critical care nursing* (3rd ed.). St. Louis: Mosby.

Veerakul, G. (2001). Coronary risk factors and modification. In O.V. Adair (Ed.), *Cardiology secrets* (2nd ed., pp. 118-123). Philadelphia: Hanley & Belfus, Inc.

Velez, D.A., Morris, C.D., Budde, J.M., Muraki, S., Otto, R.N., Guyton, R.A., et al. (2001). All blood (miniplegia) versus dilute cardioplegia in experimental surgical revascularization of evolving infarction [Electronic version]. *Circulation, 104*(12 Suppl. 1), I296-302.

Vesty, J., Rasmusson, K.D., Hall, J., Schmitz, S., & Brush, S. (2004). Cardiac resynchronization therapy and automatic implantable cardiac defibrillators in the treatment of heart failure: A review article [Electronic version]. *Journal of the American Academy of Nurse Practitioners, 16*(10), 441-450.

Weinberger, H.D. (2001a). Chest pain. In O.V. Adair (Ed.), *Cardiology secrets* (2nd ed., pp. 95-99). Philadelphia: Hanley & Belfus, Inc.

Weinberger, H.D. (2001b). Mitral valve prolapse and mitral regurgitation. In O.V. Adair (Ed.), *Cardiology secrets* (2nd ed., pp. 241-243). Philadelphia: Hanley & Belfus, Inc.

White, M.J. (2001). Anticoagulant and antiplatelet drugs. In O.V. Adair (Ed.), *Cardiology secrets* (2nd ed., pp. 264-269). Philadelphia: Hanley & Belfus, Inc.

White, T.R., & Schwartz, D.E. (2003). Valvular heart disease. In P.E. Parsons & J.P. Wiener-Kronish (Ed.), *Critical care secrets* (3rd ed., pp. 153-162). Philadelphia: Hanley & Belfus, Inc.

Wigle, E., Kitching, A., & Rakowski, H. (1998). *Atlas of heart diseases: Cardiomyopathies, myocarditis, and pericardial disease.* Current Medicine, Inc. Retrieved July 5, 2005, from http://www.imagesMD.com

Wild, D.M, Fisher, J.D., Kim, S.G., Ferrick, K.J., Gross, J.N., & Palma, E.C. (2004). Pacemakers and implantable cardioverter defibrillators: Device longevity is more important than smaller size: The patient's viewpoint [Electronic version]. *Pacing and Clinical Electrophysiology,* *27*(11), 1526-1529.

INDEX

sleep apnea, 65
smoking cessation
    hypercoagulability improved with, 74
    interventions for, 62-63
    as part of ACS management, 100
smoking risk factor, 61*b*
SNS (sympathetic nervous system), 140-141, 140-141*fig*
social support systems, 152
socioeconomic status risk factor, 61
sodium channel blockers, 219
sodium restriction, 152, 164
spironolactone, 36, 147
SSRI (selective serotonin reuptake inhibitors), 104
SSS (sick sinus syndrome), 233
stable angina
    described, 82
    long-term management of, 88
    treatment options for, 86-88
statins (or HMG-CoA reductase inhibitors), 47-48
STEMIs (ST-segment elevation myocardial infarctions)
    ACS term used to describe CHD in, 79
    anterior wall MI, 90-92*fig*, 91*fig*
    fibrin stable clot (or red clot), cause of, 49
    health statistics regarding, 90
    hemodynamic alternations after, 96
    inferior wall MI, 90
    lateral wall MI, 92-93
    left ventricular aneurysms after, 97
    mechanical complications of, 97
    MI classification of, 89
    occlusive clot producing, 91*fig*
    pathophysiology of ventricular remodeling after, 96
    pericarditis complication after, 97
    pharmacological treatment for, 95-96
    posterior wall MI, 93
    postreperfusion care in treatment of, 97-98
    reperfusion and, 93-95
    right ventricular MI, 93
    ventricular arrhythmias after, 96-97
    See also ACS (acute coronary syndrome)
stents
    drug-eluting, 123-124
    intracoronary, 122-123, 124*fig*
sternal wound infections, 116*b*
streptokinase, 49
stress
    anxiety and, 101
    oxidative, 75
    psychosocial, 73-74

stress testing
    CHD (coronary heart disease), 84-85
    chemical, 84
    chronic aortic regurgitation, 193
stroke
    atrial fibrillation and risk of, 216-217
    cardioversion and risk of, 220
stroke volume, 15, 16*fig*, 29
ST-segment elevation, 89*fig*
ST-segment elevation MI (STEMI), 118
sudden cardiac death
    HCM (hypertrophic cardiomyopathy), 174, 179*b*, 180
    heart failure, 149
    ICDs to decrease risk of, 149, 164
superior venae cavae, 2
surgical therapy
    acute aortic regurgitation, 195
    acute mitral regurgitation, 210
    aortic stenosis, 189*b*-190
    aortic valve replacement, 189*b*-190
    CABG (coronary artery bypass grafting), 55, 86-88, 109-122
    cardiac pacemakers, 149, 178, 222, 229-247
    chronic aortic regurgitation, 193-194*b*
    DCM (dilated cardiomyopathy), 164-165
    HCM (hypertrophic cardiomyopathy), 178*fig*-179*fig*
    heart failure and transplantation, 150
    Maze surgical procedure, 223
    mitral commissurotomy, 204, 205*b*
    mitral stenosis, 204*b*-205
    mitral valve replacement, 204-205
    mitral valvuloplasty, 204*b*
    PASA (percutaneous alcohol septal ablation), 178-179*fig*
    percutaneous balloon valvuloplasty, 189*b*
    RCM (restrictive cardiomyopathy), 169
    Ross procedure, 190
    ventricular septal myectomy, 178*fig*
sympathetic nervous system, 20-21
sympathomimetics
    dobutamine, 33*t*
    dopamine, 34*t*
    epinephrine, 33*t*
    for increasing/decreasing afterload, 29*t*, 30*t*
    for increasing/decreasing contractility, 30*t*
    for increasing/decreasing heart rate, 31*t*-32*t*
    for increasing/decreasing preload, 28*t*, 29*t*, 32*b*
    norepinephrine, 34*t*
    See also specific medications
symptomatic left ventricular dysfunction, 146
syncope, 173-174, 186-187, 233

PRETEST KEY

Cardiovascular Nursing:
A Comprehensive Overview

1.	c	Chapter 1
2.	d	Chapter 1
3.	a	Chapter 2
4.	a	Chapter 2
5.	c	Chapter 3
6.	b	Chapter 3
7.	b	Chapter 4
8.	d	Chapter 4
9.	a	Chapter 5
10.	b	Chapter 5
11.	c	Chapter 6
12.	c	Chapter 6
13.	d	Chapter 7
14.	a	Chapter 7
15.	c	Chapter 8
16.	c	Chapter 9
17.	a	Chapter 10
18.	d	Chapter 11
19.	b	Chapter 11
20.	c	Chapter 12